Atkins
shopping
guide

D0608597

Also available from Thorsons:

Atkins Diabetes Revolution
Atkins Made Easy

Atkins
shopping
guide
what to buy?
what to avoid?

Atkins Health & Medical Information Services

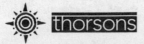

Thorsons
An Imprint of HarperCollins*Publishers*
77–85 Fulham Palace Road,
Hammersmith, London W6 8JB

The website address is www.thorsonselement.com

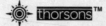

and *Thorsons* are trademarks of
HarperCollins*Publishers* Ltd

First published in the US by HarperCollins*Publishers* 2004
This edition published 2005

2

© 2005 Atkins Nutritionals, Inc.

Atkins Health & Medical Information Services
assert the moral right to be
identified as the authors of this work

A catalogue record for this book
is available from the British Library

ISBN 0 00 718134 5

Printed and bound in Great Britain by
Clays Ltd, St Ives plc

The information presented in this work is in no way intended as medical
advice or as a substitute for medical treatment. This information should
be used in conjunction with the guidance and care of your physician,
especially if you are taking medications, including diuretics or medication
for blood pressure or diabetes. Whether or not you are at your goal weight,
consult your doctor before beginning this program, as you would with any
nutritional plan. Your doctor should perform baseline laboratory tests to
allow for proper follow-up and to individualize your maintenance level of
carbohydrate intake. As with any plan, the weight-loss phases of the
Atkins Blood Sugar Control Program should not be used by patients
on dialysis or by pregnant or breastfeeding women.

Contents

Acknowledgements

This book would not have been possible without the hard work, help, expertise and enthusiasm of many people. They include our American colleagues Olivia Bell Buehl, Christine Senft, Jacqueline Eberstein and Jennifer L. Moles, who paved the way with the US edition of the *Atkins Shopping Guide* and shared their knowledge with us. In the Atkins UK headquarters, publisher Julie Philpott provided both practical and moral support and liaised with the American team, HarperCollins and the UK editorial team.

Thanks go to the multi-talented research team who tirelessly scoured supermarket shelves to select and review the products you will find in the food listing pages of this book: Stuart Penney, Jeremy Evans, Anne Stirk, Jo Forshaw, Vanessa Cotton and Elaine Lemm. Vanessa Cotton and Jo Forshaw also doubled as fact checkers and senior archivists, assisted by Andreana Austin. Senior researchers Anne Stirk, a nutritionist, and Elaine Lemm, a chef, writer, food expert and cookery school principal, advised on the product content of this book, while Elaine Lemm also wrote sections of the listings chapters and answered many impossible queries. Andrei Kiselev, assisted by Jonny Price, dealt with the vast number of products that were bought in the course of our research and organized the record-keeping and fact-checking system. Home economist Pat Peacock reviewed the research team's findings for nutritional accuracy. Food writer Lewis Esson contributed to the reference chapters of this book and provided much-appreciated advice and expertise, as did senior editors Annie Lee and Lesley Levene, who reviewed and polished the manuscript.

Daniela Soave organized and oversaw the project, wrote parts of the reference and listings sections, and assembled and edited the manuscript.

Thanks also to Wanda Whiteley and her team at HarperCollins, especially for their endless patience on a very demanding enterprise.

Introduction

When you're following the Atkins Nutritional Approach™ (ANA™), you shouldn't need a PhD to arrive at the checkout with a trolley full of healthy, delicious food. But now that the aisles of the modern British supermarket offer just about any food you could imagine, the abundance often creates confusion: how can you achieve your health and weight-control goals if you cannot be sure you're buying Atkins-appropriate foods?

Clearly, you need to be able to find the foods that will help you succeed on Atkins and avoid those that can sabotage your best intentions. This book will provide the information you need to make these informed decisions.

WHAT IS THIS BOOK ABOUT?

When Atkins followers in the US voiced their frustrations about identifying suitable foods, it became apparent that there was a need for a book that would put consumers in control by teaching them how to be smart low-carb shoppers. *The Atkins Shopping Guide*, published in the US during 2004, did exactly that.

With the number of British Atkins devotees growing by the week, it quickly became obvious that there was just as much of a need for a UK version, one that caters to British products, British shopping habits and British supermarkets. So work got under way to produce the UK edition of the *Atkins Shopping Guide*.

The typical supermarket holds tens of thousands of items, and each year thousands more new food products are introduced. The choices available to the shopper can be overwhelming, and if you're just becoming acquainted with the ANA™ your shopping trips can be doubly frustrating. Although UK food manufacturers are waking up to the demand for low-carb foods, in many cases you have to rely on your own knowledge to judge whether or not a food is suitable for Atkins – and when you multiply that by as many as a hundred items if you are doing the weekly shop, that's a lot of calculation! The information in this book will help you make the right shopping decisions by listing nutritional information about popular foods and brands so that you'll be able to compile your shopping list before you go out, in a fraction of the time.

Some people complete their entire shop at one supermarket, while others prefer to include a trip to the health-food shop, and a growing number are doing their shopping without ever leaving the house, on the Internet. So we have left it up to you where and how you buy your food, listing products alphabetically within easy-to-define sections. Whichever way you shop for groceries, this practical companion will introduce you to many of the foods you will find in the shops, offering just the information you need, at a glance.

HOW DID WE WRITE THIS BOOK?

We selected six 'real' people from various parts of the country to take part in intrepid shopping expeditions. Some of our researchers have partners or families; others live on their own. All of our team have busy lifestyles, and while some of them are already confirmed Atkins followers, others are just beginning to explore the low-carb way of eating. In other words, we believe that the variety of people we sent off on those shopping assignments reflects the diversity of readers who will use this book.

Each member of our team visited a number of shops in the area, scouring supermarkets, health-food stops, delicatessens and corner shops in the hunt for products. We asked them to scrutinize the ingredients lists and nutritional facts panels carefully, and then report their findings to us. Our aim wasn't to produce a book so comprehensive and impractical that it would be as thick as the Yellow Pages; instead we concentrated on sourcing popular products and brands to reflect what is generally available throughout the UK.

Next we asked our researchers to limit their selections to foods with a 25g carb maximum per serving (up to 30g in exceptional cases where the product is highly popular). We also gave them a list of guidelines – about which more later – and asked them to pay special attention to foods that fall within permitted carb levels but might contain ingredients that make the foods unsuitable in other ways.

An important point: this book does not *recommend* foods. We have listed the products we found on store shelves and reported the nutritional information on manufacturers' labels or websites.

When a food which might initially appear acceptable for doing Atkins has ingredients you might not be aware of, or ones that we consider unsuitable, we have pointed this out so you can make your own decision. Thus you'll find not only foods that *are* suitable for doing Atkins, but also popular foods that *aren't*. And if a popular product is missing from our pages, this generally means that its carb count or nutritional content is so far off the radar that it's completely unacceptable.

The findings of our researchers' shopping expeditions make up the main portion of the *Atkins Shopping*

Guide. It's up to you to use the information provided to determine which foods to buy to stay on track, taking into consideration the phase of Atkins you're in, your individual carbohydrate threshold and your health goals.

A NEW FOOD CATEGORY

In the last few years, scientific research has consistently validated the principles upon which Atkins is based. As a result, there has been considerable growth in the food category pioneered by Atkins Nutritionals, Inc.: products specifically created for people following a controlled-carb lifestyle. While low-carb products are widely available in the US, with entire supermarket aisles given over to them, the trend is only now gathering momentum here. Recently, major players in the food business have jumped on the low-carb bandwagon, and industry analysts predict that we are seeing just the tip of the iceberg as more and more people adopt this healthy way of eating. That said as low-carb products hit the aisles, be sure to use the lessons learned in this book to evaluate whether they live up to their claims.

Even if we were able to include every item in the supermarket on the day this book was printed, by the time you bought it there would be new products on the shelves that were not listed. Likewise, not every shop will have every item we mention. For that reason, we plan to update the *Atkins Shopping Guide* regularly – and would welcome your contributions. Do let us know when you come across products that you think should be added to new editions by emailing us at shoppingguide@atkins-uk.com. Be sure to provide the full name of the manufacturer and, if possible, a website address or other contact information.

WHAT INFORMATION IS PROVIDED?

PART ONE: REFERENCE SECTION

In the reference section there is detailed nutritional information about food groups such as cheese, fresh fish, meat, fruit and vegetables. You'll also find tips on food safety, hygiene, labelling and explanations about the many varieties of sugar. While this information is vital and you will refer to it more than once, it's not something you need to check every time you go shopping.

PART TWO: LISTINGS SECTION

In the shopping section there are alphabetical listings for basic, branded and natural foods. Here you'll find the data to help you shop wisely; information you'll refer to time and time again. Broken down into easy-to-locate categories – for example, Soups, Meat and Poultry, Ready Meals, Frozen Food – these essential listings will identify the phases of Atkins for which each food is suitable, as well as providing carb content and information about unacceptable ingredients. At the beginning of each new category we'll include advice to help you make the right shopping choices, and help you steer clear of pitfalls.

Phase Information

Each food product is coded to indicate the phases of Atkins for which it is appropriate. (See 'A Brief Look at the Atkins Nutritional Approach™', page 17.) Several factors determine the appropriate phases:

- the food itself or certain ingredients it contains

- the number of grams of carbs, based on the serving size listed on the packaging's nutritional facts panel (be aware, however, that this will not mean that the serving size is acceptable on all phases of Atkins)
- whether a product is a main dish or meal substitute, a side dish, appetizer, condiment, dessert or snack

Depending upon your individual tolerance for carbohydrates, a particular food may or may not be suitable for you. So, while some people can introduce fruits other than berries in Ongoing Weight Loss (OWL), only berries are listed as suitable for phases 2–4. (It's worth pointing out that several fruits that most people consider vegetables – avocados, olives and tomatoes, for instance – are perfectly acceptable on Induction.) On the other hand, there are foods listed for phases 3–4 that may not be suitable for you if you have a low tolerance for carbs (see 'Understanding Your Carb Threshold', page 10). Alternatively, a food may be one you can eat only rarely or in very small portions depending on the phase you are in. In the interests of space, we list phases by number, instead of by name, as follows:

- phase 1: Induction
- phase 2: Ongoing Weight Loss (OWL)
- phase 3: Pre-Maintenance
- phase 4: Lifetime Maintenance

Assuming that a food does not contain ingredients making it unacceptable for a particular phase, carb counts for phases are as follows:

Main dishes or meal substitutes:
- Induction: 0–7 grams per serving
- Ongoing Weight Loss: 0–12 grams per serving

- Pre-Maintenance and Lifetime Maintenance: 0–18+ grams per serving

Side dishes, appetizers, condiments, desserts or snacks:
- Induction: 0–3 grams per serving
- Ongoing Weight Loss: 0–9 grams per serving
- Pre-Maintenance and Lifetime Maintenance: 0–10+ grams per serving

There are certain exceptions to these categories. Although carb count is key, some foods with fewer than 3 grams of carbs per serving are not appropriate for the first two weeks of Induction, when cravings for sweets may not yet be under control. Therefore low-carb confectionery and other treats sweetened with sugar alcohols, for example, are not coded for Induction, no matter how low their Net Carb count. (Note that some people find that sugar alcohols can cause gastrointestinal distress, and may want to limit their servings.) Sugar alcohols include maltitol, isomalt, lactitol and sorbitol. Glycerine is also in the same family of ingredients, known as polyols.

Likewise, although nuts are low in carbohydrates, and some nut products contain fewer than 3 grams of carbs, they are hard to eat in moderation and are therefore not acceptable until you get to OWL. (If you stay in Induction beyond two weeks, you can add nuts and seeds back into your diet as long as you can keep your portions under control.) Note that the small amount of nuts or dried berries in Atkins Advantage™ Bars and Morning Shine™ Breakfast Bars is not enough to interfere with weight loss. However, if you are allergic to peanuts or other nuts, be aware that all Atkins Advantage™, Morning Shine™ Bars and Endulge™ Chocolate Bars either contain nuts or may contain traces of nuts.

What Carbohydrates Should You Count?

Not all carbohydrates behave the same way in your body. For example, table sugar raises your blood sugar, while others, such as fibre, sugar alcohols, glycerine or organic acids, pass through your body without any significant impact on blood sugar. When you do Atkins, you only need to count the grams of carbohydrate that impact your blood sugar (the Net Carbs).

The good news is that British food labels have done the calculation for us. The fibre is shown separately and as long as there are no sugar alcohols, glycerine and organic acids contained in the product, the grams of carbs shown is the number you count.

So, in this example (Own Brand Cannellini Beans in water) you need to count 17.4g of carbs per 100g.

Nutrition

Typical values when drained	100g
Composition	provide
Energy	466kj
	1100kcal
Protein	7.6g
Carbohydrate	17.4g
of which sugars	0.2g
Fat	1.1g
of which saturates	0.1g
Fibre	5.4g
Sodium	trace

Low-Carb Products

For low-carb products that are sweetened with glycerine or sugar alcohols, subtract the grams of sugar alcohols or glycerine from the total number of grams of carbohydrate to arrive at the Net Carb total.

So, in this example (Atkins Endulge™ Caramel Hazelnut Bar) if you subtract the 10.8g of polyols (maltitol and glycerol) from the 15g of carbohydrate you reach a total of 5g Net Carbs per serving.

Nutrition

Typical Composition	Each Serving (30g) provides	100g provide
Energy	630kj	1800kj
	152kcal	435kcal
Protein	6.5g	18.5g
Carbohydrate	15g	42.8g
of which sugars	4.1g	11.7g
of which polyols	10.8g	30.7g
of which maltitol	7.1g	20.3g
Fat	9.2g	26.2g
of which saturates	3.2g	9.2g
Fibre	0.9g	2.6g
Sodium	0.04g	0.1g

UNDERSTANDING YOUR CARB THRESHOLD

There are two calculations you must learn how to do to lose weight on Atkins and keep it off permanently.

Critical Carbohydrate Level for Losing: When you do Atkins, instead of counting calories, you count the number of grams of carbs you consume each day. Once you are past the initial Induction phase, and while you are still in the process of losing weight, the carb gram count you are aiming for each day is known as your Critical Carbohydrate Level for Losing (CCLL). This is the number of grams of carbs you can consume and still continue to lose weight. Your CCLL typically increases slightly as you deliberately slow your weight loss as you get closer to your goal.

Atkins Carbohydrate Equilibrium: Once you have reached your goal weight and are maintaining it or are doing Atkins purely for health reasons, your 'magic' number is known as your Atkins Carbohydrate Equilibrium (ACE). Your ACE represents the number of grams of carbs you can consume each day while neither losing nor gaining weight.

INGREDIENT ALERTS

The beauty of doing Atkins is that there are so many delicious foods you can eat, allowing for the variety of tasty food necessary to make it a permanent lifestyle. This book is primarily about all the things you *can* eat. However, there are certain foods and ingredients you should try to avoid. An occasional portion of any individual food will not generally do any harm, and an infrequent lapse is unlikely to set you back. Nonetheless, our goal is to provide you with this information to make it easier for you to follow the ANA™.

There are two categories of ingredient that are unacceptable at *any* phase of Atkins, even once you have achieved your goal weight. The first is added sugar in all its forms, which is at the heart of the epidemics of obesity and diabetes that are undermining the health of a growing number of Europeans. The second is manufactured trans fats in the form of hydrogenated and partially hydrogenated oils, which have been shown to lead to heart disease. Neither of these foods has any place in the Atkins lifestyle.

Added sugar: Doing Atkins is not just about cutting down on carbs; focusing on carbohydrate foods that are high in nutrients and fibre is equally important. For this reason, added sugar in any form is not acceptable in any phase of the programme (for more details, turn to the information on sugar on pages 93–5). Naturally occurring sugars, in dairy products (lactose) or in fruit (fructose), for instance, as well as in vegetables, are an organic part of the food, so they are acceptable if the carb count is within the appropriate range for a particular phase. An example: low-carb ice cream contains some naturally occurring sugars from the milk and cream used to make it. If that ice cream has strawberries (also containing natural sugars) in it, it could still be suitable for OWL and beyond. However, added fructose, sometimes used in food products in lieu of table sugar (sucrose), would make that ice cream unacceptable in any phase. When a food appears at first glance to be acceptable in terms of the Net Carb count but contains added sugars, it is marked with the 'Ingredient Alert' symbol ⚠ , indicating that it is an unacceptable food, with the words 'contains added sugar'. Phase codes are omitted because the food should not be eaten at any time on Atkins.

Trans fats: While natural fats from a variety of sources are integral to doing Atkins, and to good health in general, there is one kind of fat that is dangerous. Manufactured trans fats, which are usually listed as hydrogenated or partially hydrogenated oils on a food label, are made from inexpensive vegetable oils that have been heavily processed to make them thicker and more stable. (Humans actually produce trace amounts of naturally occurring trans fats in the intestine, as do other animals; however, when it comes to food products, we are talking about *added* trans fats – and these should be avoided at all costs.) Their use allows foods that would otherwise quickly go bad to have a long shelf-life. The hydrogenation process that transforms fats changes their chemical structure, meaning that your body cannot identify and process them. Atkins has always cautioned against added trans fats, and Atkins products do not contain hydrogenated or partially hydrogenated oils. Any food product that contains added trans fats is marked with the 'Ingredient Alert' symbol ⚠ and the words 'contains trans fats'. Unacceptable in any phase of Atkins, regardless of the carb count, these product listings again do not include phases. Consumption of saturated fats, on the other hand, is perfectly safe in the context of a controlled-carbohydrate lifestyle.

PROCEED WITH CAUTION

Certain other ingredients should be used prudently.

Monosodium glutamate: A preservative and flavour enhancer, MSG can cause water-retention and headaches in sensitive individuals. To help you avoid MSG, we have marked foods that contain it with the FYI ('For Your Information') symbol **FYI** and the words 'contains MSG'.

Nitrates: These preservatives are used in most bacon, cured ham, pepperoni and certain other meats, smoked fish and other products to produce an appealing colour and inhibit the growth of germs that could lead to food poisoning. We mark them with the FYI symbol **FYI** to alert you to their presence. Consider alternatives whenever possible. For example, instead of mortadella or salami, you could opt for sliced turkey or roast beef.

Certain other unexpected ingredients, such as cornflour, maize starch and wheat flour, that you might not be aware are in a specific product are also indicated with the FYI symbol **FYI**.

We also use the FYI symbol **FYI** in the few cases where a food may or may not contain added sugars, wheat flour or trans fats that normally would merit an ingredient alert **⚠**. In these cases, we advise you to read the label of the specific product you are considering carefully. If it contains added sugars or trans fats, pass it by.

On the positive side, we will indicate when a product is organic **⚠**.

ADVANCES IN FOOD SCIENCE

In recent years, advances in food science have helped broaden and improve the controlled-carb food category. Not only has that made doing Atkins easier, it also means that you don't have to give up certain categories of food for ever, something few people are willing to do. For example, the use of sucralose (see 'Sugar Substitutes', below) enables both commercial and home bakers to make sweets that are suitable – in moderation – for Atkins followers. Sugar alcohols such as maltitol make it possible to enjoy a chocolate bar without overloading on carbs. The development of such products is consistent with the Atkins commitment to variety and choice instead of monotony and deprivation.

Another technological breakthrough allows the use of small amounts of white flour in baked goods. As a result, we have moderated our former stance that all refined flour was unacceptable at any phase of Atkins. Just a few years ago, if you were doing Atkins your only options were to avoid bread in the weight-loss phases and to have an occasional slice of whole-grain bread when you were at or close to your goal weight. (Whole-wheat flour and products made entirely with whole grains, such as bread and breakfast cereals, are acceptable – and are so coded – for the later phases of Atkins.) Bread made with white flour was a no-go area in any phase.

Fortunately, the picture has changed. Food scientists have found out how to bake bread that tastes good and has the texture you expect, yet does not significantly make an impact on your blood sugar, meaning that even in Induction you can have a slice of toast for breakfast. One of the ways they have done this is by using flour in a variety of forms. So, for example, Atkins Bakery breads contain a small amount of unbleached enriched white flour, but the carb count is just 3 grams per slice. Compare this with the 14 or more grams of carbs in a slice of bread made completely from white flour.

Do not take this slight relaxation of the rules about white flour in a controlled-carb product as a licence to eat conventional products full of wheat flour, or to order breaded dishes in restaurants. It is only acceptable to eat food that contains a small amount of white flour if the carb count is quantified and falls within acceptable limits. Our overall recommendation continues to be to rely primarily on whole-grain flours, which contain the nutrient-rich germ and fibre-rich bran.

On a food ingredient list, unless the label says '100 per cent whole-wheat flour', you can assume when the label says 'wheat flour' the ingredient is white flour in one of its forms: it may be unbleached or bleached, or a blend of both. Our preference is for unbleached flour. To make you aware of the inclusion of wheat flour, we have identified foods that contain it with the FYI symbol **FYI** even if the carb count appears within acceptable limits.

SUGAR SUBSTITUTES

Although our sugar substitute of choice is sucralose (marketed as Splenda®), saccharin and acesulfame-K are other options. When a low-carb food contains aspartame, we have used the FYI symbol **FYI** and added the words 'contains aspartame' so that you can make your own purchasing decision.

The purpose of this book is to make it easy for you to obtain foods that are Atkins-friendly so you will find it easier than ever to succeed at living this healthy lifestyle. But we also want you to eat the best-quality foods you possibly can, and that means primarily buying whole foods. Doing Atkins is not just a numbers game. Of course, you should continue to count your carbs – at least until it becomes second nature and you are easily maintaining your weight – but *quality* is as important as quantity. We hope this book will help you to enhance the quality of your diet and your enjoyment of a variety of delicious and wholesome foods as well. Let us leave you with a crucial reminder:

- find your individual carb threshold
- then purchase foods that support your
  individualized threshold

After all, at Atkins our goal is to change the way the world eats to promote good health – including *your* health. We believe that this book will play an important part in doing just that.

A Brief Look at the
Atkins Nutritional Approach™

A FOUR-PHASE PROGRAMME

Millions of people doing Atkins confirm that Atkins works, as do a host of recent research studies. But doing Atkins is not the same as just 'doing low carb'. That's why we would like to take this opportunity to outline briefly the advantages of the Atkins Nutritional Approach™ (ANA™). As individuals, we all have our differences, our likes and our dislikes. One of the benefits of Atkins is that it can be personalized to suit your particular needs, your tastes and your activity level, among other factors. Many people confuse Induction, the first phase of Atkins, which lasts for a minimum of two weeks, with the entire ANA™. However, Atkins is actually a four-phase programme that begins with a relatively strict phase and then moves through gradual liberalization to a permanent way of eating. Here is a brief summary of each phase:

1. INDUCTION

This kick-starts your body into weight loss, switching from a glucose metabolism (fuelled by carbohydrates) to one that primarily burns fat, including your own body fat, for energy. When you stop relying on glucose for energy, you stabilize your blood sugar, which typically eliminates symptoms such as fatigue, mood swings, brain fog and cravings for high-carbohydrate foods. Do Induction for a minimum of 14 days, after which you should see significant weight-loss results.

You will eat liberal combinations of fat and protein in the form of poultry, fish, shellfish, eggs and red meat, as well as pure, natural fats in the form of butter, mayonnaise, olive oil, safflower, sunflower and other unadulterated vegetable oils. You will also eat approximately 20 grams of carbs each day, mostly in the form of salad greens and other vegetables.

Eat absolutely no wheat bread, pasta, grains, starchy vegetables or dairy products other than aged or hard cheese, cream or butter. The only fruits you can eat are avocados, olives and tomatoes. Do not eat nuts or seeds in the first two weeks. (If you stay on Induction beyond two weeks, you can add both seeds and nuts to your meals or as a snack.)

You can eat up to two servings of controlled-carb foods, such as an Atkins Advantage™ Bar or Ready-to-Drink Shake or a Morning Shine™ Breakfast Bar, or use products such as Atkins Quick Quisine™ Bake Mix, so long as your total intake does not exceed 20 grams of carbs. However, it is prudent to avoid sweets and certain desserts in the first two weeks of Induction, even if they contain fewer than 3 grams of carbs per serving. If you have a lot of weight to lose, you can safely stay on Induction for up to six months.

2. ONGOING WEIGHT LOSS

OWL lets you personalize the ANA™ to your tastes and needs, as you continue to burn fat and maintain control of your appetite to control cravings. In this phase you will gradually increase your consumption of carbs until you reach your threshold, known as your Critical Carbohydrate Level for Losing (CCLL), which will allow you to continue to lose weight. You will be able to eat a broader range of healthy foods, selecting those you enjoy most from a range of nutrient-rich carbohydrate foods as you deliberately slow your rate of weight loss to lay the groundwork for permanent weight management. To establish your CCLL, increase your daily carb intake in weekly increments of 5 grams of carbs so long as weight loss continues. When you stop losing weight for a week, drop back 5 grams and you should have found your carb threshold.

In OWL, most people can add back more vegetables, fresh cheeses, nuts and seeds, berries and low-carb speciality foods. Some people are able to add foods that are typically added in Pre-Maintenance (see below). Foods should be introduced one at a time, to ensure that they do not create cravings, increase your appetite, cause weight gain or reintroduce old symptoms that disappeared in Induction. Continue doing OWL until you have five to ten pounds left to lose.

3. PRE-MAINTENANCE

In OWL, you increase your carb intake in increments of 5 grams. In this phase, increases in daily carb count move up in 10-gram increments each week as long as weight loss continues, albeit more slowly than in OWL. If new foods are introduced and carb grams are increased gradually, your CCLL should rise slowly. During this phase most people can add beans and legumes, fruit other than berries, higher-carb vegetables such as winter squash, carrots, peas and sweet potatoes and, finally, whole grains. As you continue to make 10-gram increment additions, you'll quickly reach a point at which you will find that you are no longer losing weight. If you are at your goal weight, stay at that level for a month or so before you increase your daily carb consumption by another 10 grams to see if you can consume that level without gaining. Once you do begin to gain, drop back 5 or 10 grams and you should have established your Atkins Carbohydrate Equilibrium (ACE).

However, if, after an incremental increase, you find that you are gaining weight, or are not losing any and you are not yet at your goal weight, you'll need to go back down to the previous level. The line between gaining, maintaining and losing is a thin one and you may have to play with your revised CCLL and later your ACE for a while to understand what your body can handle.

While it may take as long as three months to drop the last few pounds and clearly establish your ACE, this leisurely pace is critical to your ultimate success. Continue to add new foods slowly and carefully so you learn good eating habits at the same time. (People with extremely low carb thresholds won't be able to add many new foods and will find Pre-Maintenance similar to OWL.)

4. LIFETIME MAINTENANCE

Once you have maintained your goal weight for a minimum of one month, you are officially in Lifetime Maintenance. You can continue to select from a greater range of foods and consume more carbs than you did in the weight-loss phases of the ANA™. If your metabolism can handle it, you can – in moderation – eat many of the foods you used to enjoy. (The exceptions are sugar, white flour and trans fats.) Stay at or around your ACE and your weight should not fluctuate beyond the natural range of two or three pounds. (Hormonal changes and other daily fluctuations in your body will account for any small seesaw effect.)

For complete information on how to do Atkins, refer to *Dr Atkins' New Diet Revolution* (Vermilion). If you have just a few pounds to lose, want to maintain your weight, or are interested in the health benefits of doing Atkins, refer to *Atkins for Life* (Pan Macmillan). The newly-published *Atkins Made Easy* (HarperCollins) focuses heavily on the first two weeks of doing Atkins. You can also find additional support at www.atkins.com/uk.

A NEW LOOK AT THE FOOD GUIDE PYRAMID

Atkins Health & Medical Information Services recently developed an alternative food guide pyramid (overleaf) which emphasizes the importance of healthy protein sources, with vegetables as the primary source of carbohydrates. It also incorporates exercise as a key component of a healthy lifestyle.

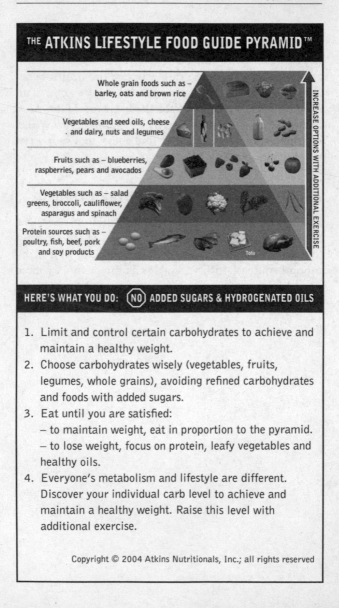

THE ATKINS LIFESTYLE FOOD GUIDE PYRAMID™

Whole grain foods such as –
barley, oats and brown rice

Vegetables and seed oils, cheese
and dairy, nuts and legumes

Fruits such as – blueberries,
raspberries, pears and avocados

Vegetables such as – salad
greens, broccoli, cauliflower,
asparagus and spinach

Protein sources such as –
poultry, fish, beef, pork
and soy products

Tofu

INCREASE OPTIONS WITH ADDITIONAL EXERCISE

HERE'S WHAT YOU DO: (NO) ADDED SUGARS & HYDROGENATED OILS

1. Limit and control certain carbohydrates to achieve and
   maintain a healthy weight.
2. Choose carbohydrates wisely (vegetables, fruits,
   legumes, whole grains), avoiding refined carbohydrates
   and foods with added sugars.
3. Eat until you are satisfied:
   – to maintain weight, eat in proportion to the pyramid.
   – to lose weight, focus on protein, leafy vegetables and
   healthy oils.
4. Everyone's metabolism and lifestyle are different.
   Discover your individual carb level to achieve and
   maintain a healthy weight. Raise this level with
   additional exercise.

PART ONE:

Reference Section

Cheese

Nutrients in cheese vary widely. Harder cheeses tend to be higher in protein and calcium and lower in carbohydrate than fresh and softer cheeses. In fact, fresh cheeses such as cottage cheese, ricotta and curd cheese are not allowed on Induction; processed cheeses can be high in carbs as well and may contain unacceptable fillers.

Up to 115g of soft, semi-soft, semi-hard and hard cheese are permitted each day. Remember that full-fat cheeses are always a better choice. Lower-fat cheese will actually have a higher carb content than full-fat cheese.

When it comes to cheese, 'fresh' means that the cheese has not been matured or ripened. These cheeses are more like milk than harder ones. They are slightly higher in carbs and are quite perishable, so it's important to look at sell-by dates.

BEL PAESE
This mild semi-soft cheese with a sweet, unctuous, buttery taste is among the most popular of Italian cheeses worldwide, as it is so versatile.

BLUE CHEESE
Blue cheeses can be mild or quite pungent. If you're cooking with them, choose a strong-flavoured variety such as Roquefort or Stilton. Milder blues, such as Gorgonzola, are ideal for crumbling over salads.

BOURSIN
This soft, creamy cheese is often seasoned with garlic and herbs, or with pepper.

BRIE AND CAMEMBERT
Brie and Camembert are covered with an edible rind that can be bitter. Both are perfectly ripe when they 'ooze'; if they're runny, they're too ripe.

CAERPHILLY
A mild but tangy cow's-milk cheese that is eaten very young, this was at one time the cheese Welsh miners snacked on while at work. There are older versions with more complex floral flavours.

CASHEL BLUE
This Irish blue cheese with an edible rind has quickly developed an international reputation. In all but the youngest examples, melt-in-the mouth creaminess is combined with an incomparable rounded, mellow flavour.

CHEDDAR
Cheddar is the most popular cheese in the UK, and for good reason: it melts beautifully and is available from mild to extra mature.

CHESHIRE
Cheshire is probably Britain's oldest cheese, as it is mentioned in the Domesday Book. This crumbly, salty cheese is sold quite young and has a clean, mild, pleasant taste. The white and blue varieties have the best and most piquant flavours, compared with the red, which is dyed with anatto.

COTTAGE CHEESE
Whether your preference is for large- or small-curd cottage cheese, skip those that are reduced-fat, flavoured with pineapple or packaged with fruit toppings. If you

like fruit mixed in with your cottage cheese – and your Critical Carbohydrate Level for Losing (CCLL) is high enough – add some berries or other low-glycaemic fresh fruit, and avoid the excessively sweetened fruit in the commercial varieties.

CREAM CHEESE, PLAIN
Only plain, full-fat, brick-style cream cheese is allowed during Induction – cream cheese spreads, reduced-fat cream cheese and fruit-flavoured cream cheese are never acceptable. Flavoured cream cheese tends to be high in additives, so check ingredient labels carefully. You might be better off adding chopped fresh chives to cream cheese rather than buying a tub of pre-flavoured cheese.

CURD CHEESE
This is a general term for fresh soft cheeses, rather like cottage cheese and Quark. They are characterized by a soft, fresh, clean, slightly acidic flavour and are often used in cooking and baking.

DERBY
Apart from Sage Derby, the version flavoured with the juice from sage leaves, this once great cheese, rather like Cheddar but closer in texture, seems to be waning in popularity and is seen less and less in the shops.

DOLCELATTE
This creamy Italian blue cheese, a mild factory-made version of the tangy Gorgonzola, lives up to the meaning of its name, 'sweet milk'.

DOUBLE GLOUCESTER
This mild hard cheese tastes like a cross between Cheddar and Cheshire but has none of the crumbliness

of the latter. Beware the many flavoured types with added carb-laden ingredients. It makes a good cooking cheese.

EDAM AND GOUDA
Hailing from Holland, these cheeses are covered with an inedible wax. They have a mellow, somewhat nutty flavour.

EMMENTAL
Resplendent with the large cherry-sized holes that characterize Swiss hard cheeses, this ancient cheese comes in huge golden wheels. The sweet, mellow flavour develops a distinctive nuttiness as the cheese ages.

FETA
Feta cheese is cured in brine, so it's actually pickled. Because it's cured it isn't considered fresh, but it is nutritionally similar to fresh cheeses. It is, however, allowed on Induction.

FONTINA
Originally from northern Italy, Fontina is now made in several European countries. It melts well and works for almost any recipe. It's worth searching for the Italian variety, though, which is much tastier.

FROMAGE FRAIS
A soft fresh cheese with a taste and texture – and carb content – rather like yoghurt or soured cream. The French versions generally taste rather more like a cheese. As with most dairy produce, be extra wary of the lower-fat and flavoured versions, as they are higher in carbs.

HALUMI
This traditional white semi-hard cheese from Cyprus is made from sheep's milk with the addition of mint. Very versatile, it can be used in salads, like feta, and can also be fried and grilled readily, as it retains its shape when heated.

HAVARTI
This mild Danish cheese is often flavoured with caraway or dill.

GOAT'S CHEESE
Sometimes called chèvre, soft goat's cheese can range in texture from smooth and spreadable to quite crumbly. Hard goat's cheese is similar in texture to Cheddar.

GRUYÈRE
This hard moderate-fat Swiss cheese, made with summer cow's milk and with only a few small holes in the curd, has a fine, sweet, nutty flavour with a sharp salty tang. It melts well and is much used in cooking.

LANCASHIRE
Developed from Cheshire cheese about 300 years ago, this crumbly, fatty white cheese starts fairly soft and mellow when young, developing a richer flavour as it ages. It cooks very well and is a favourite choice for Welsh rarebit.

LEICESTER
A striking orange-red in colour, this hard cow's-milk cheese with a loose, flaky texture has a rich, tangy flavour and a mellow aftertaste. It also melts well, so is a popular choice in cooking. It is particularly good for grilling.

MANCHEGO
Manchego has a rich yet creamy texture and is Spain's best-known cheese. It is delicious as a snack and melts beautifully.

MASCARPONE
This ultra-rich fresh Italian cheese is similar to soft butter in consistency. Mix it with mustard or anchovies and serve it with vegetables for a tasty dip. In Ongoing Weight Loss (OWL), it is delicious with berries.

MOZZARELLA
If you're lucky enough to shop somewhere with a large cheese section, you may find balls of fresh mozzarella, although most of the big supermarkets carry tubbed mozzarella in the chilled dairy section. Drizzle a slice or two with olive oil and sprinkle with fresh basil for a treat.

PARMESAN AND PECORINO ROMANO
Parmesan and Pecorino Romano are hard cheeses from Italy that are ideal for grating or shaving over stews and soups. Parmesan is made from cow's milk. Pecorino Romano, a sharply flavoured cheese similar to Parmesan, is made from sheep's milk.

PONT L'ÉVÊQUE
Made in small squares, this cow's-milk cheese from Normandy should have distinctive lattice markings on its golden rind from the straw on which it is matured. Its creamy interior has a fresh, sweet flavour with a hint of sharpness.

PROVOLONE
Young provolone is recognizable by its whitish colour and mild flavour; aged provolone has a sharp, pungent bite and is creamier, almost yellow, in hue. Aged provolone is a delicious alternative to Cheddar or Parmesan.

QUARK
This is a version of fresh soft cheese, with the flavour and texture of soured cream, that originated in Germany but has achieved wide popularity. Like all fresh cheeses, it is higher in carbs than harder cheeses. You should avoid the low-fat versions, as they are higher in carbs.

RACLETTE
Very similar to Gruyère, this French cheese has a distinctive chestnut flavour. It is often served melted or with boiled potatoes, and is also used in cooking.

RICOTTA
Originally made from the whey drained off during the making of provolone and mozzarella, ricotta has a slightly sweet flavour and a somewhat grainy texture.

STILTON
This semi-hard blue-veined cheese is often hailed as the king of British cheeses. A good Stilton should be firm rather than crumbly, but with a buttery consistency and even veining, and should have an almost floral aroma. It is worth searching out some of the unpasteurized versions stocked by the better supermarkets for their deep rich flavours.

WENSLEYDALE
Yorkshire's ancient cheese is moist and crumbly, with the addictive delicate sourish flavour of buttermilk.

Fresh Fish, Seafood and Shellfish

Fish, particularly cold-water fish, provides a host of nutritional benefits. It is an excellent source of omega-3 fatty acids, a type of polyunsaturated fat that is essential to proper cell function and has been linked to cardiovascular health. These essential fats can protect against heart disease and high blood pressure and can reduce levels of triglycerides, as well as improving autoimmune diseases such as lupus and rheumatoid arthritis. Most types of fish are high in protein, B vitamins (particularly B_{12}) and minerals like zinc and selenium, and they provide varying degrees of vitamins A, D and E. Fish, with the exception of shellfish, contains no carbohydrate.

If you're reluctant to try fish because you think it's difficult to cook, don't give up without having a try. The majority of fish cook rapidly and, unless you're roasting a whole fish or lobster, most recipes can be on the table in about 30 minutes.

Fish can be categorized in a variety of ways, such as freshwater and saltwater, or round fish and flat, but for nutritional and culinary purposes the main difference is between lean and oily. In most fish, including the white fish, which are exceptionally low in fat, the oil is concentrated in the liver. Oily fish, such as anchovies, sardines, salmon, tuna and trout, have darker flesh because their oils are distributed throughout the body, and they can contain more than 5 per cent heart-healthy fat by weight.

It's worth observing that, when it comes to fish, frozen isn't necessarily bad – in fact, it can often be preferable to fresh. Deep-sea fish like swordfish and tuna are almost always frozen at sea, since fishing boats can remain at sea for several weeks; freezing prevents them spoiling. Prawns, scallops and lobster are often frozen at sea, too.

If you plan to freeze your fish when you get it home, ask the fishmonger if the fish has been previously frozen. He may have frozen fish that you can buy instead. It's safer not to freeze any type of food more than once.

Fish spoils quickly. If you're buying fresh (or defrosted frozen) fish, avoid those on polystyrene trays in plastic wrap. These can go off more rapidly than fish that's wrapped for you. If pre-wrapped fish is your only alternative, smell it. Spoilage will be obvious, even through the plastic.

The best indicator of freshness in fish is the eyes. If you're buying whole fish, check to see that the eyes aren't sunken or cloudy. The gills should be bright red and the skin shiny and bright. If you are buying fillets, the best test is texture: the flesh should feel firm when pressed. Of course you can't poke it to see how resilient it is, but ask the fishmonger to do it and watch closely to see that the flesh springs back quickly. If the fillets pass this test, ask to smell them. Don't be shy about this request – after all, you're the one who is paying, and fish is comparatively expensive.

If you've noticed a wider variety at the fishmonger's in recent years, you're probably seeing the effects of fish farming. Fish farming helps to reduce fluctuations in availability and price and, because farm-raised fish is fed a specific diet, this helps to ensure consistency in flavour and appearance, too. Detractors, however, believe that farm-raised fish tastes blander than wild fish. Because farm-raised fish live in pens or tanks, they may be fed antibiotics to reduce disease. There is also the effect that fish farming has on the environment.

That isn't to say that all wild fish is good for you. Potentially dangerous chemicals such as PCBs and mercury can build up in fish over time, so large, long-lived predatory fish like tuna, swordfish and shark can harbour higher levels of these and other toxins.

Your best bet is to eat a variety of fish from a number of sources. If your diet includes freshwater and saltwater fish, large and small, lean and fatty, finned and shellfish, you'll lessen your exposure to harmful elements while obtaining a variety of nutrients. Advice from the UK Food Standards Agency is that, due to its healthy attributes, people should consume at least two portions of fish a week, one of which should be oily, but that no one should consume more than four portions of oily fish per week. However, pregnant and breast-feeding women are advised to eat no more than one or two portions of oily fish a week, and should not eat swordfish, marlin or shark.

FRESH FISH

ANCHOVIES
Tiny silver fish from the Mediterranean, anchovies are an excellent source of omega-3s. It's unlikely that you'll find fresh anchovies in a supermarket, as most go for salting and canning or bottling, but if you do be sure they are on ice – anchovies can go off quickly.

BREAM
There are many different varieties of bream, but those usually sold for eating are generally imported from warmer waters. Sea bream (often called porgy) is popular, especially in Japanese cuisine, but none is

more sought after than the gilthead bream or daurade, which is believed to have the best flavour and often features on the menus of both French and Italian restaurants.

CATFISH
Also known as wolf fish, rockfish, rock eel or rock salmon, this used to be a real chip-shop favourite. Fillets are white to pale pink, and may have yellow stripes on them. Catfish has a large flake and the inedible skin is usually removed.

COD
Cod flakes easily into large pieces. Salt cod, sometimes called bacalao, and dried cod or stockfish, which must be soaked in water before being cooked, are also carb-free.

COD ROE
Normally sold ready-boiled in salty water, this is most often then sliced and fried. Apart from the tinned variety, it is usually only available from November to March. Smoked roe can also be found and is a bit of a gourmet speciality.

COLEY
Also known as coalfish, saithe or rock salmon, this is a tasty fish from the cod family that has long been underrated and, as a result, is usually quite inexpensive. The flesh does tend to dry on cooking, but it is as nutritious as that of cod.

DAB
Native to northern European waters, this small lozenge-shaped fish is among the smallest of the flatfish. It is said to be at its best in autumn.

DOVER SOLE

The epithet 'Dover' has been added to the description of the sole in recent decades to differentiate it clearly from the lemon sole, which is not actually a sole at all (see below). Another reason may possibly be that even the French admit that the tastiest of this firm-textured, fine-flavoured fish, native to coastal waters between the Mediterranean and Norway, are to be found off the coast of Dover.

EEL

Once 'poor man's food', as were oysters, these long, serpentine fish with tasty omega-rich oily flesh, high in vitamins A and D, are now much less common and, as a result, are rather an expensive luxury. Smoked eel is a great delicacy.

HADDOCK

This close relation of the cod is like a smaller version of that fish. It has flaky white flesh and a fine flavour, which some say can be even better than that of cod. It is a good choice, as it is just as healthy but not as endangered a species as cod – and it is usually cheaper. Smoked haddock, or finnan haddie, is a great treat, but beware of cheaper versions that have been dyed with chemicals rather than properly smoked.

HAKE

Another member of the cod family, hake is larger than haddock but similarly flavoured, although the flesh tends to be softer and creamier. There are those, especially in the Iberian peninsula, who say that, when perfectly fresh, hake is the star of the white fish.

HALIBUT
The largest of the flatfish, halibut has a good flavour but its flesh tends to be coarse and rather dry. Smaller specimens are often called 'chicken halibut'. Whether buying steaks or fillets, look for firm, pearly-white flesh; those that are thinner than 2.5cm/1 inch will be more tender.

HERRING
There are many different varieties of this tasty oily fish, which packs as much protein, weight for weight, as beef. In addition to being as rich a source of omega-3s as salmon, herring is a good source of the anti-osteoarthritis vitamin D. A victim of over-fishing in the 1960s and 1970s, stocks in the northern Atlantic have now recovered considerably and herring are again widely available and relatively inexpensive. They are, however, still most commonly encountered in preserved form, either marinated in an aromatic vinegar as rollmops or Bismarck herrings, or salted and smoked as kippers or bloaters.

HERRING ROE
Long regarded as a bit of a delicacy, this has recently been relaunched, salted and pressed in small jars as something halfway between lumpfish roe and caviar, under the name Avruga.

JOHN DORY
Also known as St Peter's fish, this Mediterranean fish with a lobster-like flavour has become incredibly popular on restaurant menus. It is, however, very expensive, as about two-thirds of the weight of each fish is inedible head and innards.

LEMON SOLE

Not actually a sole at all but a closer relative of the dab and plaice, this is a pleasant-tasting and relatively inexpensive alternative to Dover sole.

LING

A member of the cod family, this 'poor relation' is widely available and relatively cheap, but the flesh is inclined to wateriness.

LUMPFISH ROE

The lumpfish itself makes poor eating but it is trawled in the North Sea for its roe, which, salted and pressed in small jars, makes a passable mock caviar. Check the labels for additives such as colourants and preservatives.

MACKEREL

Often sold whole, these small fish sometimes appear as fillets. Look for bright, almost vividly coloured skin. Mackerel is a wonderfully rich source of omega-3s and also contains many vitamins and minerals. It is at its best from January to June. Smoked mackerel is a great deli stand-by for snacks and pâtés, but it is becoming increasingly expensive.

MAHI MAHI (DOLPHIN FISH)

Mahi mahi, although a type of dolphin, is nothing whatsoever to do with the true dolphin, which is of course actually a mammal. It has a mild, sweet flavour and its flesh, which can be beige to rose-coloured, should be quite firm. Mahi mahi is fairly low in omega-3s.

MARLIN
This large, meaty fish has become increasingly popular in the wake of fresh tuna and swordfish. As it is a long-lived predator, it is one of those fish that health authorities are warning may carry high levels of toxic chemicals.

MONKFISH
The texture of the very fashionable monkfish is reminiscent of sea scallops or lobster, and its flavour is mild and slightly sweet. Its flesh should be creamy white. Only the meaty tail is sold.

MULLET, GREY
This silvery-grey fish is fairly high in oil content. Its firm white flesh has a distinctly nutty flavour. The roe is highly prized in the Mediterranean area. Salted, pressed and dried, it is called boutargue or botargo and is served thinly shaved on toast, in salads or over pasta.

MULLET, RED
The red mullet is not a mullet at all but a member of (or actually a couple of members of) the goatfish family. Primarily a Mediterranean fish, although those caught off the coast of Cornwall are well regarded, it has long been highly prized for its fine, full, gamey flavour. The French call it *bécasse de mer*, or sea woodcock, as it may be eaten guts and all, and its liver is a great delicacy, left in even if the fish is gutted. Use the liver for a sauce.

PLAICE
A relative of the lemon sole and the flounder, plaice needs to be ultra-fresh to be at its best, otherwise it tends towards wateriness.

SALMON

There are two main groups of salmon varieties, Pacific and Atlantic, but all are roughly similar. It is the Atlantic types that we generally see fresh, while the Pacific species like pink and sockeye (or red) are the ones we mostly come across in tins. The main difference to note in fresh salmon is between wild and farmed, the former now increasingly rare and expensive. Salmon is one of the best sources of omega-3 oils and is also high in protein and a rich source of vitamin A and the B group vitamins.

Smoked salmon was once a great luxury, but now widespread farming has made it almost everyday fare. It maintains a good level of the fish's nutritive value and is leaner.

SALMON EGGS

Previously only really enjoyed by the Finns and other northern Europeans, salmon roe has been fairly aggressively marketed in Britain over the last few years. Its luscious large, juicy, golden eggs make a delightful, fresher – and cheaper – alternative to caviar.

SARDINES

As with anchovies, fresh sardines are a rarity in most supermarkets. However, Cornish sardines are now appearing more regularly in summer to satisfy the growing barbecue market. Fresh sardines taste remarkably different from tinned ones, so if you find some, try them split and grilled. Sardines are exceptionally rich in omega-3s, even those in tins, which sometimes also actually improve in flavour with age.

SEA BASS
Sea bass has a mild, sweet flavour and is quite flaky. Look for firm flesh; its colour can range from white to a pearly beige-pink, but it should be translucent.

SKATE
Skate is the term used to describe the edible members of the ray family. It is generally the fleshy wings of skate, with a flavour of crab or scallops from the fish's seafood diet, that are sold. Like shark, they have a natural aroma of ammonia, which can be neutralized by soaking the fish in acidulated water.

SNAPPER
Red snapper has a pearly-pink flesh and a deep reddish-orange skin. If the fish is whole, you'll know it's authentic red snapper – as opposed to the many other varieties of snapper, many of which also have red skins – by its red eyes.

SWORDFISH
Fresh swordfish has a pearly, glistening sheen. Its colour indicates the fish's diet, not its quality (prawns turn the flesh a pinkish hue). Swordfish contains moderate levels of omega-3s. As with tuna and marlin, because it is a long-lived predator it is one of those fish that health authorities are warning may carry high levels of toxic chemicals.

TILAPIA
Tilapia has a white-to-pink flesh and a somewhat soft texture. Almost all tilapia sold is farmed.

TROUT
Fish from this huge family related to the salmon can be palest pink or deep orange. Whether you find freshwater trout, such as rainbow, brook or speckled, or seagoing trout, such as steelhead, they should have a firm, fine-grained flesh. Most trout are moderately high in omega-3s.

TUNA
Tuna steaks range in colour from pale pink (albacore tuna) to ruby red (yellowfin tuna) to almost maroon (big-eye tuna); darker tuna tends to be more robustly flavoured. Albacore is lower in omega-3s than other varieties. Yellowfin is the variety favoured by the Japanese for sashimi.

WHITEBAIT
These tiny fish are the fry of various oily fish, like herring, pilchard and sprats, and are usually dusted with seasoned flour and fried as a first course. As they are so young and their bones are not fully formed, they may be eaten in their entirety.

WHITING
One of the most undervalued of the cod family, the whiting's flesh is very delicately flavoured and easily digested. If not very fresh, its subtlety is lost.

SHELLFISH

Long avoided because of their high cholesterol content, shellfish are actually fine for most people to eat. This is because very few people experience a rise in blood cholesterol levels from eating foods that are high in cholesterol; it is actually your own liver that produces most of the cholesterol in your blood.

Shellfish are extremely perishable and should only be purchased on the day you plan to cook them (or buy frozen shellfish and put them in the freezer as soon as you get home). Some shellfish are purchased live – lobster, clams and mussels, for example. Choose feisty lobsters and tightly closed bivalves, and if they're packed in plastic when you buy them, remove them from the packaging once you get home so that they don't suffocate.

Smell shellfish to be sure they have a briny aroma, and avoid anything that smells musty or of ammonia. Avoid any bivalves, like mussels and clams, that are open and don't snap shut when tapped.

Clams, oysters and mussels are higher in carbs than other shellfish, so limit your portion size to 115g. Squid and scallops aren't that much lower.

FRESH SHELLFISH
Clams, Cooked
The most widely available variety of clam in Europe is the common clam – known as *palourdes* in France and *vongole* in Italy – while hard-shelled clams, or the American quahogs, now found on this side of the Atlantic, are *the* clam for chowder. Long meaty razor clams can also be found in some supermarkets and are becoming increasingly popular.

Cockles
This is a term used for several types of bivalve with a characteristic heart shape that are treated like clams.

Crab, Cooked
With the exception of soft-shell crabs, most crabmeat is sold already cooked. Even so, it's still extremely

perishable. It's usually sold in tubs, and you should ask the fishmonger to open the tub so you can smell it. It should smell of the sea. (Tinned and pasteurized refrigerated crabmeat is not as perishable.) Crab is one of the few shellfish with significant levels of omega-3s. Beware of crab or seafood sticks, or surimi, which are made from pollock or from cheaper white fish like whiting and often contain potatoes or other fillers.

Dublin Bay Prawns

Known as *langoustines* to the French and *scampi* to the Italians, these delicious 'lobsterettes' were regularly thrown back into the sea by British fishermen until recently. The best now get exported to Europe, while the rest are shelled, breaded and frozen, and sold as 'scampi'.

Lobster

A live lobster should be very active. Watch closely as it's lifted from the tank to be sure it's waving its claws and flapping its tail.

Mussels

Look for tightly closed mussel shells. If they are loose, choose ones that feel only moderately heavy (really heavy ones may be full of sand) and don't slosh around when shaken, as this may indicate that the mussel is dead. Green-lipped mussels from New Zealand are among the tastiest and best buys available, and are deemed by some to have therapeutic properties. Mussel meat is also available in tubs; these mussels should be plump and juicy-looking, beige to orange in colour. Mussels provide some omega-3s. Tinned smoked mussels make a very good storecupboard stand-by.

Oysters

Oyster shells should be tightly closed or should snap shut if tapped. The shucked meat should be beige and its liquid should be only slightly cloudy. Oysters provide some omega-3s and are packed with useful minerals.

Prawns

Ignore signs about the number of prawns to a kilo or pound – what's considered 'extra-large' at one shop may be 'medium' at another. Instead, purchase prawns by the weight, and don't forget that there's considerable waste with the shells. (Figure at least 675–900g to serve four.) Prawns should look firm and fill the shells. Prawns from the colder waters of the North Atlantic are said to have a better flavour than the larger creatures from the warm waters of the Pacific. Larger whole prawns should have the dark vein, or intestinal tract, under the back removed, as it can be gritty and harbour potentially toxic waste matter.

Scallops

Whether you choose sea scallops (up to 3.5cm in diameter) or bay scallops (about 2cm), they should be firm, with translucent flesh.

Squid (Calamari)

Choose calamari with small (no longer than 10cm), milky-white bodies and maroon tentacles; larger ones tend to be tough.

Whelks

These tiny sea snails were traditional seaside treats bathed in vinegar, but more sympathetic treatment can produce a real treat.

Prepared Fish and Shellfish

Most supermarkets sell prepared fish and shellfish behind the counter, or in a refrigerator or freezer case near the fish counter.

Sometimes these are prepared at the store, and you should be able to find out what ingredients are included by asking someone at the counter. If you get a vague answer, play it safe – skip the prepared fish and make your own.

Refrigerated or frozen fish and shellfish can vary considerably among brands. In general, though, breaded and battered fillets, fishcakes and stuffed shellfish are high in carbs and off-limits on Atkins. Pickled herring may contain sugar or another sweetener, and some salmon is coated with a sugar mixture before smoking and curing, so read the ingredients list when one is provided. Watch out for seafood salads, which may contain hidden carbs or caloric sweeteners.

Fruit

Most fruits are acceptable in the Pre-Maintenance and Lifetime Maintenance phases of the Atkins Nutritional Approach™ (ANA™). Because they are relatively low in carbohydrates (and have a high-antioxidant content), berries are among the first foods to be added back during Ongoing Weight Loss (OWL). When it's time to reintroduce other fruits to your menus, do so slowly and in small increments.

Although not traditionally considered fruits, tomatoes, olives and avocados are acceptable foods on Induction and are, botanically, deemed fruits.

BERRIES

Berries can be one of the first foods you'll add back to your menus after Induction, and for good reason: they contain fantastically high concentrations of beneficial plant compounds and antioxidants, and are fairly low in carbs.

BLACKBERRIES

High in soluble fibre, vitamin C, and phytochemicals such as anthocyanins and ellagic acid (an antioxidant), blackberries are at their peak from summer through to early autumn.

BLUEBERRIES

Among the most antioxidant-rich foods, blueberries contain generous amounts of soluble fibre, vitamins E and C and several types of anthocyanins. Cultivated blueberries are at their best in early summer, but keep an eye out for the tiny and tasty wild blueberries.

CRANBERRIES
The good news about cranberries is that they're almost as nutrient-rich as blueberries. The bad news is they are so tart that they verge on unpalatable when raw and unsweetened. Try making cranberry sauce using Splenda® to mellow their naturally sharp flavour.

GOOSEBERRIES
Like other berries, gooseberries are high in fibre and vitamin C, as well as in phytochemicals. Look for them from late May through to July. Use them in a sauce for sautéed chicken or salmon.

LOGANBERRIES
A hybrid of blackberries and raspberries, loganberries are purplish-red and somewhat tart when ripe. Look for them in June and July. They are quite perishable, so use them within a day or two of purchase.

RASPBERRIES
Exceptionally high in flavour and fibre, these are at their best from early summer to mid-autumn. Handle them gently – they are incredibly fragile and should be eaten as soon as possible after purchase. Red and black raspberries contain anthocyanins; the rarer gold ones don't.

REDCURRANTS
These tiny berries are relatives of the gooseberry and can be found from June to August. Stir them into sauces or enjoy them sweetened with Splenda® and topped with cream.

STRAWBERRIES
Gram for gram, ounce for ounce, strawberries are higher in vitamin C than oranges. They contain anthocyanins and ellagic acid (an antioxidant), as well as fibre. Locally-grown strawberries in season will be higher in flavour and freshness than imported varieties. Like all berries, strawberries are highly perishable.

TAYBERRIES
These long, thin, pale berries are a cross between a Scottish raspberry and an Oregon strain of blackberry. Developed as recently as the 1980s, they have the qualities of both antecedents and are now grown widely for their fine flavour. They're available from May to July.

CITRUS FRUITS

Choose to eat the fruit rather than juicing it: you'll get significantly more fibre and, if you eat the membranes, phytochemicals.

GRAPEFRUIT
Best known for their vitamin C content, grapefruit – the red and darker pink ones especially – are high in beta-carotene and lycopene, two of the carotenoids. The red variety is also slightly higher in fibre and in vitamin C than the white, and it tends to be sweeter.

KUMQUATS
These small citrus fruits can be eaten whole, skin and all. Most often found from late autumn through to late winter, they are high in vitamin C.

LEMONS
Fresh lemon juice is vastly superior to bottled, so it's worth keeping a few on hand at all times. Choose lemons that feel heavy for their size, as they will contain more juice, and don't forget to use the zest, or yellow part of the peel, in recipes. It's high in limonenes, a phytochemical with anti-cancer properties.

LIMES
The greener the lime, the tarter the juice. Yellower limes are riper, and their juice can be bland. As with lemons, lime zest is high in limonenes.

ORANGES
High in vitamin C, oranges supply fibre and some folate, too. The most common varieties of orange are navel and Valencia, but keep an eye out for blood oranges in the winter. They are very sweet and juicy, and their deep crimson colour comes from anthocyanins, the pigments that give berries their antioxidant punch.

TANGERINES
Tangerines, with their close cousins clementines and mandarin oranges, contain vitamin C as well as a host of carotenoids: beta-carotene, beta-cryptoxanthin, lutein and zeaxanthin.

MELONS

Melons are high in antioxidants. Avoid prepared melon at supermarkets, as its vitamin C content diminishes rapidly when exposed to oxygen. Buy whole fruits and slice them yourself to preserve the nutrients.

CANTALOUPE MELONS
These are an excellent source of vitamin C, beta-carotene, and potassium.

GALIA MELONS
These supply some beta-carotene and vitamin C.

HONEYDEW MELONS
These supply generous amounts of vitamin C and zeax-anthin.

WATERMELONS
Most people associate lycopene with tomatoes, but watermelon is actually higher in this carotenoid than uncooked tomatoes are.

TROPICAL FRUITS

AVOCADOS, HAAS
Haas avocados are small, with dark, pebbly skin. They're considerably lower in carbs than the larger, brighter Florida avocados (which have 5.5g per half-fruit) and higher in beneficial fats, making them a satisfying addition to Induction. Avocados are high in fibre, folate and iron.

BANANAS
Although an excellent source of vitamin B6, bananas are also very high in carbs. As they ripen, the starch turns to sugar. Once they are just barely ripe, store them in the refrigerator to prevent them from ripening further.

CARAMBOLA (STAR FRUIT)

Originally from Asia, star fruit is also now grown in Florida. Wait until the skin is a deep yellow-gold colour and aromatic before eating. This fruit provides some vitamin C.

CHERIMOYA

Often called custard apple, cherimoyas are wonderfully fragrant and sweet, tasting like a combination of pineapple, papaya and banana, and with the texture of a firm custard.

COCONUT

Obtaining fresh coconut flesh can be an effort, but it's worth it. These fruits supply some folate, and they're a good source of fibre and cholesterol-lowering phytoesterols.

KIWI

Exceptionally high in fibre, vitamin C and potassium, kiwis also contain lutein and cholorogenic acid, two antioxidant phytochemicals. There's no need to peel a kiwi – not only are the skins edible, they're full of nutrients. Just wash, then rub off the fuzz.

MANGOES

Mangoes range in colour from green through gold to reddish orange; the hue varies by type, not ripeness. A mango that's past its prime smells somewhat fermented and remains indented when pressed gently, so choose fruits that smell flowery and spring back when pressed.

PAPAYA OR PAWPAW

High in vitamin C, vitamin E, folate and fibre, papaya also contains beta-carotene and beta-cryptoxanthin. Don't discard the seeds – they are edible and have a spicy, somewhat peppery flavour.

PASSION FRUIT

Because passion fruit is grown all over the world, different varieties are available almost all the year round. The most common type is egg-shaped and has a purple rind. The seeds are edible and contribute a great deal of fibre to the fruit.

PINEAPPLE

Pineapples are harvested when they are on the verge of being fully ripe; the best-quality ones are shipped by air from tropical areas like Hawaii, Florida and Central America. Choose large pineapples, as they have more succulent flesh compared to the fibrous core.

PLANTAINS

Popular in Latin American countries, plantains are a larger, firmer variety of banana, which are served cooked. The flavour is mild and similar to squash.

PHYSALIS

These intriguing fruits of the tomato family are characterized by their unique appearance: a berry enshrouded in papery casing. The variety most familiar in this country is the Cape gooseberry or goldenberry, valued for its deliciously tart flavour and custardy texture, as well as for its decorative appearance.

STONE FRUIT

APRICOTS

Related to the peach, apricots are generally smaller and have a smooth, oval stone that comes away readily when the fruit is halved. They are a highly perishable fruit that doesn't travel well. Imported apricots never quite match the incomparable aroma and taste of fruit fresh from the tree. Don't settle for tinned apricots: they are lower in beta-carotene and vitamin C and higher in sugars.

CHERRIES

Cherries are in season from late June to mid-August. Bing cherries are the most prevalent variety, but they can vary considerably in quality. Choose carefully, looking for dark red fruit with unbroken skins.

NECTARINES

In season throughout the summer months, nectarines are available with familiar peachy-gold or white flesh. Choose the yellow variety, for the carotenoids contain beta-carotene and beta-cryptoxanthin.

PEACHES

At their peak in summer, the best way to determine a peach's ripeness is by feeling and smelling – many varieties are bred to have a red blush to the skins no matter how ripe they are (or aren't). In addition to the usual yellowy-pink peach, look for white peaches.

PLUMS

Plums supply some vitamin C, as well as small amounts of vitamin E. Black, purple and red plums are high in antioxidant anthocyanins.

GRAPES

Grapes, particularly those with dark skins, supply a host of phytochemicals. Eat them with caution, though, because they're high in carbs. If your preferred grape is green and seedless, consider this: seeded grapes are considered to have more flavour than seedless varieties, and red and black grapes are thought to have higher levels of flavonoids such as resveratrol and anthocyanins.

OTHER FRUITS

APPLES
If you want to get the most nutrients from an apple, choose a red one and eat the skin. Red apple skins contain anthocyanins; all apples contain quercetin.

DATES
Available both fresh and dried, dates are high in carbs: of the 16.54g carbs found per three fresh dates, 16g are sugar. Of the various types you will find in supermarkets, the best are the deglet noor and medjool varieties. Snip them with kitchen scissors (it's easier than chopping) into small pieces and use them in fruit compotes, or stir them into bulgur pilaf.

FIGS
Like dates, figs are available both fresh and dried; dried figs can get a whopping 90 per cent of their calories from sugar! Look for fresh figs in markets from late spring to late autumn.

GUAVA
When it comes to vitamin C, this tropical fruit is off the charts.

LOQUATS
Loquats have an apricot-coloured skin, but the fruit tastes more like a plum. They are very fragile and quite difficult to find. Choose large ones. They make a tasty addition to a chicken salad.

LYCHEES
If your encounters with lychees don't extend beyond the local Chinese restaurant, you might not recognize them in the supermarket. These cream-white, sweet fruits come encased in a rough, reddish-brown shell. In Europe, fresh lychees are available from November to January, but they are probably most often sold tinned, preserved in sugar syrup, making them off-limits for Atkins followers.

PEARS
Pears are quite high in sugar, but they supply good amounts of soluble (i.e. cholesterol-lowering) fibre as well as some vitamin C. Leave the skin on, though, to get the most of both nutrients.

POMEGRANATES
The pomegranate's crimson flesh is high in anthocyanins, as well as catechins and ellagic acid (an antioxidant). These compounds may make this fruit even higher in antioxidant potency than green tea or red wine. Pomegranates are in season from early autumn to early winter, but are at their best in November and December.

QUINCES
Very astringent and dry in texture, quinces are almost always served cooked. Look for them from early autumn to early winter.

RHUBARB
Unpalatably tart in its raw state, rhubarb is usually cooked with sweetener. Although rhubarb is, botanically, a vegetable, it's most commonly used as a fruit. It becomes sweeter as it's cooked, so add sweetener after it is tender.

SHARON FRUITS
In season from December to February, Sharon fruits, a type of persimmon, are ripe when they are plump, firm and glossy. They provide some vitamin C and also contain alpha-carotene, beta-carotene and beta-cryptoxanthin.

Grains and Pulses

Whole grains (as well as foods made from them), beans and legumes are rich in nutrients, including carbohydrates. During the weight-loss phases of the Atkins Nutritional Approach™ (ANA™), these foods will be absent from your eating plan. However, once you have successfully incorporated seeds and nuts, as well as berries, into your menus, you can consider adding back beans. But you should wait until after you've begun to eat fruits other than berries and starchy vegetables before you add whole grains.

GRAINS

The final rung on the Carbohydrate Ladder, whole grains are complex carbohydrates that are digested slowly and thus have less effect on blood sugar levels than refined grains. They contain varying amounts of protein, B vitamins and trace minerals.

BARLEY
Barley is used in many cultures and cuisines. In the UK it features mostly in soups. Pearl barley cooks more quickly than whole-grain barley because its husk has been removed, but it isn't technically a whole grain because the bran has been removed. However, its glycaemic index – the impact it has on your blood sugar – is relatively low. Whole-grain barley has a nuttier flavour and makes an unusual but tasty vegetarian risotto.

BUCKWHEAT

Buckwheat is rich in vitamins A and B and calcium. The grain is used in Eastern European cooking to make dumplings and blinis, while in France and America the flour is a favourite for pancakes.

BULGUR WHEAT

Also known as cracked wheat, bulgur is a form of whole wheat. The wheat berry is cooked, dried and then cracked and can either be cooked briefly or soaked in boiling water before eating. When cut fine, it is used for tabouleh.

COUSCOUS

Couscous is not a whole grain. It's similar to pasta and is made from semolina dough that has been cut into tiny pieces. It should be lightly steamed to allow the grains to swell and soften. It is a staple of North African cuisine and is served as an accompaniment to vegetable stews or to lamb, spicy sausages or chicken. When doing Atkins, only whole-wheat couscous is acceptable.

FLAXSEED

Flaxseed, also known as linseed, is an excellent source of omega-3 fatty acids and magnesium and has a delicious nutty flavour. It lowers blood pressure, helps to prevent heart disease and can even promote relaxation. Flaxseed oil is highly perishable and should be refrigerated. The seeds can be bought vacuum-packed, either whole or already ground. Once ground, they should be kept in an airtight container in the fridge. Ground flaxseed can be added to breakfast smoothies, to hot or cold cereal, or sprinkled over cooked vegetables. The seeds can be added to muffin and bread mixes.

MILLET

Millet makes a nutritious change from rice but it is not widely used in the UK. It is a good source of magnesium and zinc, and supplies thiamin and niacin as well. It can be used to thicken soups, served as an accompaniment to casseroles and cooked with milk as a breakfast cereal.

OATS

A staple of northern European cuisine, oats are extremely nutritious, containing iron, vitamin B, potassium, protein and fat. The various forms can be used to make porridge, oatcakes and crumble toppings and to coat meat or fish before frying. Be aware that old-fashioned rolled oats are acceptable on Atkins, but processed or instant oats are not.

POLENTA

Made from maize, this golden cornmeal is cooked with water to form a savoury porridge that acts as a vegetable accompaniment in Italian cuisine. It can be served with meat, game and fish dishes. It can also be left to cool after cooking, then sliced and grilled, and is delicious with grilled Mediterranean vegetables.

SEMOLINA

Semolina has many uses: it can be cooked as a milky pudding, used in savoury dishes in its couscous form, or the flour can be made into tasty breads. It is also the principal ingredient of Italian pasta. It is higher in gluten content than other flours. Pasta made from semolina is not acceptable in any phase of Atkins.

TAPIOCA

This starchy by-product of a tropical root plant is used to flesh out stews and soups, but is probably best known as a sweetened milky pudding that used to be served at school dinners.

WHEAT

Apart from flour, wheat-germ, wheat bran and wheat flakes are just some of the by-products of this universal grain. Wheat-germ can be added to cereal and soups and is very nutritious. Bleached white flour is unacceptable in any phase of Atkins.

PULSES

Although you should steer clear of pulses during Induction, and (for most people) during Ongoing Weight Loss (OWL) too, they are a valuable form of protein and provide many essential minerals and vitamins. You can use them to bulk up stews and soups or serve them as a side vegetable or puréed as a dip, but keep an eye on serving size. Depending on the type of bean you use, 50g cooked pulses yields between 6 and 20g carbs.

Some pulses, such as lentils and soya beans, have a lower glycaemic index. All pulses offer a good source of B vitamins and minerals, as well as fibre, protein and carbohydrate. Beans also contain antioxidants that can help prevent some types of cancer and protect against heart disease. To cut back on carbs, use pulses as an 'extra' rather than the main ingredient – toss a handful into salads, use in stir-fries or add to soups.

Try to eat beans with vegetables that are high in vitamin C, such as tomatoes. This helps your body absorb the iron from the beans.

Preparation: Dried beans are a storecupboard staple. They should be thoroughly rinsed and soaked before cooking: either soak them in plenty of cold water overnight or cover them with boiling water and soak for three hours. Kidney beans contain toxins in the outer skin and must be boiled for 20 minutes prior to cooking. Soya beans need to be boiled for an hour, because they contain a substance that prevents the body from absorbing protein.

Don't season your beans until the last half-hour of cooking, as salt has a hardening effect.

ADUKI BEANS

These small, rust-coloured beans are high in iron. They are a common ingredient in Japanese cooking, but they have many other uses. They make a tasty contribution to salads, are also useful in vegetarian stuffings and can be ground into a flour to make breads, cakes and pastry.

BLACK BEANS

Black beans have a creamy texture and a rich flavour. They can be used to bulk up stews, and in black bean soup their creamy flavour contrasts beautifully when combined with the sharp hints of coriander and cumin.

BLACK-EYED PEAS (BLACK-EYED BEANS)

These small white beans with black dots provide almost half the daily requirement of folate per serving. They are used in Indian and southern American cookery and are also popular in Africa.

BORLOTTI BEANS

An Italian variety of the common bean, these are a useful staple for salads, soups and stews.

BROAD BEANS
Also known as fava beans, these have a mild, floury flavour. They make a hearty addition to soups and are delicious when puréed. Look out for fresh broad beans in early summer.

BUTTER BEANS
Sometimes called lima beans, butter beans have a sweet flavour and make a good base for a bean salad or stew. They are particularly high in potassium.

CANNELLINI BEANS
Cannellini beans are another staple of Italian cookery. These white kidney beans have a creamy flavour and a light texture, making them ideal in stews, soups and salads. They form the basis of a substantial salad when combined with tinned tuna, parsley, olive oil and wine vinegar – the classic Italian *tonno e fagioli*. They also pair particularly well with bitter greens – add them to sautéed endive.

CHICKPEAS
Chickpeas (known in America as garbanzo beans) are rich in folate and iron, and in both soluble and insoluble fibre. They are a popular ingredient in many parts of the world – Greece, North Africa, Spain and India. They are delicious in spicy meat stews and are the chief ingredient in hummus, the creamy Middle Eastern dip. They may also be served with couscous, and are particularly delicious with lamb. They need to be soaked and cooked for longer than most other pulses.

FLAGEOLET
These young haricot beans have the most delicate flavour of all and care should be taken not to smother

them with stronger-flavoured ingredients. Serve them simply as a vegetable accompaniment, drizzled with olive oil or butter, or use them in a tomato and avocado salad.

HARICOT BEANS

The haricot is a small, white bean that retains its shape when cooked, which makes it the perfect ingredient for slow-cooked dishes such as cassoulet. Because haricots have a particularly mild flavour, they absorb stronger flavours easily.

KIDNEY BEANS

Large and dark red, with a firm, almost meaty texture, red kidney beans are often used in chilli. They're also a good choice for salads. If you're soaking and cooking other beans at the same time, be sure to cook kidney beans separately from paler beans, as they'll discolour them.

LENTILS

Lentils are an excellent source of folate and iron. There are many different types of this pulse, but the three most popular are green, brown and red. The tiny green Puy lentil has a delicate, distinct flavour that is very popular in its native France. It is delicious cooked with ham or fish. Brown lentils, like the Puy lentils, retain their shape when cooked and are equally good in soups and stews. Red lentils cook down into a delicious porridge-like consistency, making them ideal for soups and the Indian dhal.

MUNG BEANS

Most commonly encountered as sprouts, or ground and formed into bean threads (also called cellophane noodles and common in Chinese cookery), dried mung beans have an olive skin and yellow flesh. They have a surprisingly creamy texture.

PINTO BEANS

Pinto beans are an excellent source of cholesterol-lowering fibre, vitamins B_1 and B_6, potassium and magnesium. They are used in Mexican cookery – either refried or cooked with tomatoes, spices and cheese – and are delicious when blended with herbs and black pepper to make a versatile dip.

SOYA BEANS

Soya beans are a great source of protein and, unlike other beans, contain very little starch. Soya also helps lower cholesterol and blood pressure. Fresh soya beans take a considerable time to cook. Soya is also used to produce soya milk, tofu, miso (fermented soya bean paste) and soy sauce.

SPLIT PEAS

Available in yellow and green, split peas cook quickly and require no soaking. They are used in soups or steamed and served with roast pork.

Fresh Meat

Beef, veal, lamb and pork all supply protein, fat, B vitamins and iron, but absolutely no carbohydrate with the exception of organ meat (offal), which does contain some carbohydrate. It's only when you get into cured and prepared meat products that you need to pay careful attention to ensure you're not going to get any unpleasant surprises.

Although you needn't worry about weighing foods or obsess about counting calories when you're following the Atkins Nutritional Approach™ (ANA™), it's still wise to pay attention to portion sizes. If you consume a large steak, for instance, you may be too full to eat your vegetables, which means that you won't get enough other nutrients. Eating huge portions of protein can also cause the body to convert some of it to blood glucose, which will hinder a fat-burning metabolism. Start with about 225g of raw meat per person – that is, buy about 1kg of boneless meat to serve four people.

You should also limit portions of meat products that do include carbs, as well as cured meats. Most bacon, ham, hot dogs and the like are made with nitrates in order to preserve freshness. These compounds are harmless outside the body, but when you eat them they convert to nitrites, which have been proved to be carcinogenic when consumed over time.

BEEF

High in protein, iron and vitamin B_{12}, beef is available in almost endless variety, from quick-to-cook tender steaks to tougher cuts that require long, slow cooking. The most superior beef comes from young stock. Bright red meat indicates that it has not been well hung and will not be tender, while deep red flesh also signals that the meat will most likely be tough. Go for a colour in between the two – plum rather than maroon.

BRISKET
Brisket is the breast and can be sold on the bone or boned and rolled. The former is generally cut into smaller joints, which can be braised or pot-roasted. Rolled brisket is also good for pot-roasting. It can be bought salted too, which is ideal for boiling.

CHUCK STEAK OR BLADE BONE
A superior stewing steak, chuck and blade (also sold as braising steak) should be used in pies and stews, but never grilled or fried.

FILLET
This cut comes from below the sirloin and is sliced into steaks that are lean, tender and juicy. The fillet tapers along its length: filets mignons are generally cut from the thinner end, tournedos from further along, and fillet steaks from the middle. The thicker end makes a chateaubriand for quick roasting.

FLANK
Flank tends to be a fatty joint, which makes it good for braising, boiling or pot-roasting.

FORE RIB
A large joint ideal for roasting, fore rib can be boned and rolled prior to cooking, or cooked on the bone and then carved.

MINCED BEEF

Minced beef is quite versatile. It can be moulded into a juicy burger, made into meatballs, added to a chilli and tomato sauce or browned to make the base of a simple stir-fry.

NECK, CLOD OR STICKING

This inexpensive cut is best for stews and casseroles. Remove gristle from the meat before cooking.

RUMP STEAK

Not as expensive as sirloin or fillet steak, rump nonetheless offers excellent flavour. It is best when fried with onions or cooked under a hot grill.

SHIN

This cut has a high gelatine content and is used for brawn, stews and casseroles.

SILVERSIDE

Silverside is cut from between the rump and the leg. It can be roasted, spiced or salted for slow-cooking or boiling.

SIRLOIN

Tender and full of flavour – and thus one of the most expensive cuts – sirloin is used for the classic Sunday roast. More often than not it is sold boned and rolled, but it can be cooked on the bone as well. When sliced, sirloin provides entrecôte steaks.

SKIRT

Rump skirt must be trimmed of membrane and gristle before being minced or cubed for use in stews or casseroles.

TOP RUMP
Rump is taken from a large joint at the top of the leg. It can be stewed or braised, pot-roasted or slow-roasted.

TOPSIDE
This versatile cut, taken from the top inside of the back legs, can be roasted or braised. It is a lean, boneless joint and must be protected by larding fat if roasted.

VEAL

Veal is the flesh of calves between 16 and 20 weeks old, and is therefore very tender. It is high in protein and B vitamins; it's lower in fat and saturated fat than beef, mostly because it has very little marbling, or fat inside the muscle.

Veal, even from calves that are allowed to range freely, is quite tender; range-fed veal tends to be redder than stall-raised veal. Don't buy veal that is dark red or whitish-pink. The former will be on the old side, while the latter will lack flavour. Fat should be white, ivory or pale yellow, and the meat should be slightly moist but not mushy when you press it.

BELLY
Belly is sold in pieces for stewing.

LOIN
Veal loin is closer to the hip or leg, and is tender and flavourful. As a chop it is ideal sautéed or grilled, while larger joints – boned, rolled and stuffed or sold on the bone – make delicious roasts.

NECK
Neck is sold in pieces for stewing.

RUMP
This is the cut most usually sliced thinly and pounded into escalopes.

SHIN
This is the cut favoured by Italians for cooking as osso buco.

SHOULDER
Veal shoulder, unlike shoulder from other animals, involves only the uppermost portion of the front of the animal (breast and shank are the cuts lower on the front). Cuts from the shoulder are better if they are first browned, then braised or pot-roasted.

SILVERSIDE, ETC.
Silverside, topside and top rump are sold as joints or used to make escalopes.

LAMB

Lamb is high in iron, protein, zinc and several of the B vitamins. Choose reddish-pink cuts with pearly-white fat; dark red or purple meat and yellow fat are signs of age. Sheep are the only domesticated animals that resist all attempts to farm them intensively, so lamb remains one of the most natural and safe meats.

Next to Australians and New Zealanders, the British eat more lamb than do other nations. A good deal of the lamb we consume is home-grown, with the remainder being imported from Australia and New Zealand. Imported lamb will have been frozen and its flavour will be less subtle.

Lamb has a slightly gamey, sweet flavour that marries perfectly with strong seasonings like garlic, lemon, mint, rosemary and mustard, as well as the spices and dried fruits used in Indian and Moroccan cooking.

BEST END
Cut from between the middle neck and the loin, best end may be braised or roasted on the bone. Removing the chine or backbone and trimming away all the sinew and cartilage between the ribs produces the classic rack of lamb; two racks may be interleaved to form a guard of honour or a crown roast, which may then be filled with stuffing.

BREAST
The meat from this cut is quite fatty, which makes it a less popular and therefore cheaper option. It is ideal for roasting and braising and is usually sold boned, stuffed and rolled.

CHUMP
Chump is the lamb equivalent of beef rump steak.

CHUMP CHOPS
Because only two chops can be cut from between each leg and the loin, this is a costly cut but well worth the expense for flavour and tenderness. Each chop contains a small central bone.

FILLET
Fillets are taken from the best end of neck. They are quite small, so allow two per person. They are suitable for grilling or frying.

LEG
Leg is ideal for roasting, and joints from this cut can weigh as much as 2.75kg. It is often divided in two – knuckle and fillet – and can be roasted on the bone or boned and rolled.

LEG STEAKS
Cut from the boned leg, these steaks are extremely flavoursome.

LOIN
The loin can be ordered boned and rolled as a small roast, but generally this prime joint is sold on the bone to make a 1.8kg roast. It should have an even layer of fat under the skin. The loin is often sliced as chops.

MIDDLE NECK
Sometimes sold in one large piece with the scrag end (see below), this cut comes from between the scrag and the best end of neck. It can be quite fatty and contain bone, so is most suitable for stews, though if it is boned it can also be fried.

SADDLE
A saddle weighs about 3.65kg – an expensive but delicious roast. A saddle of lamb is the double loin joined along the backbone. A short saddle, without the chops, is considered to be possibly the best roast.

SCRAG ENG
Used for soups and stews, this cut can be quite gristly so is not suitable for anything else.

SHANKS
The lower end of the leg was, until recently, rarely sold except in specialist butchers' shops, but braised lamb shanks are now common on restaurant menus.

SHOULDER
Of all the roasting joints, this is the least expensive, largely because it is a tough cut. It is fairly fatty and more difficult to carve. Shoulder joints are fairly large. The meat may also be used for kebabs or stews.

SHOULDER CHOPS
These chops are best braised. Tenderness often depends on how they are cut.

PORK

Pork is extremely nutritious, containing more B vitamins than any other type of meat. Unlike beef, most pork is so tender that it doesn't need to be braised or pot-roasted, though some cuts can be braised or stewed with delicious results. Fresh pork doesn't keep as well as other meats, so care should be given to storage, preparation and cooking. Flesh should be pale pink, with little gristle, and smooth and firm to the touch.

BATH CHAPS
These are the bottom half of the jaw, cut in half. They are usually sold ready-boiled, skin and all.

BELLY
This is an inexpensive cut that can be roasted, stewed, grilled or salted. The thicker part of the belly is leaner, while the flank end is streakier.

BLADE BONE
A good-value joint that is taken from the shoulder, blade may be roasted on the bone or boned, stuffed and rolled for roasting.

KNUCKLE
Knuckle can be roasted or boned and stuffed. Cut from the lower portion of the leg, it is a fairly expensive joint. It is also excellent when stewed.

LEG
A whole leg can weigh in the region of 4.5–6.75kg. It is excellent roasted on or off the bone, and is one of the most expensive cuts of pork. Smaller joints of 1.35kg, sometimes part-boned, are also commonplace.

LOIN BEST END
The entire loin may be roasted whole, but it can also be cut into smaller joints or prepared by the butcher for a crown roast. It is the most expensive joint of pork, and when buying you should ask for a decent proportion of meat to fat.

LOIN CHOPS
Chops can be cut from the hind or the fore loin and, if the former, can come with the kidney.

NECK BONE
Known in Scotland as shoulder, and in northeast England as a chine, this inexpensive joint comes from the upper part of the shoulder. Apart from roasting, it can also be cut into cubes for kebabs.

SHOULDER (ALSO KNOWN AS HAND)
When boned, stuffed and rolled, this joint is ideal for roasting. It has a large proportion of rind, which makes wonderful crackling.

SPARE RIB JOINT
An upper shoulder cut that is suitable for stewing, braising or roasting.

SPARE RIB CHOPS
These chops have little bone and come from the neck end. They are best grilled or fried and have a sweet, tender flavour.

SPARE RIBS
These joints are used in East Asian cooking and can also be roasted or barbecued. Unlike the spare rib joint, they come from the rib part of the belly rather than from the shoulder.

STEAKS
Steaks are cut from the chump chop, an area that lies between the loin and the leg. They can be cut thinly and beaten flat with a rolling pin between greaseproof paper or clingfilm to form escalopes.

TENDERLOIN
Also known as fillet, this is the best cut for braising, grilling and frying. It may also be spread with a filling and rolled to form a joint for roasting.

OFFAL

Offal is rich in iron and trace minerals such as copper, zinc and phosphorus, and in B vitamins. Liver, the most common organ meat, is extremely high in vitamins A and C. Unlike other cuts of meat, it does contain some carbohydrates, so you should limit intake to 100g a day during Induction.

If you're a fan of liver, look for calves' liver rather than ox liver. Calves' liver is more tender and milder in flavour. Because the liver acts as a 'clearing house' for pesticides, fertilizers, antibiotics and other chemicals, calves' liver is likely to harbour fewer of these than the liver of an older animal.

Organ meats are highly perishable, so check that they are carefully packaged, with no holes or tears in the wrapping. Cook them on the day of purchase.

BEEF

Marrow Bones
Popular in continental cookery, beef thigh and shoulder bones contain marrow, which has a delicate flavour. Marrow can be used in dishes such as osso buco (in which veal marrow bones are used rather than beef) or poached as a spread for hors-d'oeuvres.

Ox Heart
Best used in stews and casseroles, this meat can be muscular and tough and requires slow cooking.

Ox Kidney
Suitable for slow-cooked stews, casseroles and pies, the ox kidney is large and tough.

Ox Liver
Because it is tough and has a strong flavour, this cut should not be grilled or fried. Instead, soak it in water or milk for several hours before stewing or braising.

Oxtail
Oxtail is an ideal ingredient for soups and casseroles. It is sold skinned and jointed.

Ox Tongue
Ox tongue must be cooked slowly for several hours. It can be bought fresh or salted.

Tripe
Tripe should be white, firm and thick. It comes from the lining of the stomach, and is sold bleached and partly boiled. Slice and deep-fry it; alternatively, try it boiled in milk or stewed.

VEAL

Calves' Kidney
More tender than ox kidney, this can be braised and stewed.

Calves' Liver
Calves' liver is pale and delicate. When frying it, cook it underdone. It may also be grilled.

Sweetbreads
Sold in pairs, veal sweetbreads are considered to be the most delicate of all varieties. May be braised or fried.

LAMB

Heart
Though this is the smallest and most tender of all hearts, it still requires slow cooking. It is exceedingly nutritious.

Kidneys
Lambs' kidneys are superior to any other type for frying or grilling.

Liver
Superb for grilling and frying, and less expensive than calves' liver.

Sweetbreads
These are easier to find than calves' sweetbreads and are just as tasty.

PORK

Caul fat
This is the thin, lacy layer of fat that lines the pig's stomach. It is used to wrap lean cuts of meat and dry mixtures like pâtés and terrines so that the melting fat bastes them during cooking.

Chitterlings
These are pig's intestines, sold ready-boiled. The skins are used as sausage casings.

Head
This is boiled to make the best brawn.

Heart
Stuffed and slowly braised, this makes a less expensive alternative to lambs' heart, though it is not as tender.

Liver
Best used for pâtés or in casseroles, pigs' liver may be grilled or fried, though the flavour will be stronger than calves' or lambs' liver.

Kidneys
It is essential that kidneys are halved and the cores are removed before cooking. They can be grilled, fried or diced for stews and casseroles.

Trotters
Use these as a base for soup, brawn or for making a jellied stock. Trotters can also be boned, stuffed and slow-roasted.

GAME

Game is richly flavoured despite being exceptionally lean.

GOAT

Like lamb, goat is milder in flavour and more tender when it is younger; try goat in any recipe calling for lamb.

HARE

Hare is comparable to the dark meat of chicken but has a stronger flavour. Best from October to March, young hares should be roasted whole, while older animals are best casseroled.

RABBIT

Rabbit is higher in fat than most game, but it is still lower in fat and cholesterol than beef or dark chicken meat. Rabbit shares the delicate flavour of the white meat of chicken.

VENISON

Leaner than beef, venison is an excellent alternative for red-meat lovers, supplying generous amounts of B vitamins, iron, riboflavin, niacin and zinc. Farmed venison is less gamey than wild venison. It is best from June to January.

Cold Meats, Sausages and Cured Meats

Sausages are made by grinding meats and combining them with fat, spices, seasonings and possibly a filler of some sort, such as breadcrumbs, cereals, soya-bean flour or dried-milk solids. These are used to stretch the meat further before the mixture is typically stuffed into casings. Given the range of possible fillers, it's easy to see how sausages can conceal added carbohydrates, so be sure to read ingredient labels carefully. Avoid those containing fillers and other unacceptable ingredients.

Equally, choose cured meats carefully. Curing extends storage life and is typically done using salt and/or smoke. However, if sugar is used in the curing liquid, some of it may penetrate the meat and add carbs. In addition, nitrates are frequently used in the process of curing as well as to act as a preservative (they impart a pinkish-red colour to foods such as ham and bacon). Look for fresh sausages, which are nitrate-free, and nitrate-free versions of bacon.

As with cuts of meat, it isn't necessary to weigh portions, but it's wise to pay attention to portion size.

BACON AND HAM

BACON

Bacon is pork that has been cured in salt or brine and then sometimes smoked. Unsmoked bacon is often termed 'green'. The cure can often contain added sugar or other sweet flavourings like honey, so avoid brands that contain these ingredients. Streaky bacon is made from the fatty belly of the pig, while back bacon includes the loin, and middle cut is between the two. Gammon comes from curing the hind leg of the pig in a piece, as with ham (see below).

COPPA
This raw ham from the Emilia Romagna region of Italy is made from rolled neck of pork seasoned with garlic, pepper and herbs. It is like a fattier, cheaper, more robust version of prosciutto, but is also much used as a flavouring in cooking.

HAM
Like bacon, hams are made by curing the hind legs of pigs in salt or brine; as with bacon, they are also then sometimes smoked. The cures used for ham are even more likely to contain sugar or other sweeteners and nitrate preservatives, so keep an eye on the labels. Whole hams are sold both cooked and raw, the latter usually requiring further cooking before they can be eaten, although some, like Italian Parma ham (prosciutto) and Spanish Serrano, are meant to be eaten raw (see below).

LUNCHEON MEAT AND HAM, BONELESS (TINNED OR PACKAGED)
Luncheon meats, and the sort that come vacuum-packed or in tins, are more accurately called 'ham and water products'. They are injected with a brine that cures them much more rapidly than dry-cured hams such as traditional York hams or prosciutto.

PANCETTA
Sometimes referred to as Italian bacon, pancetta is cured with salt and spices, but never smoked. It is

generally sold in a rolled piece or ready-cubed, for use as flavouring in sauces, stuffings, casseroles and other dishes.

PROSCIUTTO
Prosciutto, or Parma ham, is Italian ham that has been cured with sea salt and then hung to air-dry for several months. It is eaten raw, sliced thinly, and often served with melon or figs. Much of its delicious flavour is said to come from the pigs used, who enjoy a richly varied diet of wild treats like acorns and the whey left over from the making of local cheeses.

SPECK
This is a matured smoked ham from the northern part of Italy, where the German ham tradition prevails.

SAUSAGES

ANDOUILLE
A French sausage made from pork chitterlings and tripe, andouille is smoked and very spicy. It is a key ingredient in gumbo and jambalaya.

BLACK PUDDING
This sausage is made from pigs' blood and fat, together with some cereal like barley or rice and sometimes with added spices. The French version, boudin noir, tends to omit the cereal content and be smoother, and will obviously be lower in carbs. (See also White pudding, below.)

CHORIZO AND LINGUIÇA SAUSAGES
Popular in Portuguese and Spanish cooking, these spicy, garlicky sausages are a terrific way to add flavour

to soups and vegetable dishes. Both are deep red and look like other fully-cooked sausages, but chorizo and linguiça are fresh and need to be cooked thoroughly.

FLAVOURED SAUSAGES

Varieties such as pork, apple and cinnamon, spicy pork, polenta and tomato, and pork, apricot and lovage contain dehydrated fruits and other carb-containing ingredients, so they are not acceptable during Induction.

ITALIAN SAUSAGE, PORK

This fresh sausage comes sweet or hot, and sweet simply means not spicy rather than sweetened. Links are the most common, but you may find sausage patties, bulk sausage, meat for stuffings, etc.

POLISH SAUSAGE

Available made with pork, beef, turkey or a blend of all three, Polish sausage can vary widely in fat content (turkey is the leanest). For the best flavour, choose beef, pork or a blend.

PORK SAUSAGE

Like Italian sausage, the classic 'banger' is seasoned and often includes high-carb fillers such as bread-crumbs, oatmeal or flours.

SALAMI

These cured sausages nearly all contain nitrates; few are available in a nitrate-free form. Several of them are fairly high in carbs as well. You're best off consuming these in small portions, if at all. Rather than buy blister-packs of pre-sliced luncheon meats, stop at the deli counter for fresher meats with better flavour.

SMOKED SAUSAGES

As with Italian sausage, smoked sausages are available sweet or hot. Even if you skip the bun and sweetened condiments, you still may be surprised at the carb content of frankfurters and wurst varieties; they frequently contain cereals as filler. Skip the typical accompaniments and instead slice and pan-fry them before adding to a vegetable soup.

WHITE PUDDING

Also known as boudin blanc, this sausage can be made from a mix of pork and pork fat or may contain veal or chicken with added eggs and cream. Avoid white puddings that use breadcrumbs or oatmeal as a thickener.

OTHER PRESERVED MEAT PRODUCTS

BRAWN

This traditional preparation, which is also referred to as head cheese, is made from meat extracted from the head and trotters of the pig (or sometimes a veal calf) which is cooked and then set in a gelatinous stock pressed in a mould. Highly nutritious, it is served cut in thick slices.

BRESAOLA

This traditional Italian delicacy is made from beef fillet which has been air-dried like Parma ham. It is usually served raw and very thinly sliced, like the ham, and dressed with olive oil, lemon juice and black pepper, or perhaps with shavings of Parmesan cheese.

FAGGOTS

These meatballs are made from minced pigs' offal (traditionally liver and heart, and sometimes lungs), mixed with pork or bacon fat and chopped onions and wrapped in caul fat. Beware, as breadcrumbs are a fairly usual addition to the mixture.

JERKY

This is a traditional way of preserving meat, most commonly beef, by cutting it into strips, sometimes salting it and then drying it, usually in the sun. Popular with backpackers for its convenience, intense flavour and the protein it contains, it makes a good low-carb snack.

Poultry

Like fish, shellfish and meat, fresh poultry is one of the basic meal-builders when you're following the Atkins Nutritional Approach™ (ANA™). Poultry is high in B vitamins, iron, protein and trace minerals like zinc and selenium, and it's completely free of carbohydrates.

When cooking poultry, don't just confine yourself to chicken. Turkey, duck and game are readily available and make tasty alternatives.

If you buy a whole bird to roast, bear in mind that there's considerable waste: a 2 to 2.5kg chicken will yield a little over 500g of cooked meat – sufficient for four, with a little left over. Larger birds tend to have more meat on them in relation to the bone. Boneless cuts are more expensive, but there's virtually no waste. However, if you opt for chicken portions, don't automatically reach for boneless breasts or thighs; cuts cooked on the bone often yield more flavour.

Be especially wary of pre-seasoned poultry and ready-made meals, as these can contain hidden sugars and fillers.

CHICKEN

Chicken is an extremely versatile source of protein. Its relatively bland flavour marries well with a variety of seasonings and sauces, so much so that chicken may be used instead of pork in virtually all recipes, and in place of beef or fish in many others.

Whole chickens are categorized by weight. Chicken parts are available by part or as a cut-up chicken – that is, two breasts, two thighs, two drumsticks and two wings.

BREASTS
Skinless, boneless breasts are the most popular type of jointed chicken. Don't overlook breasts sold on the bone, however. They might take longer to cook but they are much richer in flavour.

DRUMSTICKS AND WINGS
These cuts have comparatively little meat on them and, if they're not cooked carefully, can dry out rapidly.

POUSSINS
These miniature chickens generally weigh 350–450g each, with one poussin sufficient for one portion. They're often roasted or split and then grilled.

THIGHS
Dark meat has a stronger flavour than white. You may substitute boneless, skinless thighs instead of chicken breasts in your favourite recipe.

TURKEY

There's no reason to limit turkey to the festive season – nowadays most supermarkets stock whole turkeys all year round. Even if you don't want a 7kg bird, you can find whole breasts to roast, as well as breast slices and thighs, drumsticks and wings.

Smaller turkeys can have little meat compared with the amount of bone they contain; if you are only cooking for a few people, consider a turkey breast instead of a smaller bird – you'll end up with a lot more meat.

BREAST
Whole, bone-in turkey breasts roast fairly rapidly, so they're an ideal alternative to roast chicken. Turkey breast that has been boned, skinned and sliced very thinly provides a useful alternative to chicken breast.

MINCED TURKEY
Far more common than minced chicken, minced turkey is an alternative to minced beef. Unfortunately, because it has less fat, it's not as tasty, and it's trickier to cook. Avoid packages marked 'skinless minced turkey breast' – the dark meat has more flavour, while the skin adds moisture and fat.

WHOLE TURKEY
Avoid buying a pre-basted turkey as it is injected with a salty, fatty substance that keeps it moist while roasting (and may contain sugar and trans fats). You'll get better flavour and better nutrition by choosing a plain bird and basting it yourself.

WINGS AND DRUMSTICKS
Somewhat meatier than chicken wings, turkey wings are about the size of a chicken drumstick. Wings and drumsticks make a delicious base ingredient for soups and stews.

DUCK

Duck is entirely dark meat and is high in niacin, iron, selenium and protein. This versatile bird is delicious roasted, braised or grilled. When buying duck, look for a broad, plump breast.

BREAST

Duck's rich flavour is closer to beef and dark-meat chicken than to chicken breast. Try using duck breast in place of steak in a recipe.

WHOLE DUCK

Duck doesn't contain much meat compared with bone. A bird weighing 1.3–1.8kg will feed two or three people. Whole duck is most often roasted and needs to be watched carefully, because grease can accumulate in the roasting pan and may need to be spooned off to prevent it catching fire.

GAME

GOOSE

Very rich and quite fatty, goose supplies generous amounts of B vitamins, selenium, zinc and iron. Like duck, it is entirely dark meat. It's most often available around Christmas, almost always as a whole bird.

GROUSE

Grouse shooting begins in August on the 'Glorious 12th' and continues until 10th December. The lean flesh of the red grouse is claimed by many to have the best flavour of all game birds, developed by judicious hanging according to personal taste. As with most game birds, young specimens are best simply roasted, while older birds need long, slow cooking in stews and pies, etc.

OSTRICH

Comparable in flavour, texture and colour to lean beef or duck breast, ostrich is another very lean bird – it has about one-fifth the fat of dark-meat chicken.

Spotlight on Organic Poultry

Organic livestock, including organically-raised chickens, are farmed without antibiotics, while the food they are reared on is organic, too. This means that their nourishment is free of artificial fertilizers, pesticides and other chemical additives. By eating organically-reared meat and vegetables you reduce your exposure to toxic substances that could harm your health. There are other advantages: organic foods are often more flavourful than their conventionally produced counterparts and, because they are more likely to be locally grown, they are often fresher and higher in nutrition.

Supporting organic farming goes beyond health and taste, however. By buying these products you are helping to reduce the overall use of chemical fertilizers and pesticides, which in turn protects the environment. By buying organically-produced poultry, eggs, milk and meat, you are helping to reduce the agricultural use of antibiotics and hormones. Organic farming doesn't create the toxic waste that pollutes water and disrupts ecosystems, and it helps preserve and improve farm soil.

PARTRIDGE

In season from September to January, these tasty, lean little birds have become associated with Christmas. They need only brief hanging, and it is generally accepted that the grey-legged partridge is superior in flavour to the red-legged variety.

PHEASANT

Higher in fat than most other game birds, pheasant is an excellent source of protein, B vitamins, potassium and iron. The season is from September to the end of January. Buy one bird to serve two people, and cook it carefully to prevent it from drying out, which it does readily despite its fat content.

QUAIL

These tiny birds are now mostly farmed in this country. They must be cooked very carefully to avoid drying out the tiny amount of meat. Serve two birds per person.

Spotlight on Sugar

Sugar masquerades under an array of clever names, but whether it appears as corn syrup, evaporated cane juice, honey, malt, molasses, fruit juice concentrate or one of the 'oses' (fructose, maltose, dextrose, sucrose, lactose, glucose), your body will never be fooled. It's still sugar. The same is true for sugar in all its colours and forms: from white to brown, cane to confectioner's, no incarnation of added sugar is acceptable at any phase of the Atkins Nutritional Approach™ (ANA™).

As well as the types of sugar above, you should keep an eye out for the following terms, as they will help you to negotiate the confusing minefield that is sugar.

SUGAR-FREE

The term 'free' means that a product contains no amount of – or only trivial amounts of – an ingredient, such as fat, saturated fat, cholesterol, sodium, sugars or calories. 'Sugar-free' indicates that the product contains fewer than 0.5g of sugars per serving.

NO SUGAR ADDED, WITHOUT ADDED SUGAR, NO ADDED SUGAR

Products that bear these labels contain no added sugar or other ingredients, such as fruit juice, which can be substituted for sugar. In addition, they do not contain ingredients made with added sugars, such as jam or concentrated fruit juice.

NATURALLY-OCCURRING SUGAR

You won't see this term on a package, but a product
containing naturally-occurring sugars includes sugars
found in foods in their natural state. For example, fruit
sugar, or fructose, naturally occurs in apples and other
fruits; lactose, or milk sugar, naturally occurs in milk
and other dairy products. Vegetables also contain
natural sugars. Natural sugars, in moderation, are fine
on Atkins – just remember to tally the carbs provided
by these items into your daily intake. Unfortunately,
the product's nutritional facts panel won't differentiate
between naturally-occurring sugars and added sugars.
But you can tell the difference by checking the list of
ingredients – only added sugars will be listed on the
label.

SUGAR ALCOHOLS

Also known as polyols, sugar alcohols are sugar molecules with hydroxy, or alcohol, groups attached. Sugar
alcohols, such as maltitol, isomalt, sorbitol and lactitol, have many of the characteristics of carbohydrates.
For instance, they serve to bulk up and sweeten foods.
However, they provide fewer calories and do not generally impact blood glucose in the way sugar does. When
determining the Net Carb count for foods containing
sugar alcohols, subtract the grams of sugar alcohols
from the grams of total carbs.

GLYCERINE

Like sugar alcohols, glycerine does not affect blood
sugar and is therefore not included in the Net Carb
count.

SUGAR SUBSTITUTES

As far as sugar substitutes go, sucralose (Splenda®) is the best bet. Unlike aspartame (Equal® and NutraSweet®), it is not metabolized by the body's digestive system, so it passes through quickly without affecting blood sugar levels. It also does not lose its sweetness when heated, so it can be used in cooking and baking with better results than the other sugar substitutes.

Sugar substitutes will satisfy your sweet tooth if you use them wisely. They are powerful sweeteners – most are sweeter than sugar. Except in the case of Splenda®, which can be used measure for measure as sugar, you may have to adjust your recipes to use less sugar substitute than regular sugar.

Fresh Vegetables

With few exceptions, the vast majority of vegetables can be enjoyed during any phase of the Atkins Nutritional Approach™ (ANA™). If you're not sure which ones are acceptable, as a rule of thumb choose the part of the plant that grows above ground. Roots and tubers, such as carrots and potatoes, provide energy for the growing plant so they're usually higher in carbohydrate than leaves (lettuce, kale), flowers (broccoli florets, asparagus) and fruit or seed 'containers' (tomatoes, courgettes, peppers). Vegetables that fall into the leaves, flowers and fruits categories contain the most nutrient-rich carbs and, in the early phases of the ANA™, they're the major source of carbs.

Another clue to choosing nutrient-rich vegetables is to go for those that are darker-coloured. Pigments in plants contain compounds that can promote health in a variety of ways (see Phytochemical box on page 113). If your shopping list includes a vegetable with pale flesh – courgettes, for example – leave the skin on to maximize nutrition as well as flavour.

BRASSICAS

Vegetables that fall into this group contain substances that may protect against certain cancers.

BROCCOLI
Broccoli supplies generous amounts of vitamin C, folate, beta-carotene and iron. It's also high in sulphur compounds, which fight cancer. Choose dark green

rather than bright green broccoli for higher amounts of beta-carotene and vitamin C. Avoid broccoli stems that have a white core: this is lignin, a woody substance that's hard to chew.

BROCCOLI RABE
Botanically, this Italian vegetable is closer to the turnip than to broccoli. It doesn't keep as well as broccoli and other members of the brassica family, so avoid storing it for more than a few days.

BRUSSELS SPROUTS
High in vitamin C, folate, fibre and carotenoids including lutein and zeaxanthin, Brussels sprouts are also surprisingly high in protein. Choose sprouts that are bright or deep green, as they'll be the most tender.

CABBAGE
Varieties include the large green cabbage, the crinkly-leaved Savoy and the smaller red cabbage. All are rich in indoles and isothiocyanates – powerful antioxidants that are believed to prevent certain types of breast and prostate cancer. Of the three, red cabbage is highest in vitamin C and it also contains anthocyanins, a group of antioxidant pigments.

CAULIFLOWER
Unlike most vegetables, size doesn't matter with cauliflower it comes to flavour. Select one based on how many servings you need, and avoid any with brown spots. Cauliflower is high in vitamin C and should be steamed or roasted, rather than boiled, to get the optimum amount of this nutrient.

CAVOLO NERO

With its tall stalks and long, narrow, dark-coloured leaves, the 'black cabbage' of Tuscany, central to the local classic bean and vegetable soup *ribollita*, has become increasingly popular and available in the UK over the last few years. The deep pigmentation indicates its high phytochemical content.

CHINESE CABBAGE (PE-TSAI)

Chinese or celery cabbage is characterized by its long, flat, pale ribs, which are tightly packed together and need to be peeled away from one another. It is commonly torn into pieces and added to stir-fries at the last minute, to preserve some of its satisfying crunch and delicate mustardy flavour.

KOHLRABI

Kohlrabi peaks during the summer months. The round stems can be enjoyed raw (use like cucumber, or slice thinly and spread with a soft cheese for an hors-d'oeuvre). You can also boil and mash them as you would potatoes. The leaves can be cooked like greens or kale.

PURPLE-SPROUTING BROCCOLI

These purple-headed side-shoots of broccoli appear in very early spring. Until recently their season was regarded as too short for them to be grown and distributed commercially, but their increasing popularity – due to the attractive colouration and high nutrient and phytochemical content – has led to them appearing increasingly on supermarket shelves.

RADISHES

Like other vegetables in this group, radishes are high in cancer-fighting compounds. In addition to the common red globe radish, look for daikon radishes. They're long (40cm isn't unusual), white and are sometimes shaped a bit like a rugby ball, but don't be put off by their unusual appearance – they have a sweet, fresh flavour.

SAUERKRAUT
If you've previously relied upon buying sauerkraut in tins or jars, seek out bags in the chilled salad cabinet. It's less salty, and the crisp texture is more akin to freshly made sauerkraut.

DARK LEAFY GREENS

An important source of folate, dark leafy greens are low in both carbs and calories and high in flavour and nutrients.

CHINESE MUSTARD GREENS
These cruciferous plants look like smaller, brighter kale, but their flavour is much more assertive. Mustard greens are high in calcium, folate and beta-carotene.

DANDELION GREENS
Dandelions are related to the sunflower. The dandelion greens you buy at the supermarket are indeed the same as the ones you'll find in your garden, and make a delightful addition to a salad of mixed greens. Choose small leaves; they become bitter as they grow.

KALE
There are many types of kale, but the most common is curly kale. This dark green leafy vegetable is remarkably high in beta-carotene, as well as in the carotenoids lutein and zeaxanthin. Kale tastes sweeter after it has been exposed to frost, so buy it in winter. Choose

bunches with slender stems – they're younger and milder in flavour.

PAK CHOY
This mild-tasting green is one of the many varieties of Chinese cabbage. Choose a head with lots of dark green leaves; the stems should be pearly white. Baby pak choy looks like its full-grown counterpart except that its stems are greenish, not white. This versatile vegetable can be used chopped in a salad or stir-fried until the leaves wilt and the stems are tender. For a delicious side dish, braise it with soy sauce, rice wine vinegar, root ginger and a touch of low-carb sweetener.

SPRING GREENS
These leaves provide exceptional amounts of beta-carotene, vitamin C, folate, calcium and iron.

SWISS CHARD
Chard is a member of the beetroot family, grown for its leaves and stems rather than for its roots. It is an excellent source of beta-carotene, vitamins C and E, and iron. If you're taking anticoagulant medication, opt for a different dark green leafy vegetable, since chard is also high in vitamin K, which can interfere with drugs that prevent blood clotting.

ROOTS AND TUBERS

The rule of thumb for darker-coloured vegetables is also true of roots. Beetroot and carrots come out ahead of potatoes and parsnips in the nutrition game.

BEETROOT
Beetroot is higher in sugar than any other fresh vegetable but its high fibre content helps to bring its carb levels in line, making it suitable for the later phases of Atkins. It is an excellent source of folate – considerably higher than its greens – and provides some iron. Its characteristic crimson colour comes from betacyanin, an antioxidant pigment.

CARROTS
You may work carrots into your meals as soon as you're in Pre-Maintenance – but make sure you cook or serve them with butter or oil. Carrots are sky high in beta-carotene, a fat-soluble antioxidant, so fat helps your body use and absorb it.

CELERIAC
A variety of celery grown for its root rather than its ribs, celeriac is round, rough and covered with rootlets. Its texture is not unlike the potato – use chunks in a beef stew or thin slices in a gratin. Choose comparatively smooth roots, which are easier to peel.

JERUSALEM ARTICHOKES
Neither from Jerusalem nor related to the artichoke, this member of the sunflower family is exceptionally high in iron.

JICAMA
Crisp, juicy and somewhat sweet, this tuber is becoming popular in superior supermarkets. Thin slivers add a wonderful crunch to salads – or you can add it to a beef and ginger stir-fry.

PARSNIPS
In spite of their pale colour, parsnips are fairly high in folate; they are also a source of vitamin C. Larger parsnips are fibrous, so aim for those that are 15–20cm long.

POTATOES
Although potatoes are acceptable in later phases of Atkins, their high glycaemic index can result in unstable blood sugar. So eat them rarely and in small portions.

ROOT GINGER
Like garlic, this is used more as a flavouring than a vegetable and, again like garlic, it has long been known for its medicinal properties. Look for smooth, glossy rhizomes and, unless you know you'll use a large piece within a month, choose a fairly small knob. Root ginger stays fresh for only a few weeks.

SALSIFY
Salsify has a soft, sweet flesh that tastes faintly of oysters, which explains why it is sometimes known as the oyster plant or vegetable oyster. Its leaves may be used fresh in winter salads or cooked like spinach, while the white shoots, known as chards, can be cooked as you would asparagus.

SWEDE
Fairly high in carbs, swedes (known as turnips – or neeps – in Scotland) provide vitamin C and beta-carotene. Buy the smallest ones you can find, as they're sweeter and milder in flavour.

SWEET POTATOES
An excellent provider of beta-carotene, vitamins E and C, and iron, sweet potatoes are a concentrated source of carbs. If you're craving something sweet, they're a good option (provided you're in at least Pre-Maintenance).

TARO
This tuber from the tropics is found in Caribbean and African food shops. It's very similar to the potato in flavour and texture, and supplies some vitamin A.

TURNIPS
Like swedes, to which they are closely related, turnips – known as summer turnips to the Scots – supply vitamin C, but unlike swedes they provide no carotenoids. Choose smaller turnips for sweetness.

SALAD GREENS

Whether you choose a mixture of loose greens, bagged salad blends or a head of lettuce, salad greens are your major source of carbohydrate during Induction. Avoid bagged salads that include croutons and dressings, as these extras are high in carbs and, even if the salad is pre-washed, wash it again to avoid the possibility of food poisoning.

CHICORY
Members of the endive family include frisée, curly endive, chicory and radicchio. All but chicory are good sources of vitamins C and E, folate and beta-carotene.

LAMB'S LETTUCE

Also known by the French term *mâche*, this melt-in-the mouth leaf gets its name from appearing at the same time as spring lambs. Its gentle flavour and creamy texture work well in salads.

LETTUCE

When assembling a salad, opt for darker greens, including those that are on the outside of the head of lettuce. Darker greens are higher in chlorophyll, which is linked to higher levels of beta-carotene. They tend to have more vitamin C and folate, too.

RADICCHIO

Radicchio is a member of the chicory family. It's often added to salad blends but can be cooked as well. Try braising or roasting it. Choose firm radicchio with absolutely no brown patches.

ROCKET

Rocket isn't as high in nutrients as other salad greens, but its peppery bite adds a sharp note to salads.

SORREL

Its tart flavour makes sorrel a wonderful addition to a blend of salad greens, but it also comes into its own in soups and sauces.

SPINACH

Spinach is related to chard and beetroot. High in beta-carotene, lutein and zeaxanthin, it is best served with an oil-based salad dressing or sautéed in oil – these carotenoids are fat-soluble, which means that the body is better able to absorb them in the presence of fat.

WATERCRESS
Like other cruciferous vegetables, watercress contains phytochemicals, particularly isothiocyanates and carotenoids.

BEANS AND PEAS

Beans and peas are members of the legume family – that is, vegetables with double-seamed pods containing a single row of seeds, which are the beans or peas. In some cases, however, both the seeds and the pods are eaten, as with mangetout peas and sugar snaps.

BROAD BEANS
Also called fava beans, these are similar in appearance to butter beans. Look for fresh broad beans (usually in the pods) in late spring and early summer.

GREEN BEANS
Whether you choose green beans or the less common yellow variety, the taste and texture are the same; green beans are higher in folate and beta-carotene.

PEA PODS
Mangetout peas and sugar snap peas are similar. Mangetout are flatter and sometimes broader, with smaller peas inside; sugar snaps are rounder and have larger peas. Mangetout are very high in vitamin C and supply folate, lutein and zeaxanthin.

PEAS, SHELLED
If your only experience of green peas is limited to those from the freezer, look for fresh peas from mid-spring to early summer. Don't remove them from the pod until you plan to eat them; if they're very young and fresh,

they don't even need to be cooked. As they don't store well, use them the day you buy them.

SOYA BEANS, FRESH
Sometimes called edamame, fresh soya beans are an excellent source of thiamin, folate and iron. While they are not technically a complete protein, they do supply most of the essential amino acids needed by the human body.

SUMMER SQUASH

Size matters when you're shopping for squash. Choose the smallest one you can find: it will contain smaller seeds and have a more delicate texture.

CHAYOTE
Related to cucumber and courgettes, chayote tastes like a combination of both. It goes by many names, including mirliton in Caribbean and Creole cooking, and is used in Chinese cuisine. Use it, cooked or raw, as you would courgettes (although it needs to be cooked for longer).

COURGETTE
This most common summer squash is a good source of vitamin C and fibre. Leave the skin intact to obtain carotenoids – courgette peel is very high in lutein and zeaxanthin.

PATTYPAN SQUASH
Sometimes called scallop squash, pattypan squash is about the size of a tennis ball, with scalloped edges. Pale green in colour, it turns white as it matures. There are also yellow varieties.

YELLOW SQUASH

Yellow squash supplies about one-tenth of the lutein and zeaxanthin that courgettes do. Look for crookneck and straightneck, which are similar to yellow courgettes.

WINTER SQUASH

Most varieties of winter squash are superb sources of fibre, potassium, beta-carotene and vitamin C. They also supply respectable amounts of folate, vitamin E and B vitamins, as well as alpha-carotene and lutein.

ACORN SQUASH

High in fibre and beta-carotene, acorn squash also supplies generous amounts of thiamin, vitamin C, iron, potassium, folate and vitamin E.

BUTTERNUT SQUASH

Butternut squash is an excellent source of beta-carotene and vitamin C.

PUMPKIN SQUASH

Use pumpkins as you would any other winter squash. They are very high in carotenoids, particularly beta-carotene, alpha-carotene and lutein.

SPAGHETTI SQUASH

The similarity of spaghetti squash to strands of spaghetti is astonishing. Cook some at the weekend and have it with your favourite pasta sauce.

OTHER VEGETABLES

We've included common vegetables here that don't fall neatly into previously mentioned categories.

ASPARAGUS

High in fibre, folate and flavour, asparagus comes into season in early spring. To choose the best, look at the bottoms of the stalks – avoid oval spears, which can be woody or tough, and go for those that are rounder. Thicker spears are actually more tender and juicy than thin ones.

AUBERGINES

Aubergines, though a good source or fibre and potassium, don't provide significant amounts of most vitamins. Choose small yet heavy specimens.

BAMBOO SHOOTS

Bamboo must be cooked to be edible, but once done it can be used in place of jicama or water chestnuts in stir-fried dishes or salads.

CARDOONS

Although cardoons are shaped like large celery, they aren't as bright or as crisp. Because large ones can be stringy, look for the smallest bunch with the most slender stalks you can find. They appear in the shops from autumn and winter to spring.

CELERY

For the freshest, least stringy celery, look for sprightly leaves and pale green stalks. Celery is low in calories and carbs – one stalk has a mere 6 calories – but don't believe the myth that it has 'negative' calories. Eating celery burns about 2 calories a minute.

CORN
More than 20 varieties of sweetcorn are grown; choose corn with yellow, not white, kernels and you'll get lutein and zeaxanthin, two carotenoids that can protect against age-related eye disorders.

CUCUMBERS
Relatives of summer squash, cucumbers are mostly water, so take care not to store them in a very cold refrigerator or else they'll freeze. Don't peel them, as cucumber skins are high in lutein.

FENNEL
Fennel's subtle anise flavour and crisp texture make it ideal for using raw (slice and treat as dippers for a crudité platter) or cooked (sautéed, braised or roasted). The entire plant – seeds, fronds, stalks and bulb – can be eaten. Fennel is best from early autumn to spring.

GLOBE ARTICHOKES
At their peak from March until May and in October, the best artichokes are compact and squeak when pressed or squeezed. They are very high in fibre and provide iron, magnesium and folate, too.

MUSHROOMS
Mushrooms are an excellent way to add a range of flavours to many foods. They contain glutamic acid, a natural compound upon which the flavour-enhancer monosodium glutamate (MSG) is based. Explore beyond plain white mushrooms: portabello, chestnut, oyster and shiitake mushrooms will all add extra zest to dishes.

OKRA
High in vitamin C, lutein, zeaxanthin and soluble fibre, okra has become easier to find in supermarkets. If the pods are longer than 8cm/3 inches, they'll probably be less tender.

PEPPERS, CHILLI
Basically there are two types of fresh chilli on sale: unripe green ones and ripe red ones, such as the little red Thai bird's-eye chillies. In specialist suppliers, some chillies are sold by their variety, like the fiercely hot lantern-shaped, orange Scotch Bonnet or habanero chillies, the torpedo-like serranos and the mild anchos, looking a little like small sweet peppers. Chilli peppers get their heat from capsaicin, a phytochemical so caustic that even one drop diluted in a million drops of water can blister the tongue. Peppers vary considerably in the amount of capsaicin they contain. As a very general rule, the smaller the pepper, the hotter it is.

PEPPERS, SWEET
If you can, choose red rather than green peppers, as they supply more than twice the vitamin C. They also contain beta-carotene and beta-cryptoxanthin. Orange, yellow and red peppers are all slightly different forms of ripe peppers, while green peppers are unripe and contain fewer carbs, which is what you'd expect with sugars concentrating as the vegetable develops.

SPROUTS
Known as micro-food, sprouts are full of fantastic enzymes. Be sure to buy only sprouts that have been refrigerated, are crisp-looking and have their buds attached. Refrigerate them when storing at home, and rinse them thoroughly before using to remove surface dirt.

TOMATILLOS
These look like green cherry tomatoes in a papery husk. They are related to Cape gooseberries and are commonly used in salsa verde.

TOMATOES
High in vitamin C, tomatoes contain generous amounts of the carotenoid lycopene. Cherry and plum tomatoes provide some vitamin E. While they are technically considered fruit, tomatoes are commonly thought of as vegetables.

ALLIUMS

These members of the onion family are high in antioxidant sulphur compounds, which also give them their distinctive flavours.

CHIVES
The slender green tubular stalks of this culinary herb have a pleasant mild onion flavour much favoured in salads and in egg and cheese dishes. If using in cooking, the stalks should be added only at the last minute and cooked very lightly, otherwise the flavour is lost.

GARLIC
Garlic has been used as a medicine since ancient times. Modern science proves that it has remarkable antioxidant powers. It contains allicin, a compound that develops when the vegetable is exposed to oxygen but not in the presence of heat. Try to chop or crush garlic 10 minutes before you cook it so the allicin has time to develop, as once this has happened heat won't destroy it.

LEEKS

Though they're available all year round, leeks are at their best from autumn to spring. To ensure they're thoroughly cleaned before cooking, split them in half lengthways and rinse them under cold running water, holding the split end down to prevent driving the dirt deeper into the layers. Smaller leeks are more tender. Try them baked: arrange 2.5 to 5cm lengths on a foil square before drizzling with olive oil, herbs, salt and pepper. Seal the packet well and bake at 180–200°C/350–400°F/Gas Mark 4–6 for 15–20 minutes, until tender.

ONIONS

During Induction, onions should be used primarily as a garnish or in moderate amounts in cooked dishes. Sweet onions, such as Valencia, are slightly lower in sugar than regular storage onions (they're milder in flavour because they're lower in the compounds that make onions so pungent).

SHALLOTS

Shallots look and taste like a cross between onions and garlic. They can be used as you would onions, but note that a little goes a long way.

SPRING ONIONS

Also known as scallions and green onions, spring onions are actually immature onions. Their flavour is milder as a result, and they are much more perishable, but they come with a nutritional bonus: their green tops contain beta-carotene.

Phytochemicals

Phytochemicals are compounds in plants ('phyto' is from the Greek word for plant), and although thousands of these compounds have been identified, researchers are still discovering more, and what they are capable of doing.

Some phytochemicals are antioxidants, which means that they prevent unstable oxygen molecules from damaging cells. Some are thought to prevent cancer cells from forming, and others are thought to produce enzymes that neutralize carcinogens. Still others are thought to lower blood cholesterol or boost the immune system.

Many phytochemicals are found in the pigments of plants: carotenoids give foods an orange or deep yellow hue. Some green vegetables are high in carotenoids too, but the orange is masked by chlorophyll, while anthocyanins give food a blue or reddish colour. Other phytochemicals come from elements such as nitrogen or sulphur.

All About Herbs

Herbs contain generous amounts of nutrients, but they're rarely eaten in sufficient quantity to provide significant amounts. Likewise, when used as seasoning or garnish, herbs add virtually no grams of carbs to foods, so they can be used in all four phases of Atkins.

In addition to adding flavour to recipes, fresh herbs can be added to salads. Toss basil or parsley leaves into a green salad, for instance, and notice the difference. Consider making herb sauces such as pesto to maximize the vitamins these plants contain. Herbs also are a good source of folate, vitamin C and beta-carotene. Some supply iron.

Experiment with the following herbs to enhance your favourite dishes without boosting carbs:

Basil	Oregano
Chives	Parsley
Coriander	Rosemary
Dill	Sage
Mint	Thyme

Safe Handling

Animal products, such as meat, poultry and seafood, require special care during preparation and cooking. So too do vegetables – even those that come pre-washed and pre-packed – and dairy produce. Yet, with the demise of domestic science classes in our schools, simple common sense in preparing and storing food has all but disappeared. As a result, incidences of food poisoning have dramatically increased. To prevent illnesses from bacteria found in food, follow these simple guidelines.

FOOD PREPARATION

Wash hands, chopping boards, dishes and utensils with hot soapy water, using anti-bacterial washing-up liquid, before and after contact with raw food, especially meats.

Use one chopping board for raw meats and one for fresh fruits and vegetables.

Keep raw meats away from other foods in your shopping trolley. When you get home, transfer them to a dish, which you should cover with clingfilm, and keep meats separately on the lowest shelf in the refrigerator. While cooking meals, keep raw meats away from other foods as they are being prepared.

Pre-washed, bagged salad can often be a cause of salmonella. Always rinse leaves under cold running water before removing excess moisture in a salad spinner. Likewise, always rinse pre-washed fruit and vegetables.

Place cooked meats on a clean plate; do not use the same plate used for the food in its raw state. Do not reapply a marinade used on raw meats to the cooked item, unless the marinade has been boiled beforehand.

FRIDGE AND FREEZER TIPS

Always cover food in the refrigerator, using clingfilm or foil. Regularly clean your fridge, mopping up any spills as soon as they happen, and defrost the freezer at frequent intervals to ensure it runs at maximum efficiency.

Make sure food is cold before you freeze it. This allows it to freeze faster and reduces the likelihood that it will develop freezer burn.

When shopping, stop by the freezer aisle last. If food thaws, even briefly, before you put it in the freezer at home, its texture and flavour will suffer when you thaw it completely to cook it.

Your freezer temperature should remain constant at –32°C/0°F. Changes in temperature can ruin food. If your low-carb ice cream forms ice crystals, for example, this is an indication that your freezer's temperature is fluctuating.

For food safety, defrost foods in the refrigerator. Put meats and poultry on a plate to catch any liquid.

When storing cooked food in the refrigerator, let the food cool properly before transferring it to a clean dish and covering with film or foil. Never place warm food in the fridge.

Be vigilant about sell-by dates, discarding foodstuffs that have gone past their limit. Take special care with ready meals.

COOKING

When it comes to reheating food, make sure it is thoroughly cooked through, especially if you are using a microwave. Reheated soups and stews should be cooked vigorously to kill off any bacteria.

Use a meat thermometer. Cook these raw meats to the following safe internal temperatures:

Minced meat: 71°C/160°F
Pork: 71°C/160°F (medium); 77°C/170°F (well done)
Poultry, breasts: 77°C/170°F
Poultry, whole: 82°C/180°F

Cook fish until it is opaque and flaky. If searing rare tuna, make sure the fish is at optimum freshness first.

Making Sense of Labelling

Whether you shop for food at a supermarket, a natural-foods store, an independent grocer's or a farmers' market, you'll often come across product labels bearing a baffling number of terms and acronyms. The good news is that most of these words are legally defined – that is, the Government has developed a set of criteria that foods bearing a label must meet. Here's a quick rundown of what it all means.

ORGANIC

Organic food has become one of the fastest growth areas in the UK. All major supermarket chains carry an ever-increasing organic range of fruit, vegetables, meat, poultry and fish, dairy produce, cooking ingredients, teas, juices, etc.

To be certified organic, producers have to meet a strict set of guidelines set by the UK region of the Organic Food Standards Agency. Organic farming restricts the use of artificial chemicals and pesticides. Animals are reared without the routine use of drugs and antibiotics, and the food they consume must be organic as well; fruit and vegetables must be grown without the use of chemicals and pesticides. The use of genetically modified technology is banned.

NON-GMO OR NON-GEO

GMO and GEO stand for genetically-modified or genetically-engineered organisms. When a food is genetically modified or engineered, its genes have been rearranged.

FREE-RANGE

This means that the animals and poultry are not penned up in cages or small spaces, and are instead allowed to move around and graze in a way that is natural for their species. Depending on the animals, these areas may be indoors.

GLUTEN-FREE

Gluten is a component of grains found in greatest concentrations in wheat, barley and rye. Gluten causes allergic reactions in certain people (Coeliac Disease is a condition defined by an intolerance of gluten). However, a gluten-free diet may also be beneficial in the treatment of a host of other problems, ranging from skin conditions to mental illness.

DAIRY-FREE

Dairy-free means that a product contains no milk, cheese, butter, cream cheese, cottage cheese, soured cream or ice cream. The most common reason for following a dairy-free diet is an allergy to dairy products, whether it's due to lactose-intolerance or an allergy to or intolerance of dairy protein. Some people who are extremely lactose-intolerant may also be unable to tolerate other dairy products.

PART TWO:

Listings Section

Introduction

In the following pages you will find product information that will help you shop wisely while doing Atkins. Although you might believe you have a firm grasp on the Atkins Nutritional Approach™, sometimes, when you are faced with shelf upon shelf of products, it's all too easy to become confused. Are trans fats always unacceptable or can you exercise discretion when shopping for products that contain them? Which phase is a tin of tomato soup suitable for? If a ready meal contains fewer than 25g carbs is it acceptable, even though it has added sugars? With the product listings section of the *Atkins Shopping Guide*, help is at hand.

The information within the following pages is presented in a straightforward, easy-to-locate way. Each product entry lists carb counts and phase information, as well as warning you against ingredients that are unacceptable and those which, while not off-limits, you might wish to avoid.

Within each listings chapter you'll find advice on how to negotiate the vast assortment of products on the aisle shelves. To do Atkins successfully you have to be aware of the products that are suitable and, equally important, those that are not.

Because we want to make your shopping experience as simple as possible, where appropriate we have repeated product listings in more than one chapter. For example, if planning which meat products you are going to buy, you might turn to the Meat and poultry chapter, where you will find listings for fresh meat, tinned meat, frozen meat and deli meat. If you are compiling a shopping list for a buffet party, however, you might consult the Delicatessen chapter because you will be buying a range of salads, dips, cold fish and cold meat. The same deli meat listings will be found here, to save you flicking back and forth throughout the book.

There are other devices that will help make your shopping expeditions as simple as possible.

INGREDIENT ALERTS

There are three symbols you will come to recognize. These icons help you quickly identify certain types of product:

⚠ Unacceptable

Foods containing added sugars and/or trans fats, both of which are unacceptable on any phase of Atkins. No phasing information, therefore, will be given.

(FYI) FYI

Products containing one or more of the following ingredients: aspartame, cornflour, maize flour, maize starch, modified maize starch, monosodium glutamate (MSG), nitrates and wheat flour. While these ingredients are not off-limits, you might wish to exclude them from your diet. Because they are not forbidden, phasing information is included. You may sometimes find the term cornstarch listed within the nutritional information. This is the American term for cornflour. Food labels refer variously to cornflour, cornstarch, maize flour and maize starch, sometimes in modified forms. In UK food production, only basic native starch is used. This is a standard ingredient added to improve texture and structure. When we describe it as modified, it has been altered by manufacturers to improve shelf life, heat tolerance or the appearance of convenience foods.

There is a second use for the FYI icon FYI. In certain chapters it is used to draw your attention to the ingredients or nutritional information panel. This could be because the product might contain trace elements of carbs where you would expect to find none, and it is up to your discretion whether or not you wish to buy it. It could also alert you to the fact that there might be discrepancies in Own Brand ingredients – see below for further clarification.

⚠ Organic

Denotes an organic product.

OWN BRANDS

Every supermarket offers its Own Brand range of popular foodstuffs. We shopped at all major British supermarkets and health-food chains in the course of our research for this book and where we have included an Own Brand listing for a product, we have bought at least two, and more often three, versions of the same food and compared the number of carbs contained in each of them. If we use Own Brand Thick Pork Sausages as an example, one supermarket version has 9.6g carbs per 100g, the second 11g per 100g and the third 12.9g carbs per 100g. This would be reported as 9.6–12.9g carbs per 100g.

Sometimes, though, not all of the three products contain exactly the same ingredients. In the case of an ingredient alert, two might contain trans fats, but the third might not. If all three versions contained trans fats, we would use an unacceptable food alert ⚠ and use the phrase *contains trans fats*. In a case where not all three products contained trans fats, we would modify this to an FYI **(FYI)** and use the wording *some may contain trans fats*. It would be up to you to examine the nutritional information.

NATURALLY OCCURRING CARBS

We encourage you to scrutinize nutritional labels when doing Atkins. The more you do it, the better you will come to understand the composition of foods. Initially this might be confusing, especially when you come across a trace carb listing for a food that you believed to have zero carbs. Where do the carbs in a tin of green beans in brine come from, for example? Does it contain hidden ingredients?

The simple answer is that all foods are made of ingredients that were once alive, whether in the form of animal or vegetable. All living things are composed of protein, fat and carbohydrate. When foods are chemically analysed, some food components always end up in the carbohydrate category because the analysis is imprecise. Scientifically speaking, there are virtually no carb-free foods but the level may be too low to significantly affect blood sugar levels. In America, if the trace element is less than half a gram, it is permissible to list it as zero carbs. In the UK, the rules are more stringent and we have to report the food as containing carbs, no matter how small. In instances where you would expect to find a zero carb reading and we have reported a trace, we will alert you with a FYI symbol **(FYI)** .

PORTION SIZES

Most, but not all, products offer two types of nutritional information on the labelling. You will always find protein, carbohydrate, fat, fibre, sodium and sugar content measured against 100g or 100ml. You will also often find the same information relating to a serving size.

With few exceptions, we follow standard procedure and list carbohydrate content against 100g or 100ml. This is not to be confused with a serving size. In some cases, 100g would be too large a portion – for example, if you ate 100g of Branston pickle you would feel sick! In other cases, 100g would be too small a helping, such as with a Quorn fillet. So, while we list carbohydrate content against 100g, when we code our phasing information, we do so against a serving size. For example, while you might read that New Covent Garden Co. Wild Mushroom Soup contains 3.8g carbs per 100g, we have phased it 3–4 because you would have a 200g serving.

Pay attention to portion sizes and be aware that when you start to reintroduce foods into your menu, as you would with berries once you reach Ongoing Weight Loss (OWL), you should do so cautiously. When in doubt, always use your kitchen scales to check the weight of a portion size. In doing so, you'll soon become accustomed to visually recognizing a portion.

HOW TO READ A FOOD LABEL

What Carbohydrates Should You Count?

Not all carbohydrates behave the same way in your body. For example, table sugar raises your blood sugar, while others, such as fibre, sugar alcohols, glycerine and organic acids, pass through your body without any significant impact on blood sugar. When you do Atkins, you only need to count the grams of carbohydrate that impact your blood sugar (the Net Carbs).

The good news is that British food labels have done the calculation for us! The fibre is shown separately and as long as there are no sugar alcohols, glycerine or organic acids contained in the product, the grams of carbs shown is the number you count.

So, in this example (Organic Crunchy Cereal) you need to count 33.4g of carbs per serving.

Nutrition

Typical Composition	Each Serving (50g) provides	100g provide
Energy	888kj	1777kj
	211kcal	422kcal
Protein	3.8g	7.6g
Carbohydrate	33.4g	66.7g
of which sugars	12.8g	25.6g
Fat	7.0g	13.9g
of which saturates	2.3g	4.5g
monounsaturates	3.2g	6.5g
polyunsaturates	1.5g	2.9g
Fibre	2.7g	5.2g
Salt	0.1g	0.2g
of which Sodium	trace	0.09g

Low-Carb Products

For low-carb products that are sweetened with glycerine or sugar alcohols, subtract the grams of sugar alcohols or glycerine from the total number of grams of carbohydrate to arrive at the Net Carb total.

So, in this example (Atkins Advantage™ Chocolate Hazelnut Crunch Bar), if you subtract 15.2g of polyols (maltitol and glycerine) from 17.4g of carbohydrate you reach a total of 2g Net Carbs per serving.

Nutrition

Typical Composition	Each Serving (60g) provides	100g provide
Energy	987kj	1637kj
	236kcal	392kcal
Protein	19.4g	32.2g
Carbohydrate	17.4g	28g
of which sugars	1.1g	1.9g
of which polyols	15.2g	25.2g
of which maltitol	5.2g	8.7g
of which glycerine	10g	16.5g
Fat	12.2g	20.2g
of which saturates	5.4g	9g
Fibre	5.0g	8.3g
Sodium	0.1g	0.2g

Bakery

As manufacturers wake up to consumer demand for low-carbohydrate products, you'll be able to enjoy an ever-widening range of acceptable foods to help you do Atkins, including biscuits, bread and bagels. At the moment, however, you'll have to keep an eye on the nutrition facts panel and ingredients list of bakery products, because many contain ingredients that are off-limits on Atkins, such as sugar in its many guises, including honey, molasses and high-fructose corn syrup.

You'll also need to take account of the particular phase of Atkins you're in to know which breads are acceptable for you. As a general guideline, look for those breads made with whole grains and, once you're in Pre-Maintenance and Lifetime Maintenance, seek out sandwich-style breads that have no more than 16 grams of carbs per slice – those with 10 or fewer are even better. You should also keep an eye on portions. For example, some wheat-free loaves are small but dense with whole grains, so more than one slice will rack up the carbs.

Bringing Home the Bread

If you know about flours, you'll have a better idea of which breads to reach for and which to avoid.

White, wheat, whole-wheat

The first two are refined white flour. Unless the loaf's label specifies '100%' whole-wheat or wholemeal, there's no telling how much of the whole-grain flour you're getting.

100% wholemeal, whole grain, rye, sprouted, sourdough, pumpernickel

Whole grains, including whole wheat, are lower in carbs and higher in nutrients than refined breads. Rye (including pumpernickel) is too dense to make a palatable bread, so it's often blended with refined wheat flour. Instead, look for ryes blended with whole-wheat flour. Pumpernickel bread contains both rye and wheat flour and usually contains molasses to darken it.

Reduced-carb or low-carb

This type of bread will be the lowest in carbs, but even so, keep your consumption low to ensure you are not exceeding your daily carb allowance. Allow yourself only one piece of low-carb bread a day during Induction.

Why Rye?

Rye is high in fibre, which makes it lower in carbs than most wheat bread. Depending on how much rye flour is used, rye bread can be comparatively low in carbs. But watch out for commercial brands, as these might be made with hydrogenated oils.

Breaking Bread

Until low-carb and controlled-carb bread is more readily available in the UK, use the few that exist or wait until Pre-Maintenance, when you can eat wholemeal bread.

Low-Carb Coating Mixes and Breadcrumbs

Many commercial coating mixes, breadcrumbs and stuffings add unnecessary carbs to your meal and often contain hydrogenated oils. Instead of using these, dry out slices of controlled-carb bread or toast them lightly, then give them a quick blast in a food processor. Add dried herbs or other seasonings for variety. After Induction, when you can add back nuts, grind them finely to make a tasty and crunchy coating for chicken and fish. Nuts can burn easily, however, so watch the pan carefully and adjust the heat as necessary.

BREAD

Brown Sliced

⚠ Kingsmill Brown Thick Sliced
17.8g carbs per slice
Contains added sugars and wheat flour

Ⓕ Own Brand Brown Medium Sliced
13.8–15.1g carbs per slice
Some may contain added sugars and wheat flour

Ⓕ Weight Watchers Brown Bread (Phases 3–4)
4.9g carbs per slice
Contains wheat flour

Hi Bran

⚠ Allinson Hi Bran Sliced
7.9g carbs per slice
Contains added sugars and wheat flour

⚠ Burgen Hi Bran Sliced
14.7g carbs per slice
Contains added sugars and wheat flour

Low Carb

Ⓕ Atkins Sliced White Loaf (Phases 1–4) (COMING SOON)
2g carbs per slice
Contains maize starch and wheat flour

Ⓕ Hovis Best with Less Reduced Carbohydrate (Phases 3–4)
13.4g Net Carbs per slice
Contains wheat flour

(FYI) **Marks & Spencer Low Carb White (Phases 3–4)**
7.6g Net Carbs per slice
Contains wheat flour

(FYI) **Nimble Carbs So Low (Phases 3–4)**
7.6g Net Carbs per slice
Contains wheat flour

(FYI) **Tesco Only 6.0g Carbohydrate per slice White Bread (Phases 3–4)**
6g Net Carbs per slice
Contains wheat flour

Malted
⚠ **Hovis Granary Thick Sliced**
17.9g carbs per slice
Contains added sugars and wheat flour

⚠ **Kingsmill Gold Malted Wheat Sliced**
12.2g carbs per slice
Contains added sugars and wheat flour

⚠ **Nimble Amazing Grain**
10.1g carbs per slice
Contains added sugars and wheat flour

⚠ **Weight Watchers Malted Danish Sliced**
8.5g carbs per slice
Contains added sugars and wheat flour

Multi Grain
⚠ **Dietary Specials Multigrain Gluten/Wheat/ Egg Free Sliced Loaf**
6.8g carbs per slice
Contains added sugars

⚠ **Hovis Country Grain Multi Grain Wholemeal**
16.7g carbs per slice
Contains added sugars

Rolls

⚠ **Hovis 6 Wholemeal Square Rolls**
18.9g carbs per roll
Contains added sugars

⚠ **Own Brand Wholemeal Rolls**
22.8–26.5g carbs per roll
Contains added sugars

Rye

⚠ **Sunnyvale Organic Rye Bread with Sunflower
Seeds (Phases 3–4)**
15.2g carbs per slice

⚠ **Village Bakery Organic Baltic Wheat and Rye**
⚠ **Bread**
16.8g carbs per slice
Contains added sugars and wheat flour

Sourdough

**Sunnyvale Gluten Free Mixed Grain
Sourdough Bread (Phases 3–4)**
14.1g carbs per slice

Speciality Bread

⚠ **Burgen Soya and Linseed**
11.4g carbs per slice
Contains added sugars

⚠ **Duchy Originals Organic Malted Oat Bread**
⚠ 17.4g carbs per slice
Contains added sugars and wheat flour

(FYI) **Duchy Originals Organic Mixed Seed Bread**
⚠ **(Phases 3–4)**
15.6g carbs per slice
Contains wheat flour

⚠ **Duchy Originals Organic Sunflower Seed and**
⚠ **Honey Bread**
17.5g carbs per slice
Contains added sugars and wheat flour

(FYI) **Vogels Original Mixed Grain Brown Bread**
(Phases 3–4)
18.8g carbs per slice
Contains wheat flour

(FYI) **Vogels Soya and Linseed Brown Bread**
(Phases 3–4)
15g carbs per slice
Contains wheat flour

(FYI) **Vogels Sunflower and Barley Bread (Phases 3–4)**
17.7g carbs per slice
Contains wheat flour

Wheat-free/Gluten-free

⚠ **Barkat Brown Rice Bread Wheat and**
Gluten Free
20g carbs per slice
Contains added sugars and trans fats

⚠ **Barkat White Rice Bread Wheat and Gluten Free**
21g carbs per slice
Contains added sugars and trans fats

EnerG Brown Rice Bread Gluten Free and Wheat Free (Phases 3–4)
18.9g carbs per slice

⚠ **Glutafin Sliced Fibre Loaf Gluten Free**
11g carbs per slice
Contains added sugars

⚠ **Glutafin Sliced White Loaf Gluten Free**
12.3g carbs per slice
Contains added sugars

Glutano Wholemeal Sliced Wheat Free and Gluten Free (Phases 3–4)
19g carbs per slice

⚠ **Stamp Collection Organic and Wheat Free with Sunflower Seed Topping (Phases 3–4)**
19.8g carbs per slice

Wheatgerm

(FYI) Hovis Brown Original Wheatgerm Medium Sliced (small loaf) (Phases 3–4)
15.8g carbs per slice
Contains wheat flour

⚠ **Hovis Wheatgerm Medium Sliced (small loaf)**
13.2g carbs per slice
Contains trans fats and wheat flour

Wholemeal

⚠ **Allinson Wholemeal Large**
16.4g carbs per slice
Contains added sugars

⚠ **Allinson Wholemeal Small**
8.8g carbs per slice
Contains added sugars

🔠 **Hovis Best of Both Thick Sliced (Phases 3–4)**
19.8g carbs per slice
Contains wheat flour

⚠ **Hovis Best of Health**
13.2g carbs per slice
Contains added sugars

⚠ **Hovis Hearty Wholemeal Medium Sliced**
13.8g carbs per slice
Contains added sugars

⚠ **Hovis Hearty Wholemeal Thick Sliced**
16.9g carbs per slice
Contains added sugars

**Hovis Wholemeal Farmhouse Thick Sliced
(Phases 3–4)**
16.3g carbs per slice

⚠ **Kingsmill Gold Wholemeal**
17.3g carbs per slice
Contains added sugars

⚠ **Kingsmill Tasty Wholemeal Medium Sliced**
14.3g carbs per slice
Contains added sugars

⚠ **Kingsmill Tasty Wholemeal Square**
10g carbs per slice
Contains added sugars

⚠ **Kingsmill Tasty Wholemeal Thick Sliced**
15.8g carbs per slice
Contains added sugars

⚠ **Nimble Wholemeal Sliced**
7.4g carbs per slice
Contains added sugars

Own Brand Wholemeal Longlife Medium Sliced (Phases 3–4)
13–14g carbs per slice

FYI **Own Brand Wholemeal Medium Sliced**
13.5–14g per carbs per slice
Some may contain added sugars

⚠ **Warburtons Wholemeal**
9.8g carbs per slice
Contains added sugars

Wholemeal Organic

⚠ **Cranks Organic Wholemeal Loaf (small and large) (Phases 3–4)**
17.7g carbs per slice

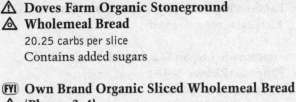

⚠ **Doves Farm Organic Stoneground**
⚠ **Wholemeal Bread**
20.25 carbs per slice
Contains added sugars

(FYI) Own Brand Organic Sliced Wholemeal Bread
⚠ **(Phases 3–4)**
16.7–17.7g carbs per slice
Some may contain added sugars

FANCY BREADS

Breadsticks
⚠ **Kallo Organic Original Breadsticks (Phases 3–4)**
3.6g carbs per breadstick

Chapattis
Pataks Original Chapatti Wraps (Phases 3–4)
17.9g carbs per chapatti

Poppadoms (Ready-to-eat)
**Sharwoods Indian Garlic and Coriander
Puppodums (Phases 3–4)**
4.7g carbs per poppadom

**Sharwoods Indian Mildly Spiced
Puppodums (Phases 3–4)**
4.4g carbs per poppadom

Sharwoods Indian Plain Puppodums (Phases 3–4)
4.9g carbs per poppadom

Poppadoms (Require Cooking)
Pataks Original Pappadums Garlic (Phases 3–4)
4.4g carbs per poppadom

Pataks Original Pappadums Plain (Phases 3–4)
4.32g carbs per poppadom

Sharwoods Indian Garlic and Green Chilli Pappads (Phases 3–4)
5.41g carbs per poppadom

Sharwoods Indian Plain Puppodums (Phases 3–4)
5.25g carbs per poppadom

Taco Shells

(FYI) **Old El Paso Crunchy Taco Shells (Phases 3–4)**
6.86g carbs per shell
Contains cornflour

Tortillas (Corn)

⚠ **Discovery Gluten Free Corn Tortillas**
8.6g carbs per tortilla
Contains added sugars

BISCUITS, CRACKERS & CRISPBREADS

Added sugars and refined wheat flour are no strangers to the biscuits and crackers aisle, so both areas can be particularly challenging when you're searching for Atkins-friendly products. Additionally, virtually all major brands use dangerous hydrogenated oils – heart-damaging trans fats that are absolutely forbidden on Atkins – and these should be avoided at all costs, no matter what your dietary regime. Be careful: even sugar-free biscuits, for example, can contain hydrogenated oils.

During Induction, don't waste your time by venturing into this aisle. In Ongoing Weight Loss, the selection will increase slightly, but only in the latter

phases of Atkins will you find more options here. Keep
in mind that your choices will still be limited even
when your carb threshold increases, since trans fats
and sugars must always be avoided. To make the best
selection, look for items that offer lots of flavour and
great texture – products with these qualities will be
more likely to satisfy you in fewer bites.

Your best bets include crispbreads, since many of
them are made with rye and some are exceptionally
high in fibre. You need to take care as they can contain
sugar; however, you won't have to worry about trans
fats. For biscuits, look for sugar-free meringues, wafers
and treats made from healthy whole grains such as oats
and barley.

SAVOURY BISCUITS

Crackers

⚠ **Doves Farm Organic Wheat Free Rye Crackers
(Phases 3–4)**
4.1 carbs per cracker

⚠ **Duchy Originals Organic Oaten Biscuits**
 9.7g carbs per biscuit
Contains added sugars and wheat flour

⚠ **Glutafin Gluten Free Wheat Free High Fiber
Crackers**
4g carbs per cracker
Contains added sugars and cornflour

Millers Damsel Celery Wafer Thins (Phases 3–4)
2.4g carbs per cracker

Millers Damsel Original Wafer Thins (Phases 3–4)
2.2g carbs per cracker

Millers Damsel Poppy Wafer Thins (Phases 3–4)
2.7g carbs per cracker

Millers Damsel Sesame Wafer Thins (Phases 3–4)
2.9g carbs per cracker

⚠ **Nairn's Organic Wholemeal Crackers (Phases 3–4)**
4.4g carbs per cracker

FYI **Own Brand Cream Crackers (Phases 3–4)**
5–6.2g carbs per cracker
Contains wheat flour

Paterson's Oat Crackers (Phases 3–4)
3.7g carbs per cracker

⚠ **Trufree Herb & Onion Crackers**
4.5g carbs per cracker
Contains added sugars and cornflour

⚠ **The Village Bakery Melmerby Organic Savoury Seed Biscuits (Phases 3–4)**
6.5g carbs per biscuit

Crispbreads

⚠ **Allinson Organic Wholemeal Crispbread (Phases 3–4)**
3.3g carbs per crispbread

⚠ **DS (Dietary Specials) Snackers Crispbread**
5.5g carbs per crispbread
Contains added sugars

Ⓕ **Finn Crisp Multigrain (Phases 3–4)**
4g carbs per crispbread
Contains wheat flour

⚠ **Kallo Organic Wholemeal Rye Crispbread**
(Phases 3–4)
5.8g carbs per crispbread

Orgran Corn Crispbreads (Phases 3–4)
4.2g carbs per crispbread

⚠ **Ryvita Breaks**
10.1g carbs per crispbread
Contains added sugars

Ryvita Dark Rye Rye Crispbread (Phases 3–4)
5.9g carbs per crispbread

Ryvita Multi Grain Rye Crispbread (Phases 3–4)
6.4g carbs per crispbread

Ryvita Original Rye Crispbread (Phases 3–4)
6g carbs per crispbread

Ryvita Sesame Rye Crispbread (Phases 3–4)
5.4g carbs per crispbread

Scandinavian Bran Crispbread (Phases 2–4)
2.4g carbs per crispbread

Oat Cakes

Nairn's Cheese Oat Cakes (Phases 3–4)
4.4g carbs per oat cake

Nairn's Fine Milled Oat Cakes (Phases 3–4)
5.6g carbs per oat cake

Nairn's Mini Oat Cakes (Phases 3–4)
2.4g carbs per oat cake

⚠ Nairn's Organic Oat Cakes (Phases 3–4)
7.2g carbs per oat cake

Nairn's Scottish Oat Cakes (Phases 3–4)
6.9g carbs per oat cake

ⓕⓨⓘ Own Brand Oat Cakes (Phases 3–4)
7–7.4g carbs per oat cake
Some may contain added sugars

Rice & Corn Cakes

Clearspring Rice Cakes Sesame Garlic Wheat Free (Phases 3–4)
6.2g carbs per rice cake

Clearspring Rice Cakes Sesame Teriyaki Wheat Free (Phases 3–4)
6.2g carbs per rice cake

⚠ Kallo Gluten Free Thick Slice Rice Cakes Caramel
7.9g carbs per rice cake
Contains added sugars

⚠ **Kallo Organic Corn Cakes Thin Slice Lightly Salted (Phases 3–4)**
3.4g carbs per corn cake

⚠ **Kallo Organic Thick Slice Rice Cakes No Added Salt (Phases 3–4)**
6g carbs per rice cake

⚠ **Kallo Organic Thick Slice Rice Cakes Savoury (Phases 3–4)**
6.1g carbs per rice cake

⚠ **Kallo Organic Thick Slice Rice Cakes Slightly Salted with Sesame (Phases 3–4)**
6g carbs per rice cake

⚠ **McVitie's Go Ahead! Sour Cream & Herbs Flavour Crispy Rice Crackers**
1.4g carbs per cracker
Contains added sugars and MSG

⚠ **Orgran Organic Rice Cakes Unsalted with Sesame (Phases 3–4)**
6.2g carbs per rice cake

Orgran Rice Crispbreads (Phases 3–4)
4.1g carbs per crispbread

Own Brand Rice Cakes (Phases 3–4)
3.5–5.7g carbs per rice cake

Real Foods Corn Thins Original (Phases 3–4)
4.7g carbs per slice

Real Foods Corn Thins Sesame (Phases 3–4)
4.5g carbs per slice

SWEET BISCUITS

 **Duchy Originals Organic Chocolate Coconut
Biscuits**
6.5g carbs per biscuit
Contains added sugars and wheat flour

 **Duchy Originals Organic Chocolate Ginger
Biscuits**
7.5g carbs per biscuit
Contains added sugars and wheat flour

**Duchy Originals Organic Chocolate & Orange
Biscuits**
7.5g carbs per biscuit
Contains added sugars and wheat flour

Duchy Originals Organic Lemon Biscuits
9.9g carbs per biscuit
Contains added sugars and wheat flour

 **Green & Black's Organic Dark Chocolate
Coated Butter Biscuits**
7.1g carbs per biscuit
Contains added sugars and wheat flour

 **Green & Black's Organic Dark Chocolate
Coated Butter Biscuits with Ginger**
7.1g carbs per biscuit
Contains added sugars and wheat flour

⚠ **Green & Black's Organic Milk Chocolate**
⚠ **Coated Butter Biscuits**
7.1g carbs per biscuit
Contains added sugars and wheat flour

⚠ **Green & Black's Organic Milk Chocolate**
⚠ **Coated Butter Biscuits with Chopped**
Hazelnuts
6.4g carbs per biscuit
Contains added sugars and wheat flour

⚠ **Wheat Free Raspberry Cookies**
13g carbs per biscuit
Contains added sugars and cornflour

⚠ **Wheat Free Stem Ginger Cookies**
12g carbs per biscuit
Contains added sugars and cornflour

Breakfast Food and Bars

Recent research confirms what mothers have been telling their offspring for generations: breakfast is the most important meal of the day. A satisfying breakfast that's high in protein and low in carbohydrates will give you plenty of energy until lunchtime and help you think more clearly. Even better, eating breakfast also makes it easier to curb your intake of high-carb snacks, helping you to lose weight.

The question, of course, is what constitutes a 'good' controlled-carb breakfast when you're doing Atkins? A cooked breakfast can offer the perfect solution, but what if this isn't your natural choice? If you usually opt for cereal and toast, you will have to shop wisely.

Once you are in the maintenance phases, look for natural cereals that do not contain added sugars of any kind (including honey) and are high in fibre, which will help you to stay fuller for longer. Conventional cakes and pastries are obviously out of the question, as are most regular and low-fat muffins, frozen waffles and pancakes. The same applies to bagels.

You may prefer to start your day with a shake, low-carb cereal or breakfast bar. If you go down this route, make sure that your choice of shake or breakfast bar is a low-carb option. If either the bar or the shake doesn't contain adequate protein, make a point of getting your protein from another acceptable source

COLD CEREAL

When it comes to cold cereals, most are loaded with sugars. Even those that are marketed as 'healthy' and don't taste sweet, including many bran cereals, usually contain at least some added sugars. This makes them unacceptable on any phase of Atkins. Refined flour, sugars and hydrogenated oils packed into one convenient box – almost all of the foods in this aisle qualify as products to avoid. Your best bets are multi-grain cereals, which typically have the highest amount of fibre. In particular, organic brands came out well in our research. Check to see that your multi-grain choice has at least 5 grams of fibre per serving. But you will also need to scrutinize the ingredients list, since sugar in all its forms (cane juice, concentrated fruit juice, honey) may still be lurking inside.

Don't be fooled by serving sizes either. Bran cereals, for example, are so dense that you probably wouldn't want to sit down to a large heaped bowl. Puffed wheat, on the other hand, is full of air, so although a large bowlful might keep the carbs in line it won't be enough to provide you with the nutrients you need to start your day. When it comes to muesli, look for sugar-free, organic or controlled-carb versions.

HOT CEREAL

Whole grains are among the last foods you add back to your eating plan on Atkins because of their relatively high carb count. Even then, you should consume them in smaller portions and less frequently.

If you are in Induction, enjoy low-carb hot cereal with double cream diluted with water or unsweetened soya milk (remember to include the additional carbs in your tally). If you prefer your hot cereal sweet, sprinkle with Splenda®.

There is nothing more comforting on a cold winter morning than a bowl of hot cereal. If you're in the later phases of Atkins and your carb threshold is high enough, you can enjoy whole-grain, old-fashioned porridge. Oats are one of the most nutritious grains, because the hull and germ are not removed when they are rolled. Dress up your porridge with a tablespoon or two of nuts, double cream or butter. Avoid processed oat products, sticking instead to old-fashioned and rolled oats. Also try hot flax meal mixed with ricotta cheese – it tastes just like creamy hot cereal.

THINK BEFORE YOU POUR

As if the carbs listed in this chapter weren't high enough, they climb even *higher* when you add milk. So, for example, 225ml of whole milk increases the total grams of carbs by 11 grams. Whole milk is fine in moderation in Pre-Maintenance and Lifetime Maintenance, but a carb-rich breakfast can send your blood sugar soaring, then bring it crashing well before lunchtime. At that point you'll be hungry and irritable – and all too ready to eat whatever food is most convenient, not the smartest choice. Opt, therefore, for no-added-sugar soya milk or double cream that has been mixed with water.

CEREALS
Cold Cereals
⚠ **Alpen Crunchy Bran**
  16.9g carbs per 30g serving
  Contains added sugars

Alpen No Added Sugar (Phases 3–4)
19.4g carbs per 30g serving

⚠ Alpen Original
20.2g carbs per 30g serving
Contains added sugars

⚠ Alpen Wheat Flakes
21.6g carbs per 30g serving
Contains added sugars

Atkins Morning Shine™ Cinnamon Breakfast Flakes (COMING SOON)

(FYI) Grape-nuts® (Phases 3–4)
21.5g carbs per 30g serving
Contains wheat flour

⚠ Jordans Country Crisp
19.4g carbs per 30g serving
Contains added sugars

Jordans Natural Muesli (Phases 3–4)
18.7g carbs per 30g serving

⚠ Jordans Organic Muesli (Phases 3–4)
17.8g carbs per 30g serving

⚠ Jordans Swiss Style Organic Muesli (Phases 3–4)
18.8g carbs per 30g serving

⚠ Kelloggs All-Bran Bran Flakes
20g carbs per 30g serving
Contains added sugars

Kelloggs All-Bran Original
14.4g carbs per 30g serving
Contains added sugars

 Kelloggs All-Bran Sultana Bran
20.4g carbs per 30g serving
Contains added sugars

 Kelloggs Special K
22.2g carbs per 30g serving
Contains added sugars and wheat flour

 Kelloggs Special K with Red Berries
22.5g carbs per 30g serving
Contains added sugars and wheat flour

Mornflake Original Pure Oat Bran (Phases 3–4)
14.1g carbs per 30g serving

Nestlé Bitesize Shredded Wheat (Phases 3–4)
20.9g carbs per 30g serving

 Nestlé Bitesize Triple Berry Shredded Wheat
21.2g carbs per 30g serving
Contains added sugars

 Nestlé Fibre 1
14.8g carbs per 30g serving
Contains added sugars, maize starch and wheat
flour

 Nestlé Force Whole Wheat Flakes
20g carbs per 30g serving
Contains added sugars

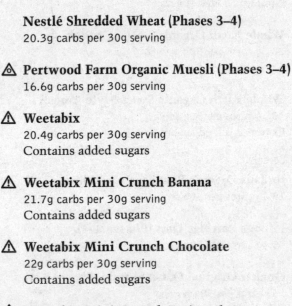

⚠ **Nestlé Fruitful Shredded Wheat**
20.6g carbs per 30g serving
Contains added sugars

Nestlé Shredded Wheat (Phases 3–4)
20.3g carbs per 30g serving

⚠ **Pertwood Farm Organic Muesli (Phases 3–4)**
16.6g carbs per 30g serving

⚠ **Weetabix**
20.4g carbs per 30g serving
Contains added sugars

⚠ **Weetabix Mini Crunch Banana**
21.7g carbs per 30g serving
Contains added sugars

⚠ **Weetabix Mini Crunch Chocolate**
22g carbs per 30g serving
Contains added sugars

⚠ **Weetabix Mini Crunch Fruit and Nut**
21g carbs per 30g serving
Contains added sugars

⚠ **Weetabix Mini Crunch Honey**
22g carbs per 30g serving
Contains added sugars

**Weight Watchers Luxury Fruit Muesli
(Phases 3–4)**
20.1g carbs per 30g serving

⚠ **Weight Watchers Toasted Multi-Grain Flakes with Apple**
20.2g carbs per 30g serving
Contains added sugars

⚠ **Whole Earth Organic Cocoa Crunch**
 20.5g carbs per 30g serving
Contains added sugars

⚠ **Whole Earth Organic Swiss Style Muesli**
 18.3g carbs per 30g serving
Contains added sugars

Hot Cereals
⚠ **Jordans Organic Porridge Oats (Phases 3–4)**
18.4g carbs per 30g serving

Jordans Porridge Oats (Phases 3–4)
18.4g carbs per 30g serving

Quaker Original Oatso Simple (Phases 3–4)
18g carbs per 30g serving

⚠ **Ready Brek®**
17.6g carbs per 30g serving
Contains added sugars

CEREAL BARS & FRUIT ROLLS

You can't beat the convenience of a bar for a fast, nutritious breakfast. Unfortunately, muesli bars, once considered the quintessential health food, are often held together with honey or corn syrup. That fact, on top of the grains themselves, means that finding a low-carb selection is practically an impossible task. Think

of these more as grain-based confectionery rather than
health food, so choose a low-carb breakfast or nutrition
bar instead. When choosing a nutrition bar as a meal
replacement, if it does not contain adequate protein
make sure you have some protein along with it.

**Atkins Advantage™ Bar Chocolate Decadence
(Phases 1–4)**
2g Net Carbs per bar

**Atkins Advantage™ Bar Chocolate Hazelnut
Crunch (Phases 1–4)**
2g Net Carbs per bar

**Atkins Advantage™ Bar Chocolate Orange
Sensation (Phases 1–4) (COMING SOON)**
3g Net Carbs per bar

**Atkins Advantage™ Bar Fruits of the Forest
(Phases 1–4)**
3g Net Carbs per bar

**Atkins Morning Shine™ Breakfast Bar Apple
Crisp (Phases 1–4)**
3g Net Carbs per bar

**Atkins Morning Shine™ Breakfast Bar
Chocolate Chip Crisp (Phases 1–4)**
3g Net Carbs per bar

**Atkins Morning Shine™ Mixed Berry Granola
Cereal Bar (Phases 1–4) (COMING SOON)**
3g Net Carbs per bar

**Atkins Morning Shine™ Breakfast Bar
Strawberry Crisp (Phases 1–4)**
3g Net Carbs per bar

⚠ **CarboLite Breakfast Bars Blueberry Flavour**
4g Net Carbs per bar
Contains added sugars, modified maize starch and
wheat flour .

⚠ **CarboLite Breakfast Bars Strawberry Flavour**
4g Net Carbs per bar
Contains added sugars, modified maize starch and
wheat flour

⚠ **Carb Count High Protein Bar Crispy
Chocolate Marshmallow**
2g Net Carbs per bar
Contains added sugars and trans fats

⚠ **Carb Count High Protein Bar Crispy
Chocolate Roasted Peanut**
3g Net Carbs per bar
Contains added sugars and trans fats

⚠ **Carb Count High Protein Bar Crispy Yoghurt
Lemon**
4g Net Carbs per bar
Contains added sugars and trans fats

⚠ **Carb Minders Crispy Delicious High Protein
Bar Crispy Chocolate Peanut**
3g Net Carbs per bar
Contains added sugars

⚠ **Carb Minders Crispy Delicious High Protein Bar Crispy Chocolate S'Mores**
2g Net Carbs per bar
Contains added sugars

⚠ **Carb Solutions Good Mornings! Breakfast & Lunch Bar Cinnamon Apple Crisp**
2.5g Net Carbs per bar
Contains added sugars and trans fats

⚠ **Carb Solutions Good Mornings! Breakfast & Lunch Bar Pecan Cinnamon Bun**
2g Net Carbs per bar
Contains added sugars and trans fats

⚠ **CarbWise Delicious Crispy High Protein Bar Crispy Chocolate Peanut**
3g Net Carbs per bar
Contains added sugars, trans fats and wheat flour

⚠ **CarbWise Delicious Crispy High Protein Bar Crispy Chocolate Raspberry**
3g Net Carbs per bar
Contains added sugars, trans fats and wheat flour

⚠ **Lyme Regis Foods Fruit 4U Cherry**
20.6g carbs per 28g bar
Contains added sugars

⚠ **Lyme Regis Foods Fruit 4U Raspberry**
20.6g carbs per 28g bar
Contains added sugars

⚠ **Lyme Regis Foods Kidz Organic Fruit Bar Blackcurrant Buzz (Phases 3–4)**
13.5g carbs per 20g bar

Lyme Regis Foods La Fruit Blackcurrant (Phases 3–4)
19.9g carbs per 25g serving

Lyme Regis Foods La Fruit Raspberry (Phases 3–4)
18.8g carbs per 25g serving

⚠ **Lyme Regis Foods Organic Fruitus Chewy Apricot Cereal Bar (Phases 3–4)**
21.4g carbs per 35g bar

⚠ **Lyme Regis Foods Organic Fruitus Chewy**
⚠ **Mixed Berry Cereal Bar**
22.3g carbs per 35g bar
Contains added sugars

⚠ **Lyme Regis Organic Seven Seeds and Nut Bar (Phases 3–4)**
17.4g carbs per 40g bar

Lyme Regis Zaps Apricot Fruit Bar (Phases 3–4)
16.6g carbs per 25g bar

Lyme Regis Zaps Orange Fruit Bar (Phases 3–4)
17.4g carbs per 25g bar

⚠ **Village Bakery Fruit Nut and Seed Bar**
18.4g carbs per 25g bar
Contains added sugars

RICE & CORN CAKES

⚠ **Kallo Organic Corn Cakes Thin Slice Lightly Salted (Phases 3–4)**
3.6g carbs per 4.8g corn cake

⚠ **Kallo Organic Rice Cakes Milk Chocolate**
⚠ 6.2g carbs per 11g rice cake
Contains added sugars

⚠ **Kallo Organic Rice Cakes Snack Size Caramel**
⚠ 15.8g carbs per 20g serving
Contains added sugars

⚠ **Kallo Organic Rice Cakes Snack Size Plain – No Added Salt (Phases 3–4)**
15.7g carbs per 20g serving

⚠ **Kallo Organic Rice Cakes Snack Size Savoury (Phases 3–4)**
17.8g carbs per 25g serving

⚠ **Kallo Organic Rice Cakes Thick Slice Savoury (Phases 3–4)**
6.5g carbs per 9g rice cake

⚠ **Kallo Rice Cakes Snack Size Apple and Cinnamon**
16.6g carbs per 20g serving
Contains added sugars

⚠ **Kallo Rice Cakes Thick Slice Caramel**
7.5g carbs per 10g rice cake
Contains added sugars

Real Foods Corn Thins Original (Phases 3–4)
4.7g carbs per slice

Real Foods Corn Thins Sesame (Phases 3–4)
4.5g carbs per slice

MILK

When you are able to reintroduce milk into your diet,
make sure that you use whole milk or controlled-carb
dairy products only.

Cow's Milk

**Gold Top Jersey & Guernsey Whole Milk
(Phases 3–4)**
4.7g carbs per 100ml

⚠ **Organic Whole (Phases 3–4)**
4.8g carbs per 100ml

Whole (Phases 3–4)
4.7g carbs per 100ml

UHT Milk

Whole (Phases 3–4)
4.8g carbs per 100ml

Goat's Milk

Whole (Phases 3–4)
4.3g carbs per 100ml

Low-carb Milk

**Atkins Low-Carb Semi-Skimmed Milk
(Phases 1–4) (COMING SOON)**
2.5g Net Carbs per 100ml

Oat & Rice Milk

⚠ **Oat Supreme**
3.3g carbs per 100ml
Contains added sugars

⚠ **Oatly Organic Oat Drink**
⚠ 6.5g carbs per 100ml
Contains added sugars

⚠ **Provamel Alpro Rice Organic**
⚠ 9.9g carbs per 100ml
Contains organic rice syrup

ⒻⓎⒾ **Rice Dream Original (Phases 3–4)**
9.4g carbs per 100ml
Contains partially milled brown rice

ⒻⓎⒾ **Rice Dream Original with Added Calcium
(Phases 3–4)**
9.4g carbs per 100ml
Contains partially milled brown rice

Soya Milk

**Holland & Barrett Unsweetened Soya
(Phases 1–4)**
0.6g carbs per 100ml

⚠ **Provamel Alpro Chilled Soya**
2.8g carbs per 100ml
Contains added sugars

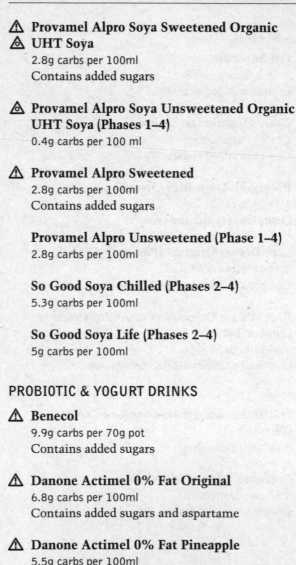

⚠ **Provamel Alpro Soya Sweetened Organic**
⚠ **UHT Soya**
2.8g carbs per 100ml
Contains added sugars

⚠ **Provamel Alpro Soya Unsweetened Organic UHT Soya (Phases 1–4)**
0.4g carbs per 100 ml

⚠ **Provamel Alpro Sweetened**
2.8g carbs per 100ml
Contains added sugars

Provamel Alpro Unsweetened (Phase 1–4)
2.8g carbs per 100ml

So Good Soya Chilled (Phases 2–4)
5.3g carbs per 100ml

So Good Soya Life (Phases 2–4)
5g carbs per 100ml

PROBIOTIC & YOGURT DRINKS

⚠ **Benecol**
9.9g carbs per 70g pot
Contains added sugars

⚠ **Danone Actimel 0% Fat Original**
6.8g carbs per 100ml
Contains added sugars and aspartame

⚠ **Danone Actimel 0% Fat Pineapple**
5.5g carbs per 100ml
Contains added sugars and aspartame

⚠ **Danone Actimel Multifruit**
16g carbs per 100ml
Contains added sugars and modified starch

⚠ **Danone Actimel Orange**
15.9g carbs per 100ml
Contains added sugars

⚠ **Danone Actimel Original**
14.3g carbs per 100ml
Contains added sugars

⚠ **Danone Actimel Strawberry**
15.9g carbs per 100ml
Contains added sugars and modified starch

⚠ **Müller Vitality Low Fat Raspberry Yoghurt Drink**
12.8g carbs per 100ml
Contains added sugars and modified starch

⚠ **Ocean Spray Cranberry and Raspberry Yogurt Drink**
15.2g carbs per 100ml
Contains added sugars

⚠ **Yakult**
7.9g carbs per 65ml pot
Contains added sugars

⚠ **Yakult Light**
5.4g carbs per 65ml pot
Contains added sugars

SHAKES

**Atkins Advantage Ready-to-Drink Shake
Chocolate Flavour (Phases 1–4)**
2g Net Carbs per serving

**Atkins Advantage Ready-to-Drink Shake
Strawberry Flavour (Phases 1–4)**
2g Net Carbs per serving

**Atkins Advantage Ready-to-Drink Shake
Vanilla Flavour (Phases 1–4)**
2g Net Carbs per serving

SHAKE MIXES

**Atkins Advantage Shake Mix Chocolate
Flavour (Phases 1–4)**
2g Net Carbs per serving

**Atkins Advantage Shake Mix Strawberry
Flavour (Phases 1–4)**
3g Net Carbs per serving

**Atkins Advantage Shake Mix Vanilla Flavour
(Phases 1–4)**
3g Net Carbs per serving

⚠ **Carb Solutions High Protein Shake Mix
Creamy Vanilla**
3g Net Carbs per serving
Contains added sugars and trans fats

Carb Solutions High Protein Shake Mix Rich Chocolate

4g Net Carbs per serving

Contains added sugars and trans fats

Condiments

Clever cooks know that the difference between meals bursting with flavour and bland food often comes down to condiments. Whether your dish needs the kick of Tabasco, the zest of a Caesar dressing or the tangy bite of mustard, condiments add punch – and they usually have modest carb counts.

However, there are a few classic condiments that will contribute too many carbs in their traditional formulations – especially regular ketchup. If you generally pour it on to your plate with no thought to quantity, squeeze some into a measuring spoon before putting it on your plate. How does it compare to what you normally eat? Most ketchup is full of sugars, so if you always squirt a generous dollop to accompany your food, you might want to think carefully in future!

Other red flags in the salad-dressing aisle are honey mustards and fruity vinaigrettes, which are almost always high in sugars.

MAYONNAISE & SALAD CREAM

Mayonnaise is made primarily from oil and eggs, but vegan versions can be found in most supermarkets. All major brands of regular mayonnaise contain small amounts of added sugars; reduced-fat, light and fat-free versions contain even more sugars, as well as other fillers to compensate for the flavour and texture provided by oil, making them higher in carbohydrates and less tasty.

⚠ Benedicta La Mayonnaise à la Moutarde de Dijon
1.4g carbs per 100g, 0.2g carbs per 15g
Contains added sugars and modified cornflour

⚠ Heinz Salad Cream
20.3g carbs per 100g, 2g carbs per 10ml serving
Contains added sugars and modified cornflour

⚠ Hellmann's Olive Oil Mayonnaise
1.3g carbs per 100g, 0.2g carbs per 15g
Contains added sugars

⚠ Hellmann's Real Mayonnaise
1.3g carbs per 100g, 0.2g carbs per 15g
Contains added sugars

⚠ Simply Delicious Organic Mayonnaise
2.2g carbs per 100g, 0.3g carbs per 15g
Contains added sugars

⚠ Weight Watchers Mayonnaise Dressing
7.3g carbs per 100g, 1.1g carbs per 15g
Contains added sugars

MUSTARDS

You'll find an enormous range of mustards in supermarkets, but be sure to steer clear of the sweet varieties, whether they're made with honey or brown sugar. Confusingly, many mustards might list ingredients but not nutritional content, and this makes your task difficult when determining carb counts. In those cases, you may prefer to put the jar back on the supermarket shelf and choose one that does provide information. As a rule, smooth mustard contains 9.7g carbs per 100g, while wholegrain has 4.2g carbs per 100g. In cases where information about ingredients is not provided, you would be wise to avoid that product in case it contains added sugars. (Source: Food Standards Agency)

⚠ Burgess French Mustard
12g carbs per 100g, 1.8g carbs per 15g
Contains added sugars and wheat flour

⚠ Colmans Mild Mustard
9g carbs per 100ml, 1.3g carbs per 15ml
Contains added sugars

Dijon Original Maille Mustard (Phases 1–4)
6g carbs per 100g, 1.3g carbs per 15g

⚠ Simply Delicious Organic Coarse Grain ⚠ Mustard
11.5g carbs per 100g, 1.7g carbs per 15g
Contains added sugars

OILS & VINEGARS

As long as you stick with unflavoured oils and vinegars, you can be confident that your oil will be free of carbs and your vinegar quite low. However, if you start adding fruits, vegetables and even some herbs, you may gradually boost the carb count, so take care.

Keep a variety of oils on hand and look for unrefined, cold-pressed fresh vegetable and nut varieties. While they tend to be more expensive, these oils have not been heated and treated with harsh chemicals (which strip away their nutrients), so they still have a rich flavour, essential fatty acids and lots of vitamins.

Expeller-pressed oils are exposed to heat, but they do retain more of the natural flavour and aroma of the seeds from which they were mechanically pressed than refined oils. Buy in small quantities and store in a cool, dark cupboard away from direct heat.

Cooking Oils

⚠ **Again and Again**
0g carbs per 100ml
Contains trans fats

Crisp 'n' Dry (Phases 1–4)
0g carbs per 100ml

Fry Light Butter Flavour Oil Spray (Phases 1–4)
Trace carbs per 100ml

Fry Light Sunflower Oil Spray (Phases 1–4)
Trace carbs per 100ml

Own Brand Sun Olive Oil (Phases 1–4)
0g carbs per 100ml

⚠ **Pura Light Touch**
0g carbs per 100g
Contains trans fats

Sharwoods Vegetable Ghee (Phases 1–4)
Trace carbs per 100g

Sharwoods Wok Oil (Phases 1–4)
1.5g carbs per 100ml

Vegalene Spray 'N' Cook (Phases 1–4)
0g carbs per 100ml

Flavoured Oils

Filippo Berio Extra Virgin Oil Flavoured with Basil (Phases 1–4)
0g carbs per 100ml

Filippo Berio Extra Virgin Oil Flavoured with Garlic (Phases 1–4)
0g carbs per 100ml

Filippo Berio Extra Virgin Oil Flavoured with Lemon (Phases 1–4)
0g carbs per 100ml

Napolina Basil Flavoured Olive Oil (Phases 1–4)
0g carbs per 100ml

Napolina Garlic Flavoured Olive Oil (Phases 1–4)
0g carbs per 100ml

Napolina Lemon & Dill Flavoured Olive Oil (Phases 1–4)
0g carbs per 100ml

Napolina Sundried Tomato Flavoured Olive Oil (Phases 1–4)
0g carbs per 100ml

Own Brand Basil Flavoured Olive Oil (Phases 1–4)
0g carbs per 100ml

Own Brand Chilli Flavoured Olive Oil (Phases 1–4)
0g carbs per 100ml

Own Brand Garlic Flavoured Olive Oil (Phases 1–4)
0g carbs per 100ml

Own Brand Italian Style Herb Dipping Oil (Phases 1–4)
0.9g carbs per 100ml

Own Brand Lemon Flavoured Olive Oil (Phases 1–4)
0g carbs per 100ml

Vinegars

While most vinegars are a safe zero-carb bet, there are some exceptions – primarily those that are flavoured and seasoned. If you use more than the serving size, you might be consuming more carbs than you bargained for.

Remember, too, that balsamic vinegar contains some sugars and should be limited, especially during the Induction Phase. Not all labels list nutritional information or ingredients, so use common sense when selecting vinegar.

Aspall Cyder Vinegar (Phases 1–4)
0.1g carbs per 100ml

⚠ Aspall English Apple Balsamic Vinegar (Phases 3–4)
23.1g carbs per 100ml
Contains added sugars

⚠ Aspall Organic Balsamic Vinegar (Phases 3–4)
17.5g carbs per 100ml
Contains added sugars

⚠ **Aspall Organic Red Wine Vinegar (Phases 1–4)**
0.6g carbs per 100ml

⚠ **Aspall Organic White Wine Vinegar
(Phases 1–4)**
0.6g carbs per 100ml

Boromeo Sherry Vinegar (Phases 1–4)
0g carbs per 100ml

⚠ **Carlo Magno Balsamic Vinegar (Phases 3–4)**
12.5g carbs per 100ml
Contains added sugars

⚠ **Fattorie Giacobazzi White Balsamic Vinegar
(Phases 3–4)**
12.5g carbs per 100ml
Contains added sugars

**Mitsukan Rice Vinegar Light & Mild
(Phases 1–4)**
2.6g carbs per 100ml

⚠ **Mitsukan Seasoned Rice Vinegar (Phases 3–4)**
30.9g carbs per 100ml
Contains added sugars

⚠ **Own Brand Balsamic Vinegar of Modena
(Phases 3–4)**
25.5g carbs per 100ml
Contains added sugars

Own Brand Cider Vinegar (Phases 1–4)
0.6–0.8g carbs per 100ml

Own Brand White Wine Vinegar (Phases 1–4)
0.6g carbs per 100ml

 Salad Light Balsamic Vinaigrette
15.3g carbs per 100ml
Contains added sugars

SALAD DRESSINGS, SAUCES & GRAVIES

Whipping up a simple vinaigrette with your favourite oil and vinegar or lemon juice is a cinch, and will ensure that your dressing is as low in carbs as possible. Nevertheless, there are times when you want the convenience of a bottled dressing, perhaps with exotic ingredients and flavourings. Always avoid fat-free and reduced-fat varieties – they're invariably loaded with corn syrup (it has the same consistency as oil and is a cheap substitute). When you're doing Atkins, the benefits of healthy fats, such as olive oil, are many: consuming enough fat helps you stay satisfied, moderates blood sugar and can help control cravings for carbs. When you're controlling carbs, getting adequate dietary fat also accelerates a fat-burning metabolism.

None of the salad dressings below came out well in our research. Bottled dressings may be convenient, but you pay a price in terms of carbs and unacceptable ingredients.

Salad Dressings

⚠ **English Provender Co. More Than a Dressing Sundried Tomato & Smoked Paprika Dressing**
8.3g carbs per 100g, 1.2g carbs per 15g
Contains added sugars

⚠ **English Provender Co. Thai Lime & Coriander Dressing**
22.3g carbs per 100g, 3.3g carbs per 15g
Contains added sugars

⚠ **Kraft Classics French Vinaigrette Dressing**
7.3g carbs per 100ml, 1.1g carbs per 15ml
Contains added sugars

⚠ **Kraft Classics Italian Vinaigrette Dressing with Garlic**
5.6g carbs per 100ml, 1g carbs per 15ml
Contains added sugars

⚠ **Kraft Classics Thousand Island Dressing**
19.5g carbs per 100ml, 4g carbs per 15ml
Contains added sugars

⚠ **Kraft Fat Free Italian Vinaigrette Style Dressing**
6.8g carbs per 100ml, 1g carbs per 15ml
Contains added sugars

⚠ **Kraft Get Dressed Caesar Dressing**
7.9g carbs per 100ml, 1.2g carbs per 15g
Contains added sugars

⚠ **Kraft 10% Fat Balsamic Dressing**
8.1g carbs per 100ml, 1.2g carbs per 15ml
Contains added sugars

⚠ **Loyd Grossman Green Thai with Coconut Dressing**
15.3g carbs per 100g, 2.3g carbs per 15g
Contains added sugars and modified maize starch

Newman's Own Balsamic Vinaigrette
3.9g carbs per 100g, 0.6g carbs per 15g
Contains added sugars

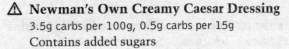 **Newman's Own Creamy Caesar Dressing**
3.5g carbs per 100g, 0.5g carbs per 15g
Contains added sugars

⚠ **Pizza Express Balsamic Dressing**
10.3g carbs per 100g, 1.5g carbs per 15g
Contains added sugars

⚠ **Pizza Express Olive Oil Dressing**
3.4g carbs per 100g, 0.5g carbs per 15g
Contains added sugars

⚠ **Pizza Express Reduced Calorie Light Olive Oil Dressing**
3.6g carbs per 100g, 0.5g carbs per 15g
Contains added sugars

⚠ **Salad Light 1 Calorie Dressing Spray Balsamic Vinaigrette**
15.3g carbs per 100ml, 0.1g carbs per spray
Contains added sugars

⚠ **Schwartz Creamy Garlic & Herb Dressing**
4.9g carbs per 100ml, 0.7g carbs per 15ml
Contains added sugars and modified maize starch

⚠ **Schwartz French Vinaigrette with Cracked Black Pepper**
7.2g carbs per 100ml, 1.1g carbs per 15ml
Contains added sugars

⚠ **Schwartz Italian Dressing with Olives & Oregano**
25.4g carbs per 100ml, 3.1g carbs per 15ml
Contains added sugars

⚠ **Schwartz Roasted Red Pepper & Chilli Dressing**
15.8g carbs per 100ml, 2.4g carbs per 15ml
Contains added sugars

Sauces & Gravy Mixes

Instant gravy mixes, gravy granules and stock cubes nearly all contain high levels of unacceptable ingredients. If possible make your own. Tartare sauce is made by combining mayonnaise with capers and gherkins, all of which add carbs. In addition, most brands of tartare sauce contain sugars. If you can't find one that is suitable, the best solution is to make your own.

(FYI) **Bisto Original Gravy Powder (Phases 3–4)**
61.9g carbs per 100g, 2.2g carbs per 50ml serving
Contains wheat starch

Colmans Fresh Garden Mint Sauce (Phases 1–4)
3.1g carbs per 100ml, 0.5g carbs per 15ml

⚠ **Colmans Tartare Sauce**
17g carbs per 100ml, 2.5g carbs per 15ml
Contains added sugars and modified starch

English Provender Co. Freshly Grated Hot Horseradish (Phases 1–4)
17.9g carbs per 100g, 2.7g carbs per 15g

⚠ **English Provender Co. Seafood Sauce with Dill & Balsamic Vinegar**
15.9g carbs per 100g, 2.4g carbs per 15g
Contains added sugars

⚠ **English Provender Co. Tartare Sauce**
3.6g carbs per 100g, 0.5g carbs per 15g
Contains added sugars

⚠ **Heinz Tomato Ketchup**
24.7g carbs per 100g, 2.7g carbs per 10ml serving
Contains added sugars

⚠ **HP Sauce**
27.1g carbs per 100g, 4.1g carbs per 15g
Contains added sugars and modified maize starch

PICKLES

⚠ **Baxters Beetroot Pickle**
26g per 100g, 3.9g carbs per 15g
Contains added sugars and modified cornflour

⚠ **Baxters Beetroot Slices in Vinegar**
6g carbs per 100g, 0.9g carbs per 15g
Contains added sugars

FYI **Cooks & Co. Green Peppers Stuffed with Feta Cheese (Phases 3–4)**
2.6g carbs per 100g, 0.4g carbs per 15g
Contains modified cornflour

ⒻⓎⒾ **Cooks & Co. Red Peppers Stuffed with Feta Cheese (Phases 3–4)**
2.6g carbs per 100g, 0.4g carbs per 15g
Contains modified cornflour

⚠ **Crosse & Blackwell Branston Original**
34.2g carbs per 100g, 5.1g carbs per 15g
Contains added sugars and modified starch

Haywards Crisp & Crunchy Traditional Onions (Phases 2–4)
4.7g carbs per 100g, 0.7g carbs per 15g

Haywards Mixed Pickle (Phases 1–4)
2.4g carbs per 100g, 0.4g carbs per 15g

⚠ **Haywards Sliced Dill Gherkins**
5.5g carbs per 100g, 0.8g carbs per 15g
Contains added sugars

⚠ **Heinz Ploughmans Pickle**
26.7g carbs per 100g, 4g carbs per 15g
Contains added sugars and modified cornflour

⚠ **Mrs Elswood Cucumber Spears with Dill**
7.7g carbs per 100g, 1.1g carbs per 15g
Contains added sugars

⚠ **Opies Cocktail Gherkins in Vinegar**
5.6g carbs per 100g, 0.8g carbs per 15g
Contains added sugars

⚠ **Opies Cocktail Onions in Vinegar**
8.3g carbs per 100g, 1.3g carbs per 15g
Contains added sugars

Opies Pickled Onions in Balsamic Vinegar (Phases 1–4)

1.7g carbs per 100g, 0.2g carbs per 15g

Opies Pickled Walnuts in Malt Vinegar

27.5g carbs per 100g, 4.1g carbs per 15g
Contains added sugars

Patak's Lime Pickle (Phases 1–4)

4g carbs per 100g, 0.6g carbs per 15g

STOCK CUBES & POWDER

Kallo Organic Beef Flavour Stock Cubes (Phases 1–4)

0.4g carbs per 100ml of stock

Kallo Organic Chicken Stock Cubes (Phases 1–4)

0.4g carbs per 100ml of stock

Kallo Organic Vegetable Stock Cubes (Phases 1–4)

0.4g carbs per 100ml of stock

Marigold Organic Vegan Dairy Free Swiss Vegetable Bouillon Powder (Phases 1–4)

0.4g carbs per 100ml stock serving

Confectionery and Desserts

CONFECTIONERY

The concept of low-carb confectionery seems like a dream come true – and it can be, if you enjoy such treats in moderation. Luckily, many manufacturers have started to offer sugar-free or low-carb versions of their best-selling products.

You'll often find such low-carb confectionery mixed in with ordinary brands in the sweets aisle. If you don't see them there, take a look for diabetic foods in the sugar-free section, or by the slimming products. But even if they are low in carbs you should still approach these products with caution, as they can still contain added sugars and hydrogenated oils, which are unacceptable on any phase of Atkins. No packaged sweets are suitable in the Induction phase. But protein bars, which are also full of nutrients, can satisfy the desire for a sweet snack.

It's also important to note that certain controlled-carb products contain sugar alcohols, which at higher levels can cause gastrointestinal symptoms and a laxative effect in some individuals. Be wary of products with more than 15g of sugar alcohols.

While you may indulge in the occasional treat, such foods can be hard to eat in small quantities. And just because it's low-carb, that doesn't mean you can eat as much as you want. Primarily burning fat for energy in the early phases of Atkins has the effect of naturally controlling your appetite. However, as you move through the phases and begin switching back and forth from fat-burning to glucose-burning, you'll have to rely more on self-control to avoid over-indulging. Set out the appropriate portion and be firm with yourself about not going back for more. If you find that you are incapable of practising moderation, it may be easier to steer clear of these things altogether and satisfy sweet cravings with berries and whipped cream.

CONFECTIONERY

Diabetic

Boots Barley Sugars (Phases 2–4)
0g carbs per 100g

⚠ **Boots Belgian Chocolate Coated Wafer**
5.7g carbs per 30g bar
Contains trans fats and wheat flour

Boots Belgian Milk Chocolate (Phases 2–4)
5g carbs per 44g bar

Boots Belgian Milk Chocolate with Hazelnuts (Phases 2–4)
4g carbs per 44g bar

Boots Belgian Plain Chocolate (Phases 2–4)
1.8g carbs per 44g bar

Boots Fruit Gums (Phases 2–4)
0g carbs per 100g

Boots Mint Humbugs (Phases 2–4)
1g carbs per 100g

Boots Toffees (Phases 2–4)
2g carbs per 100g

⚠ **Ernest Jackson Praline Filled Chocolate**
12.2g carbs per 25g
Contains added sugars

⚠ **Holex Peppermint Cream**
13.5g carbs per 25g
Contains added sugars

⚠ **Holex Strawberry Cream Bar**
11.5g carbs per 25g
Contains added sugars

**Stretch Island Fruit Leather Bar Apple
(Phases 3–4)**
10.9g carbs per 14g bar

**Stretch Island Fruit Leather Bar Apple and
Mango (Phases 3–4)**
11g carbs per 14g bar

**Stretch Island Fruit Leather Bar Apple, Pear
and Raspberry (Phases 3–4)**
10.7g carbs per 14g bar

Low-Carb

⚠ **Advant Edge Chocolate Fudge Carb Control Bar**
1.5g Net Carbs per 50g bar
Contains trans fats and aspartame

Advant Edge Strawberry Flavour Carb Control Bar
1g Net Carbs per 50g bar
Contains added sugars, trans fats and aspartame

Atkins Advantage™ Bar Chocolate Decadence (Phases 1–4)
2g Net Carbs per 60g bar

Atkins Advantage™ Bar Chocolate Hazelnut Crunch (Phases 1–4)
2g Net Carbs per 60g bar

Atkins Advantage™ Bar Chocolate Orange Sensation (Phases 1–4) (COMING SOON)
3g Net Carbs per bar

Atkins Advantage™ Bar Fruits of the Forest (Phases 1–4)
3g Net Carbs per 60g bar

Atkins Endulge™ Caramel Hazelnut Bar (Phases 2–4)
5g Net Carbs per 35g bar

Atkins Endulge™ Caramel Wafer Crisp (Phases 2–4)
4g Net Carbs per 24g wafer

Atkins Endulge™ Chocolate Creme Wafer Crisp (Phases 2–4)
3g Net Carbs per 28g wafer

Atkins Endulge™ Crispy Milk Chocolate Bar (Phases 2–4)
1g Net Carbs per 30g bar

Atkins Endulge™ Milk Chocolate Bar (Phases 2–4)
2g Net Carbs per 30g bar

Atkins Endulge™ Mint Wafer Crisp (Phases 2–4)
2g Net Carbs per 28g wafer

Carbolite Chocolate Flavour Bar (Phases 2–4)
0.2g Net Carbs per 28g bar

Carbolite Chocolate Flavour Coconut Bar (Phases 2–4)
0.4g Net Carbs per 28g bar

Carbolite Chocolate Flavour Crisp Bar (Phases 2–4)
1.3g Net Carbs per 28g bar

⚠ Carbolite Chocolate Flavour Truffle Bar
0.8g Net Carbs per 28g bar
Contains trans fats and modified cornflour

⚠ Carbolite Crisp Wafer
0.9 Net Carbs per bar
Contains trans fats

⚠ Carbolite Crispy Caramel Flavour Bar
3.7g Net Carbs per 28g bar
Contains trans fats

⚠ **Carb Count High Protein Bar Crispy Chocolate Marshmallow**
2g Net Carbs per bar
Contains added sugars and trans fats

⚠ **Carb Count High Protein Bar Crispy Chocolate Roasted Peanut**
3g Net Carbs per bar
Contains added sugars and trans fats

⚠ **Carb Count High Protein Bar Crispy Yoghurt Lemon**
4g Net Carbs per bar
Contains added sugars and trans fats

⚠ **Carb Minders Crispy Delicious High Protein Bar Crispy Chocolate Peanut**
3g Net Carbs per bar
Contains added sugars

⚠ **Carb Minders Crispy Delicious High Protein Bar Crispy Chocolate S'Mores**
2g Net Carbs per bar
Contains added sugars

⚠ **Carb Solutions Taste Sensations Coconut Almond Clusters**
1g Net Carbs per bar
Contains trans fats

⚠ **Carb Solutions Taste Sensations High Protein Bar Chocolate Fudge Almond**
3g Net Carbs per bar
Contains added sugars

⚠ **Carb Solutions Taste Sensations High Protein
Bar Chocolate Toffee Hazelnut**
3g Net Carbs per bar
Contains added sugars

⚠ **Carb Wise High Protein Bar Crispy Chocolate
Marshmallow Flavour**
2g Net Carbs per bar
Contains trans fats

⚠ **Carb Wise High Protein Bar Crispy Chocolate
Peanut Flavour**
3g Net Carbs per bar
Contains trans fats

⚠ **Carb Wise High Protein Bar Crispy Chocolate
Raspberry Flavour**
3g Net Carbs per bar
Contains trans fats and wheat flour

⚠ **Dietline Slimmers Biscuit**
6g carbs per cake
Contains added sugars and wheat flour

FYI **Nestlé Low Carb Kit Kat (Phases 3–4)**
4g carbs per two-finger bar
Contains wheat flour

Nestlé Low Carb Rolo (Phases 2–4)
3.5g carbs per packet

DESSERTS

Most of the great British puddings are strictly out of bounds during all phases of Atkins, as many of them are simply too high in carbs to make them acceptable. As a result, the dessert aisles of supermarkets are off-limits.

This doesn't mean you have to abandon puddings, however. While shop-bought products, with their sugars, trans fats, white flour and other unacceptable ingredients, should definitely become a thing of your past, those made with Splenda® and Atkins™ Bake Mix would be acceptable, for example. Check out the Food & Recipes section of the Atkins website (www.atkins.com/uk) for other delicious options.

After Induction, berries and other acceptable fruits make delicious desserts when accompanied by crème fraîche, cream or fresh custard (made with eggs, not cornflour); add nuts and you have not only a delicious dessert but a nutritious end to a meal, too.

Ice Cream

There's no doubt about it: ice cream is even more popular with adults than it is with children – just look at the vast selection on offer in the supermarket freezer cases. But while some of the ice creams we reviewed did come within acceptable carb limits, all of them contained sugars, which means they are unacceptable on any phase of Atkins.

At the moment, there is no ice cream sold in the UK that is acceptable on Atkins. If you cannot live without ice cream, consider making your own. It's not as difficult as you might imagine, nor is it necessary to have an ice cream machine. Mix equal quantities of natural yogurt and fromage frais, and sweeten to taste with Splenda®. Mash a handful of your favourite berries and stir through the mixture. Place in a freezer-proof polythene tub and freeze, stirring every 30 minutes or so to break up any ice crystals that may have formed. Not only will you have a delicious, low-carb ice cream, but if you make a large batch it will ensure you have a scrumptious, convenient dessert waiting for you in the freezer when you fancy a treat.

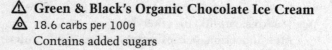

⚠ Duchy Originals Organic Vanilla Ice Cream
⚠ 15.8g carbs per 100g
   Contains added sugars

⚠ Green & Black's Organic Chocolate Ice Cream
⚠ 18.6 carbs per 100g
   Contains added sugars

⚠ Green & Black's Vanilla Ice Cream
⚠ 15.2g carbs per 100g
   Contains added sugars

⚠ Hill Station Dark Roast Coffee Ice Cream
17.3g carbs per 100g
   Contains added sugars

⚠ Hill Station Mango and Lime Ice Cream
19.9g carbs per 100g
   Contains added sugars

⚠ Hill Station Stem Ginger Ice Cream
20.2g carbs per 100g
   Contains added sugars

⚠ Hill Station Vanilla Bean Ice Cream
17.8g carbs per 100g
   Contains added sugars

⚠ **Mackie's of Scotland Traditional Luxury Dairy**
⚠ **Ice Cream**
  18g carbs per 100g
  Contains added sugars

⚠ **Minghella Dolce Vita Real Vanilla Ice Cream**
  17g carbs per 100g
  Contains added sugars

⚠ **Yeo Valley Organic Vanilla Dairy Ice Cream**
⚠ 21.3 carbs per 100g
  Contains added sugars

⚠ **Yorkshire Dales Natural Flavour Old**
  Fashioned Luxury Dairy Ice Cream
  18.6g carbs per 100g
  Contains added sugars

⚠ **Yorkshire Dales Old English Sticky Toffee**
  Crunch Luxury Dairy Ice Cream
  10.9g carbs per 100g
  Contains added sugars

⚠ **Yorkshire Dales Triple Chocolate Chunk**
  Luxury Dairy Ice Cream
  12.5g carbs per 100g
  Contains added sugars and modified maize starch

FROZEN DESSERTS

⚠ **Slim-Fast Chocolate and Caramel Stick Bars**
  14.5g carbs per stick
  Contains added sugars

⚠ **Slim-Fast Vanilla and Strawberry Mini Tubs**
18g carbs per 60g tub
Contains added sugars

⚠ **Viennetta Vanilla**
22.9g carbs per 100g
Contains added sugars

⚠ **Weight Watchers Chocolate with Honeycomb Pieces**
15.2g carbs per 100ml pot
Contains added sugars and modified maize starch

⚠ **Weight Watchers Vanilla with Raspberry Swirl**
13.3g carbs per 100ml pot
Contains added sugars and modified cornflour

⚠ **Weight Watchers Vanilla with Strawberry Swirl**
13.3g carbs per 100ml pot
Contains added sugars and modified cornflour

Dairy, Eggs and Fresh Juice

From nutrient-rich cheese to sugar-laden puddings, this aisle contains some of the best and worst food choices in the supermarket. When you're doing Atkins, common sense will tell you to avoid dairy desserts such as regular cheesecake, chocolate mousse, fresh custard and crème brûlée. But even if you push your trolley straight past temptation, you can still slip up when you think you're choosing something virtuous and nutritious. For example, although regular fruit-flavoured yogurt is marketed as a healthy choice, it is full of sugars, and probiotic drinks and smoothies are equally hazardous.

But there are also many good choices on offer in the dairy section. Cheese and eggs are valuable sources of protein, while butter, whole milk and cream also have an important part to play in your diet. Ensure you pay attention to the nutritional information on product labels and you won't go wrong!

BUTTER, MARGARINE & SPREADS

Natural, creamy and unmistakable in flavour, butter remains the spread of choice for people following a controlled-carb lifestyle. Butter provides a mix of saturated and unsaturated fats, and its taste is inimitable. Unsalted butter is often fresher than salted – salt is a preservative, so salted butter may stay on warehouse or refrigerator shelves longer.

Butter is comprised of 80 per cent fat, and most Atkins recipes are formulated with the assumption that you'll be using butter. Never choose a soft, tub-style margarine or spread, or one that's reduced-fat. Also, avoid margarine–butter blends, which contain hydrogenated oils.

Margarine labelling can be tricky: even though you'll see labels trumpeting 'cholesterol-free', don't be fooled. While margarine does not contain cholesterol, it is usually made with artery-damaging hydrogenated oils. Look instead for trans-fat-free margarine. (If the ingredients panel doesn't list trans fats, look for the words 'hydrogenated oils' or 'partially hydrogenated oils' instead.)

Butter & Spreads

Anchor Butter (Phases 1–4)
Trace carbs per 100g

Anchor Spreadable (Phases 1–4)
0.3g carbs per 100g

⚠ **Benecol**
0.2g carbs per 100g
Contains trans fats

⚠ **Bertolli with Olive Oil**
1g carbs per 100g
Contains trans fats

Clover (Phases 1–4)
0.9g carbs per 100g

Country Life English Butter (salted) (Phases 1–4)
Trace carbs per 100g

Country Life Spreadable (Phases 1–4)
0.5g carbs per 100g

Duchy Originals Organic Butter with Sea Salt (Phases 1–4)
Trace carbs per 100g

 I Can't Believe It's Not Butter
0.3g carbs per 100g
Contains trans fats

Kerrygold Pure Irish Butter (salted) (Phases 1–4)
Trace carbs per 100g

Kerrygold Pure Irish Butter Spreadable (Phases 1–4)
Trace carbs per 100g

Lurpak Butter (Phases 1–4)
0.8g carbs per 100g

Lurpak Butter (unsalted) (Phases 1–4)
0.8 carbs per 100g

Lurpak Lighter Spreadable (Phases 1–4)
0.5g carbs per 100g

Lurpak Spreadable (Phases 1–4)
0.75g carbs per 100g

 Original Flora
Trace carbs per 100g
Contains trans fats

President Unsalted French Butter (Phases 1–4)
Trace carbs per 100g

⚠ **St Ivel Gold Low Fat**
3.3g carbs per 100g
Contains trans fats

⚠ **Willow Traditionally Churned**
0.9g carbs per 100g
Contains trans fats

Yeo Valley Organic Butter (Phases 1–4)
Trace carbs per 100g

CHEESE

With so many different types of cheese available, it should be impossible to tire of the many varieties that you can choose from. Whether you enjoy slices of cheese with a salad or grated over steamed vegetables, it is a tasty, versatile ingredient. There are only a few points to remember. Steer clear of reduced-fat varieties and, unless you are pressed for time, avoid ready-sliced and grated cheeses as these often contain additives. After all, how long does it take to slice or shred a lump of cheese! Likewise, buy a pot of plain cottage cheese and stir in chopped chives, prawns or berries, which will certainly taste fresher than a shop-bought variety. Remember that you are allowed no more than 100g of cheese per day.

Boursin Ail & Fines Herbes (Phases 1–4)
2g carbs per 100g

Boursin with Crushed Pepper (Phases 1–4)
4.2g carbs per 100g

Boursin with Garlic and Herbs (Phases 1–4)
5g carbs per 100g

Brie (Phases 1–4)
0.9g carbs per 100g

Cambozola (Phases 1–4)
0.1g carbs per 100g

Camembert de Normandie (Phases 1–4)
Trace–0.2g carbs per 100g

**Cheddar (Mild, Medium, Mature, Extra
Mature) (Phases 1–4)**
0.1g carbs per 100g

**Cottage Cheese with Added Flavourings (e.g.
Onion, Chives, Vegetables) (Phases 2–4)**
3.7–8.3g carbs per 100g

Crème de Saint Agur (Phases 1–4)
2.3g carbs per 100g

Danish Blue (Phases 1–4)
0.7g carbs per 100g

Double Gloucester (Phases 1–4)
0.1g carbs per 100g

(FYI) **Edam (Phases 1–4)**
Trace carbs per 100g
Contains nitrates

Emmental (Phases 1–4)
0–0.5g carbs per 100g

Feta (Phases 1–4)
0.7g carbs per 100g

Goat's Cheese, Hard (Phases 1–4)
0.1g carbs per 100g

Goat's Cheese, Soft (Phases 1–4)
1–5g carbs per 100g

Goat's Cheese, Spreadable (Phases 1–4)
3.4g carbs per 100g

Gorgonzola (Phases 1–4)
0g carbs per 100g

(FYI) **Gouda (Phases 1–4)**
Trace carbs per 100g
Contains nitrates

Gruyère (Phases 1–4)
Trace–0.8g carbs per 100g

Halloumi (Phases 1–4)
2.5g carbs per 100g

(FYI) **Jarlsberg (Phases 1–4)**
0.1g carbs per 100g
Contains nitrates

Lancashire (Phases 1–4)
0.1g carbs per 100g

Leerdammer (Phases 1–4)
0g carbs per 100g

Manchego (Phases 1–4)
0.1g carbs per 100g

Mascarpone (Phases 1–4)
3.5–5.2g carbs per 100g

Mozzarella (Phases 1–4)
0.6–1.5g carbs per 100g

Mozzarella Bocconcini (Phases 1–4)
0.9–1.2g carbs per 100g

Parmigiano Reggiano (Phases 1–4)
0–0.1g carbs per 100g

Pecorino (Phases 1–4)
2g carbs per 100g

Quark (Phases 2–4)
4.1g carbs per 100g

Red Leicester (Phases 1–4)
0.1g carbs per 100g

Ricotta (Phases 2–4)
2.8–3.8g carbs per 100g

Roquefort (Phases 1–4)
Trace carbs per 100g

Saint Agur Blue (Phases 1–4)
0.2g carbs per 100g

Stilton, Blue (Phases 1–4)
0.1g carbs per 100g

Taleggio (Phases 1–4)
0g carbs per 100g

Wensleydale (Phases 1–4)
0.1g carbs per 100g

Yorkshire Blue (Phases 3–4)
9.3g carbs per 100g

Cheese Slices

Cathedral City Slices (Phases 1–4)
0.1g carbs per 100g

Cheddar Slices (Phases 1–4)
0.1 carbs per 100g

[FYI] Dairylea Thick Slices (Phases 3–4)
9.5g carbs per 100g
Contains modified starch

[FYI] Dairylea Thick Slices Light (Phases 3–4)
8.6g carbs per 100g
Contains modified starch

[FYI] Edam Slices (Phases 1–4)
1.5g carbs per 100g
Contains nitrates

[FYI] Kraft Singles (Phases 3–4)
7.6g carbs per 100g
Contains modified starch

Cheese Spreads

Dairylea Cheese Spread Triangles (Phases 2–4)
6g carbs per 100g

Primula Cheese & Shrimp Spread (Phases 1–4)
1.8g carbs per 100g

Primula Light Cheese Spread (Phases 2–4)
4.1g carbs per 100g

Primula Original Cheese Spread (Phases 2–4)
3.3g carbs per 100g

The Laughing Cow Cheese Spread Triangles (Phases 2–4)
6.5g carbs per 100g

The Laughing Cow Cheese Spread Triangles Light (Phases 2–4)
6.5g carbs per 100g

Grated Cheese

Grated cheese spoils more rapidly than do blocks of cheese; if properly wrapped, a block of cheese may keep for several months, but once you've opened a bag of grated cheese, you have only a week or so before it begins to deteriorate. Be aware that certain types of grated cheese often contain potato starch to help with texture.

(FYI) Cheddar, Extra Mature (Phases 3–4)
0.9–1.4g carbs per 100g
Contains potato starch

Edam (Phases 1–4)
1.5g carbs per 100g

Emmental (Phases 1–4)
0g carbs per 100g

Leerdammer (Phases 1–4)
1.6g carbs per 100g

FYI **Mozzarella (Phases 3–4)**
0.6g carbs per 100g
Contains potato starch

FYI **Own Brand Mozzarella and Mild Cheddar
(Phases 3–4)**
0.9–2.5g carbs per 100g
Contains potato starch

Miscellaneous

**Benecol Light Cream Cheese Style Spread
(Phases 2–4)**
3.8g carbs per 100g

**Heartily Healthy Proven to Reduce
Cholesterol Cheese Alternative (Phases 2–4)**
Trace carbs per 100g

**Kraft Philadelphia Extra Light Soft Cheese
(Phases 1–4)**
3g carbs per 100g

**Kraft Philadelphia Full Fat Soft Cheese
(Phases 2–4)**
3.2g carbs per 100g

**Kraft Philadelphia Light Soft Cheese
(Phases 2–4)**
3.5g carbs per 100g

Vegetarian Cheese

**The Redwood Co. Cheezly Lactose & Dairy
Free Cheddar Style (Phases 3–4)**
16.9g carbs per 100g

MILK, CREAM & MILK SUBSTITUTES

Milk is high in carbs and is not acceptable on the weight-loss phases of Atkins. If you do decide to use milk during the maintenance phases, opt for whole milk or controlled-carb dairy products rather than a lower-fat variety. The less fat that dairy products contain, the higher they are in carbohydrate. The same principle holds true for creams: whipping cream is lower in carbs than half-fat. On Atkins, you should always opt for the higher-fat or controlled-carbs choices.

Cow's Milk

Gold Top Jersey & Guernsey (Phases 3–4)
4.7g carbs per 100ml

⚠ **Organic Whole (Phases 3–4)**
4.8g carbs per 100ml

Whole (Phases 3–4)
4.7g carbs per 100ml

UHT Milk

Whole (Phases 3–4)
4.8g carbs per 100ml

Goat's Milk

Whole (Phase 3–4)
4.3g carbs per 100ml

Low-Carb Milk

Atkins Low-Carb Semi-Skimmed Milk (Phases 1–4) (COMING SOON)
2.5g Net Carbs per 100ml

Oat & Rice Milk

⚠ Oat Supreme
3.3g carbs per 100ml
Contains added sugars

⚠ Oatly Organic Oat Drink
⚠ 6.5g carbs per 100ml
Contains added sugars

⚠ Provamel Alpro Rice Organic
⚠ 9.9g carbs per 100ml
Contains organic rice syrup

ⓕⓨⓘ Rice Dream Original (Phases 3–4)
9.4g carbs per 100ml
Contains partially milled brown rice

ⓕⓨⓘ Rice Dream Original with Added Calcium (Phases 3–4)
9.4g carbs per 100ml
Contains partially milled brown rice

Soya Milk

Often touted as a healthy alternative to cow's milk, some brands of soya milk can contain twice the grams of carbs of cow's milk. Soya beans contain carbohydrate, and even though you won't often see 'sugar' or 'high-fructose corn syrup' in the ingredients list, the overwhelming majority of soya drinks are sweetened with barley syrup, rice syrup or cane juice. Look for the word 'unsweetened' on the label, or choose one with no more than 5 grams of carbs per 100ml.

Holland & Barrett Unsweetened Soya (Phases 1–4)
0.6g carbs per 100ml

 Provamel Alpro Chilled Soya
2.8g carbs per 100ml
Contains added sugars

 Provamel Alpro Soya Sweetened Organic
 UHT Soya
2.8g carbs per 100ml
Contains added sugars

 Provamel Alpro Soya Unsweetened Organic UHT Soya (Phases 1–4)
0.4g carbs per 100 ml

 Provamel Alpro Sweetened
 2.8g carbs per 100ml
Contains added sugars

Provamel Alpro Unsweetened (Phases 1–4)
2.8g carbs per 100ml

So Good Soya Chilled (Phases 2–4)
5.3g carbs per 100ml

So Good Soya Life (Phases 2–4)
5g carbs per 100ml

CREAM

Cream can slow down weight loss, so limit your intake of double cream to 50g a day. If you are on Induction and you're not progressing as quickly as you'd like, you may wish to avoid cream altogether and re-introduce it when you move into Ongoing Weight Loss.

You may have up to 50g of soured cream per day in place of full-fat cream during Induction. Crème fraîche is an aged, thickened cream with a tangy-nutty flavour and the texture of soured cream; it's terrific for adding creaminess to soups and sauces since it doesn't curdle.

Crème Fraîche

Own Brand Crème Fraîche (Phases 1–4)
2.8g carbs per 100g

Fresh Cream

Own Brand Clotted Cream (Phases 1–4)
2.2g carbs per 100ml

Own Brand Double Cream (Phases 1–4)
2.6–2.7g carbs per 100ml

Own Brand Extra Thick Double Cream (Phases 1–4)
2.6–2.7g carbs per 100ml

Own Brand Fresh Soured Cream (Phases 1–4)
3.9–4g carbs per 100ml

Own Brand Single Cream (Phases 1–4)
3.9–4.3g carbs per 100ml

Own Brand Whipping Cream (Phases 1–4)
3–3.1g carbs per 100ml

⚠ **Yeo Valley Organic Double Cream (Phases 1–4)**
2.8g carbs per 100ml

Yeo Valley Organic Really Thick Cream (Phases 1–4)
3.6g carbs per 100ml

Fromage Frais

Atkins Fromage Frais Peaches & Cream (Phases 2–4) (COMING SOON)
5g Net Carbs per serving

Atkins Fromage Frais Raspberries & Cream (Phases 2–4) (COMING SOON)
4g Net Carbs per serving

Atkins Fromage Frais Strawberries & Cream (Phases 2–4) (COMING SOON)
4.1g Net Carbs per serving

Own Brand Fromage Frais (Phases 1–4)
3.7–3.9g carbs per 100g

Processed Cream

⚠ Anchor Real Dairy Cream UHT
1.4g carbs per 100ml
Contains added sugars

⚠ Elmlea Double
3.9g per 100ml
Contains trans fats

⚠ Elmlea Single
4.6g carbs per 100ml
Contains trans fats

⚠ **Elmlea Whipping**
3.5g carbs per 100ml
Contains trans fats

Nestlé Extra Thick Cream (Phases 2–4)
3.6g carbs per 100ml

**Scottish Life Longlife Double Cream Ultra
Heat Treated (Phases 1–4)**
2.6g carbs per 100ml

**Scottish Life Longlife Single Cream Ultra Heat
Treated (Phases 2–4)**
3.9g carbs per 100ml

Cream Alternatives
Nestlé Carnation Light (Phases 3–4)
10.5g carbs per 100ml

⚠ **Nestlé Tip Top**
9g carbs per 100ml
Contains added sugars, trans fats and modified starch

YOGURT & SMOOTHIES

Yogurt is comparable to milk in grams of carbohydrate.
It's high in calcium, protein, vitamins and minerals, and
in moderation it can be a nutritious choice. But
flavoured yogurts are a different matter altogether: some
contain the equivalent of 4 tablespoons of sugar per 500g
pot, and it isn't unusual for fruit-flavoured yogurts to
contain 40 grams of carbs! Typical drinkable yogurts and
yogurt smoothies can contain up to 60 grams of carbs in
a standard bottle. Even sugar-free flavoured yogurts can
provide close to 20 grams of carbs.

Because fruit takes up space in a yogurt pot, fruit–flavoured yogurt contains less calcium. A 500g tub of plain yogurt contains nothing but yogurt, but a similar tub of the fruit-flavoured variety contains yogurt, sugar, fruit, corn syrup, cornflour, and a host of emulsifiers and enhancers. *Not* a very nutritious combination at all!

If you choose regular yogurt when you are doing later phases of Atkins, buy plain yogurt made with whole milk. Stir in berries and wheat germ for a little crunch.

Yogurt

FYI **Ann Forshaw's Diet Health Style Yogurt (Phases 3–4)**
9.2g carbs per 100g
Contains apple sweetener, cornflour and modified maize flour

⚠ **Benecol Low Fat Bio Flavoured Yogurt**
14.3–14.9g carbs per 100g
Contains added sugars

Danone Activia Low Fat Natural Bio Yogurt (Phases 3–4)
6.1g carbs per 100g

Danone Activia Natural Bio Yogurt (Phases 3–4)
6g carbs per 100g

⚠ **Müller Blueberry Fruit Corner**
15.5g carbs per 100g
Contains added sugars

Onken Natural Biopot Set Yogurt (Phases 3–4)
5.3g carbs per 100g

⚠ **Rachel's Organic Fat Free Bio-live Natural Yoghurt (Phases 3–4)**
4.8g carbs per 100g

⚠ **Rachel's Organic Greek Style Bio-live Natural Yoghurt (Phases 3–4)**
4.6g carbs per 100g

⚠ **Rachel's Organic Low Fat Bio-live Rhubarb**
⚠ **Yoghurt**
11g carbs per 100g
Contains added sugars

St Helen's Farm Bio Goatsmilk Yogurt Natural (Phases 3–4)
4.3g carbs per 100g

Total 0% Fat Free Greek Yoghurt (Phases 3–4)
4g carbs per 100g

Total Greek Yoghurt (Phases 3–4)
4g carbs per 100g

Total Sheeps' Yoghurt (Phases 3–4)
4.8g carbs per 100g

⚠ **Yeo Valley Organic Fat Free Natural Bio Live Yogurt (Phases 3–4)**
8.4g carbs per 100g

⚠ **Yeo Valley Organic Natural Bio Live Yogurt (Phases 3–4)**
6.6g carbs per 100g

Smoothies

⚠ **Benecol Yogurt Drink**
9.9g carbs per 70g pot
Contains added sugars

⚠ **Danone Actimel 0% Fat Original**
6.8g carbs per 100ml
Contains added sugars and aspartame

⚠ **Danone Actimel 0% Fat Pineapple**
5.5g carbs per 100ml
Contains added sugars and aspartame

⚠ **Danone Actimel Multifruit**
16g carbs per 100ml
Contains added sugars and modified starch

⚠ **Danone Actimel Orange**
15.9g carbs per 100ml
Contains added sugars

⚠ **Danone Actimel Original**
14.3g carbs per 100ml
Contains added sugars

⚠ **Danone Actimel Strawberry**
15.9g carbs per 100ml
Contains added sugars and modified starch

⚠ **Müller Vitality Probiotic Low Fat Raspberry
Yogurt Drink**
12.8g carbs per 100ml
Contains added sugars and modified starch

⚠ **Ocean Spray Plus Probiotic Cranberry & Raspberry Yogurt Drink**
15.2g carbs per 100ml
Contains added sugars

⚠ **PJ Smooothie Oranges, Mangoes & Bananas**
13.6g carbs per 100ml
Contains added sugars

⚠ **PJ Super Smooothie Daily Detox**
11.9g carbs per 100ml
Contains added sugars

⚠ **Yakult**
7.9g carbs per 65ml pot
Contains added sugars

⚠ **Yakult Light**
5.4g carbs per 65ml pot
Contains added sugars

⚠ **Yoplait Yop Strawberry Flavoured Yogurt Drink**
14g carbs per 100ml
Contains added sugars

JUICES

If you're hankering after the taste of fruit, always try to eat a piece of fruit rather than filling up on fruit juice. Whole fruit contains fibre, while the juice, more often than not, contains added sugars. If you must have juice, stick to tomato or grapefruit, or dilute juice with mineral water for a refreshing fruit-flavoured drink.

Atkins Apple & Cranberry Flavoured Drink (Phases 1–4)
1g Net Carbs per serving

Atkins Grapefruit & Lime Flavoured Drink (Phases 1–4)
1g Net Carbs per serving

Atkins Morning Shine™ Tropical Fruit Drink (Phases 3–4) (COMING SOON)
2g Net Carbs per serving

Copella Apple & Elderflower (Phases 3–4)
10.2g carbs per 100ml

Copella Apple & Mango (Phases 3–4)
10.1g carbs per 100ml

Copella Apple & Raspberry (Phases 3–4)
9.4g carbs per 100ml

Ocean Spray Cranberry & Blackcurrant Light (Phases 2–4)
5.7g carbs per 100ml

Ocean Spray Cranberry Classic Light (Phases 2–4)
5.5g carbs per 100ml

Ocean Spray Cranberry & Mango Light (Phases 3–4)
5.9g carbs per 100ml

⚠ **Ocean Spray Cranberry Select**
14.3g carbs per 100ml
Contains added sugars

Ocean Spray Orange & Cranberry (Phases 3–4)
11g carbs per 100ml

**Tropicana Pure Premium Fibre – 4 Fruits &
Carrot Juice (Phases 3–4)**
15.8g carbs per 100ml

**Tropicana Pure Premium Golden Grapefruit
(Phases 3–4)**
8g carbs per 100ml

**Tropicana Pure Premium Original Orange
(Phases 3–4)**
9g carbs per 100ml

**Tropicana Pure Premium Pink Grapefruit
Phases 3–4)**
8g carbs per 100ml

**Tropicana Pure Premium Purely Pineapple
(Phases 3–4)**
12.5g carbs per 100ml

EGGS

Eggs are a valuable source of protein, vitamins and
minerals. Most of the carbohydrate, cholesterol, fat and
fat-soluble vitamins are in the yolk; the white contains
the protein, water and most of the minerals.

Whether you choose hen's, duck's or quail's eggs,
they all have the same carb count. That goes for free
range, organic, barn and battery eggs too.

Eggs (Phases 1–4)
Trace–0.1g carbs per egg

Delicatessen

THE DELICATESSEN

The deli is one of the most popular departments in any supermarket, with the fresh counter usually boasting the longest queue. This should come as no surprise, because keeping a range of deli meats, fish, salads and dips in your fridge can be a fail-safe shortcut to producing a quick lunch or supper. But though you will find many Atkins-friendly foods both at the deli counter and in the chilled cabinets, there are also some dangers lurking among the enticing treats.

Note that we have used the FYI symbol **FYI** to draw your attention to foods in which you would not normally expect to find carbohydrates, such as cold fish and meat. While most of these foods should have a zero carb rating, because of the rules that dictate the way in which we report naturally occurring carbs we have to indicate the possible carb content. For further information, see Naturally Occurring Carbs on page 126 of the Listings Section introduction.

DELI FISH

Fish and seafood are both healthy and nutritious, and, with the exception of shellfish, are virtually carb-free. However, fish and seafood products from the deli counter are often combined with high-carb ingredients. 100g of sushi, for example, contains a massive 30g carbs in total, thanks to the white rice, which is unacceptable on Atkins. Seafood salads, prawn spring rolls, sweet and sour prawns and many other products are also high in carbs and can contain added sugars.

Smoked salmon is a lovely addition to any meal and with 0g carbs is perfect for Atkins. Gravadlax, however, while it may look similar, has been cured with sugar (as well as salt and dill) and is therefore unacceptable on any phase.

Read labels carefully (or ask the deli manager) and avoid any products cured in sugar, with added sugars or starches. When a product *may* contain such ingredients, we have not indicated that it is unacceptable, but we have alerted you with the FYI symbol **FYI** to the fact that you should proceed with caution.

Mackerel

FYI **Own Brand Peppered Mackerel Fillets (Phases 1–4)**
0.6–1.6g carbs per 100g

FYI **Own Brand Smoked Mackerel Fillets (Phases 1–4)**
0.3–0.7g carbs per 100g

Salmon

John West Mild Oak Smoked Salmon (Phases 1–4)
0.5g carbs per 100g

FYI **Own Brand Poached Salmon (Phases 1–4)**
Trace carbs per 100g
Some may contain maize starch

FYI **Own Brand Smoked Salmon (Phases 1–4)**
0.1–0.8g carbs per 100g
Some may contain trace added sugars

(FYI) Own Brand Smoked Salmon Parcels
1.2–3.5g carbs per 100g
Some may contain trace added sugars and
modified maize starch

Trout
**Own Brand Smoked Rainbow Trout Fillets
(Phases 1–4)**
0.1g carbs per 100g

**(FYI) Own Brand Smoked Rainbow Trout Slices
(Phases 1–4)**
0.1g carbs per 100g
Some may contain trace added sugars

⚠ RR Spink Arbroath Smoked Trout
0.1g carbs per 100g
Contains trace added sugars

Other Deli Fish
**Own Brand Marinated Anchovy Fillets
(Phases 1–4)**
2g carbs per 100g

⚠ Own Brand Marinated Seafood Salad
5.5g carbs per 100g
Contains added sugars

⚠ Own Brand Rollmop Herrings
17.3g carbs per 100g
Contains added sugars

⚠ **Own Brand Sushi Fish Selection Pack**
25.8–27.9g carbs per 100g
Contains added sugars, maize starch and wheat flour

Paté

FYI **Own Brand Crab Paté (Phases 3–4)**
5.5–5.9g carbs per 100g
Contains modified maize starch and wheat flour

⚠ **Own Brand Mackerel Paté**
0.6–1g carbs per 100g
Contains added sugars

⚠ **Own Brand Smoked Salmon Paté**
0.2–3.4g carbs per 100g
Contains added sugars and modified maize starch

⚠ **Own Brand Tuna Paté**
Trace–0.9g carbs per 100g
Contains added sugars and modified maize starch

COLD MEATS

Cold meats are always useful to have in your fridge, but you need to be discriminating while shopping. For a start, you should avoid pre-packed chilled meat because it tends to contain more preservatives, so opt instead for meats from the deli counter. Even then, you'll still have to be choosy.

Steer clear of honey-baked hams and sugar-cured meats and ask the counter assistant about the ingredients in marinated meats – chicken and turkey may be basted with a sauce that contains added sugars. Store-roasted pork, beef and turkey breast are sensible options, as they are free of additives and flavour enhancers such as MSG.

Cold cuts, smoked and cured meats can be high in nitrates, which the body converts to nitrites. These are potential carcinogens if consumed regularly and in excess; while small amounts are unlikely to be harmful, you should choose alternatives whenever possible.

MEATS & PATÉS

Cold Cuts

Atkins Gourmet Chargrilled Chicken Strips (Phases 1–4)
1g Net Carbs per serving

(FYI) Own Brand Carved Roast Beef (Phases 1–4)
0–0.4g carbs per 100g

(FYI) Own Brand Chicken Slices (Phases 1–4)
2.1g carbs per 100g
Some may contain added sugars and maize starch

(FYI) Own Brand Roast Chicken Fillet (Phases 1–4)
Trace–0.7g carbs per 100g
Some may contain trace added sugars

(FYI) Own Brand Roast Pork (Phases 1–4)
0.1–0.7g carbs per 100g
Some may contain nitrates

(FYI) Own Brand Sliced Chicken Breast (Phases 1–4)
0.1–0.5g carbs per 100g
Some may contain trace added sugars and nitrates

🕅 **Own Brand Sliced Corned Beef (Phases 1–4)**
Trace carbs per 100g
Some may contain trace added sugars

Own Brand Sliced Ham, Boneless (Phases 1–4)
0g carbs

🕅 **Own Brand Sliced Gammon (Phases 1–4)**
0.1g–0.2 carbs per 100g
Contains nitrates

Own Brand Sliced Luncheon Meat (Phases 1–4)
1g carbs per 100g serving

🕅 **Own Brand Sliced Turkey Breast (Phases 1–4)**
Trace–0.2g carbs per 100g
Some may contain trace added sugars

🕅 **Own Brand Turkey Slices (Phases 3–4)**
Trace– 1.3g carbs per 100g
Some may contain MSG and maize starch

Continental meats

🕅 **Own Brand Black Pudding (Phases 3–4)**
14.6–17.8g carbs per 100g
Contains nitrates and wheat flour

⚠ **Own Brand Bresaola**
0.1g carbs per 100g
Contains added sugars and nitrates

⚠ **Own Brand Garlic Sausage**
Trace–1.4g carbs per 5g slice, 0.7–1.4g carbs per 100g
Contains added sugars, nitrates and wheat flour

Own Brand Mortadella
Trace carbs per 13g slice, 0.1–1g carbs per 100g
Contains added sugars and nitrates

⚠ Own Brand Pancetta
Trace–0.1g carbs per 100g
Contains added sugars and nitrates

⚠ Own Brand Pepperoni
0.1–2.4g carbs per 100g
Contains added sugars and nitrates

⚠ Own Brand Prosciutto di Parma/di Speck – Parma Ham
Trace–1g carbs per 100g
Contains added sugars and nitrates

⚠ Own Brand Salt Beef
0.1–2.2g carbs per 100g
Contains added sugars and nitrates

⚠ Peperami Grab the HOT Meat Snack
0.6g carbs per 25g stick, 2.5g carbs per 100g
Contains added sugars, MSG and nitrates

⚠ Peperami Grab the SPICY Meat Snack
0.4g carbs per 25g stick, 1.7g carbs per 100g
Contains added sugars, MSG and nitrates

⚠ Rocking JC Original Flavour Beef Jerky
5.5g carbs per 28g serving, 19.4g carbs per 100g
Contains added sugars, MSG and nitrates

Paté

⚠ Own Brand Ardennes Paté
0.5–2.4g carbs per 100g
Contains added sugars, nitrates and wheat flour

⚠ Own Brand Brussels Paté
2.8–8.4g carbs per 100g
Contains added sugars and nitrates

⚠ Own Brand Chicken Liver Paté
1.9–6.4g carbs per 100g
Contains added sugars, nitrates and wheat flour

⚠ Own Brand Duck Paté
1.7–9.3g carbs per 100g
Contains added sugars and nitrates

⚠ Own Brand Duck & Orange Paté
3.0–3.9g carbs per 100g
Contains added sugars and nitrates

PREPARED SALADS

Always proceed with caution when selecting prepared salads, as many may be bulked out with potato or grains or with refined carbohydrates in the form of rice and regular pasta. All will be high in carbs, but those with potatoes or whole grains are acceptable in the maintenance phases (assuming they do not have added sugars in them), while the white rice and pasta are not suitable in any phase. Even salads that you might assume are fine – such as tuna, tomato and cucumber salad, as well as white fish salad and coleslaw – can contain hidden carbohydrates. There are many acceptable salads to choose from as long as you pay a little attention: Greek salad with delicious olives and feta cheese; grilled Mediterranean vegetables; crisp green salad with grilled chicken pieces and baby vegetables. Don't be afraid to ask the counter assistant about ingredients to ensure you're not getting too many carbs, or choose a self-serve salad bar and create your own salad bowl.

(FYI) Atkins Gourmet Chargrilled Chicken Salad (Phases 3–4)
3g Net Carbs per serving
Contains modified maize starch and nitrates

(FYI) Atkins Gourmet Chargrilled Chicken & Bacon Salad (Phases 3–4)
2g Net Carbs per serving
Contains modified maize starch and nitrates

(FYI) Atkins Gourmet Chicken & Bacon Wrap (Phases 3–4)
4g Net Carbs per serving
Contains modified maize starch and nitrates

(FYI) Atkins Gourmet Crayfish & Salsa Salad (Phases 3–4)
5g Net Carbs per serving
Contains modified maize starch

(FYI) Atkins Gourmet Prawn & Poached Salmon Salad (Phases 3–4)
1g Net Carbs per serving
Contains modified maize starch

FYI Atkins Gourmet Roast Chicken & Salad Wrap (Phases 3–4)
2g Net Carbs per serving
Contains modified maize starch

⚠ Own Brand Beetroot Salad
11.5–14.8g carbs per 100g
Contains added sugars

FYI Own Brand Coleslaw (Phases 3–4)
5.3–6.1g carbs per 100g
May contain added sugars and modified maize starch

⚠ Own Brand Couscous Salad
21.5–23.7g carbs per 100g
Contains added sugars and modified maize starch

FYI Own Brand Low Fat Coleslaw (Phases 3–4)
6.7–7.9g carbs per 100g
Some may contain added sugars and modified maize starch

Own Brand Marinated & Grilled Aubergines (Phases 1–4)
3g carbs per 100g

Own Brand Marinated Peppers (Phases 2–4)
5.4g carbs per 100g

Own Brand Marinated Sun Dried Tomatoes (Phases 3–4)
20g carbs per 100g

⚠ **Own Brand Potato Salad**
8.3–10.7g carbs per 100g
Contains added sugars and wheat flour

⚠ **Own Brand Three Bean Salad**
10.2–11.6g carbs per 100g
Contains added sugars

⚠ **Own Brand Waldorf Salad**
11.3–12.3g carbs per 100g
Contains added sugars

Fresh & Marinated Olives

Own Brand Green Olives (Phases 1–4)
0.1–0.6g carbs per 100g

Own Brand Italian Olives with Herbs (Phases 1–4)
Trace carbs per 100g

Own Brand Kalamata Olives (Phases 1–4)
1.9g carbs per 100g

Own Brand Olive Selection (Green, Black and Kalamata Olives) (Phases 2–4)
3.9–11.4g carbs per 100g

Own Brand Pitted Black Olives (Phases 1–4)
0.1g carbs per 100g

DIPS

Packaged dips can be full of sweeteners and partially hydrogenated vegetable oil, a form of manufactured trans fat, which means that those with such ingredients are never acceptable on any phase of Atkins. You'll get much more flavour and fewer additives if you buy sour cream and stir in your own seasonings.

Hummus, the Middle Eastern dip made of chickpeas and seasonings, is high in fibre and makes a tasty snack or light meal. Even better, it doesn't take too long to make from scratch – a tin of chickpeas, a heavy dash of sesame oil or tahini, a clove of garlic, a sprinkling of sea salt and freshly ground pepper blended together in a food processor takes only a few minutes and costs a fraction of the price of shop-bought hummus.

Other tasty, nutritious dips: Greek yogurt with a handful of freshly chopped mint and diced cucumber; avocado blended with lime juice and fresh coriander; crème fraîche with diced chilli and a teaspoon of harissa; natural yogurt, a teaspoon of curry paste, black pepper and ground coriander – quick, easy and cost-effective!

Flavoured dips

FYI Own Brand Guacamole (Phases 2–4)
3.2–5.1 carbs per 100g
Some may contain added sugars

⚠ Own Brand Sour Cream and Chives
5.4–5.6g carbs per 100g
Contains added sugars and modified maize starch

⚠ Pringles Cool Curry Dip
9.4g carbs per 100g
Contains added sugars, modified starch and wheat flour

⚠ **Pringles Sour Cream and Chive Dip**
5.6g carbs per 100g
Contains added sugars, modified starch and wheat
flour

Greek dips

Own Brand Houmous (Phases 3–4)
8.9–9.8g carbs per 100g

⚠ **Own Brand Organic Houmous (Phases 3–4)**
10.7g carbs per 100g

⚠ **Own Brand Taramasalata**
7.5–10.5g carbs per 100g
Contains added sugars and wheat flour

Own Brand Tzatziki (Phases 3–4)
3.7–4.9g carbs per 100g

Salsa

Own Brand Fresh Salsa (Phases 2–4)
5–7.8g carbs per 100g

⚠ **Doritos Extra Hot Salsa Dippas Dip**
8.5g carbs per 100g
Contains added sugars

⚠ **Doritos Hot Salsa Dippas Dip**
8.5g carbs per 100g
Contains added sugars

⚠ **Doritos Mild Indian Dippas Dip**
9g carbs per 100g
Contains added sugars

⚠ **Doritos Mild Salsa Dippas Dip**
8.5g carbs per 100g
Contains added sugars

⚠ **Doritos Sweet & Zesty Dippas Dip**
8g carbs per 100g
Contains added sugars

⚠ **Pringles Fiery Salsa Dip**
5.8g carbs per 100g
Contains added sugars and modified starch

⚠ **Pringles Salsa Heaven Dip**
6.2g carbs per 100g
Contains added sugars and modified starch

OTHER DELICATESSEN ITEMS

⚠ **Cauldron Organic Spicy Middle Eastern Falafel**
⚠ 5.8g carbs per falafel
Contains added sugars and wheat flour

FYI **Own Brand Falafel (Phases 3–4)**
23.3g carbs per 100g
Some may contain added sugars and wheat flour

FYI **Own Brand Onion Bhaji (Phases 3–4)**
7.8–13.6g carbs per bhaji, 22.2–29.2g carbs per 100g
Contains wheat flour

⚠ **Own Brand Pork Pie**
11.3–16.3g carbs per 50g pork pie, 22.6–32.6g carbs
per 100g
Contains added sugars, trans fats, nitrates and
wheat flour

⚠ **Own Brand Sausage Rolls**
6.9–8.8g carbs per roll, 21–26.7g carbs per 100g
Contains added sugars, trans fats and wheat flour

⚠ **Own Brand Scotch Eggs**
16–18g carbs per Scotch egg, 14.2–16g carbs per 100g
Contains added sugars, trans fats and wheat flour

⚠ **Own Brand Chicken Spring Rolls**
11.4g carbs per roll, 22.8g carbs per 100g
Contains added sugars and wheat flour

⚠ **Own Brand Duck Spring Rolls**
7.9g carbs per roll, 26.2g carbs per 100g
Contains added sugars, trans fats, maize starch and
wheat flour

⚠ **Own Brand Prawn Spring Rolls**
6.9g carbs per roll, 23g carbs per 100g
Contains added sugars and wheat flour

⚠ **Own Brand Vegetable Spring Rolls**
8.9–14g carbs per roll, 22.8–29.5g carbs per 100g
Contains added sugars, trans fats, cornflour,
modified maize starch and wheat flour

⚠ **Own Brand Vegetable Samosa**
12.3–20.4g carbs per samosa, 24.5–32.7g carbs per 100g
Contains added sugars, maize starch and wheat flour

Vegetarian paté

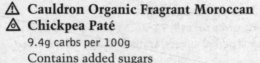

 Cauldron Organic Aromatic Herb & Soya Bean Paté (Phases 3–4)
14.1g carbs per 100g

⚠ **Cauldron Organic Fragrant Moroccan**
⚠ **Chickpea Paté**
9.4g carbs per 100g
Contains added sugars

⚠ **Cauldron Organic Soft & Creamy Mushroom Paté (Phases 2–4)**
4.3g carbs per 100g

⚠ **Cauldron Organic Spinach, Cheese & Crunchy Almond Paté (Phases 2–4)**
6.3g carbs per 100g

⚠ **Cauldron Organic Sweet Roasted Parsnip &**
⚠ **Carrot Paté**
9.8g carbs per 100g
Contains added sugars

⚠ **Own Brand Mushroom Paté**
4.8g–9.8g carbs per 100g
Contains added sugars, modified maize starch and wheat flour

Quorn Deli Farmhouse Style Paté (Phases 2–4)
7.8g carbs per 100g

Quorn Paté Brussels Style (Phases 2–4)
5.7g carbs per 100g

Delicious Meal Shortcuts from the Deli

Do you sometimes crave food that tastes like it's home-cooked but doesn't require the time or the fuss? Do you need a fast yet elegant hors d'oeuvre to kick off your supper party? These shortcuts, using items found at the deli counter, can help:

- **Spicy beef-wrapped asparagus:** Slather thinly sliced roast beef with a blend of horseradish and mayonnaise, then wrap around two lightly steamed asparagus spears. (Phases 1–4; 2g carbs)
- **Italian ham roll-ups:** Spread thinly sliced prosciutto with a tablespoon of garlicky hummus or a mixture of pesto and mayonnaise; roll up. (Phases 3–4; 2g carbs)
- **Speedy cannellini bean soup:** Take 250g of thickly sliced ham and cut into cubes. Make broth with 250ml of boiling water and an organic chicken stock cube. Add the ham and 50g of tinned cannellini beans. Simmer for 20 minutes. (Phases 3–4; 8.5g carbs)
- **Almost-instant chicken soup:** Make a chicken broth with 250ml of boiling water and an organic chicken stock cube. Shred a roast chicken breast and add to the broth. Add 25g of tinned organic green lentils and a handful of chopped fresh parsley and coriander. Simmer for 5 minutes. (Phases 3–4; 6g carbs)
- **Almost-instant Italian-inspired soup:** Combine 2 tablespoons tomato purée with chicken broth made from 250 ml of boiling water and an organic chicken stock cube. Add coarsely chopped salami,

55g of cubed mozzarella and a handful of slivered
basil. Heat to serving temperature. (Phases 1–4; 3g
carbs)

- **Zesty beef salad:** Cut thinly sliced roast beef into
strips. Toss with mixed salad greens, a handful of
mint and coriander leaves and your favourite low-
carb dressing. (Phases 1–4; 2g carbs)

- **Grilled chicken tossed salad:** Combine a sliced,
grilled chicken breast, mixed salad greens, 2
tablespoons of crumbled blue cheese and 2
tablespoons sliced almonds, toasted; toss with your
favourite low-carb salad dressing. (Phases 2–4; 3g
carbs)

- **Creamy curry chicken salad:** Remove the skin from
a roast chicken; pull the meat off the bone and
shred. In a large bowl, combine mayonnaise, curry
powder and thinly sliced spring onions. Add the
chicken and a few sliced water chestnuts. (Phases
2–4; 4g carbs)

Dried, Cooking and Preserves

A storecupboard with everyday basics is a must in any household, but especially important when you're doing Atkins. Having core ingredients within reach makes cooking and preparing meals on a day-to-day basis much easier, and if you run out of fresh produce you are less likely to snack on forbidden foods. However, extra vigilance must be used when examining nutritional labelling to ensure the foods that you're buying are acceptable.

DRIED LEGUMES, PASTA & VEGETABLES

It is always a good idea to keep your storecupboard stocked with a range of pulses, dried vegetables and legumes, as these are a perfect stand-by when fresh is not an option. As well as being highly nutritious, pulses, dried vegetables and legumes all have an extended shelf-life – so you can always be assured of cooking with healthy ingredients no matter how busy you are. Though many of these products are high in carbs, if you use them sparingly once you are in the maintenance phases, you can reap the benefits without exceeding your daily carb count.

All dried pasta is high in carbs. Avoid pasta made completely from white flour as it is unacceptable on any stage of Atkins and use whole-wheat varieties instead in the later phases of the ANA™. Don't forget that whole-wheat is still very high in carbs, so think carefully about your portion size. Instead, replace some of the pasta with added vegetables and protein, such as grilled chicken or tuna.

You should apply the same degree of caution to rice, noodles and grains; brown is always better than refined varieties, and choose buckwheat instead of rice-based noodles.

BEANS & LEGUMES (BY 50g COOKED WEIGHT)

Aduki Beans (Phases 3–4)
20g carbs per 50g cooked

Black Beans (Phases 3–4)
13g carbs per 50g cooked

Black-eyed Peas (Phases 3–4)
12.5g carbs per 50g cooked

Butter Beans (Phases 3–4)
13g carbs per 50g cooked

Cannellini Beans (White Kidney Beans) (Phases 3–4)
17g carbs per 50g cooked

Chickpeas (Phases 3–4)
16.5g carbs per 50g cooked

Fava Beans (Broad Beans) (Phases 3–4)
12g carbs per 50g cooked

Flageolet Beans (Phases 3–4)
8.2g carbs per 50g cooked

Haricots Blancs
4.7g carbs per 50g cooked

A Better Way with Beans

Beans and legumes are rich in fibre and nutrients but they're also high in carbs. When you're ready to add them back to your meal plans, use them sparingly and you'll reap the benefits without using up all your carbs. Here are some ideas:

- Scatter beans over a salad; use dark greens like rocket, watercress and cos lettuce and toss with sliced red peppers.
- Add 100g of puréed beans to a litre of soup to thicken it and give it a rich, creamy texture.
- Make your own dips, but don't just stop at hummus, which is made with chickpeas. Purée black beans with chilli powder and lime juice, or purée white beans with sage or rosemary and a splash of white wine vinegar. Serve alongside broccoli florets, strips of peppers, blanched cauliflower florets and cherry tomatoes.
- Stir small cooked beans into fresh salsa for a terrific topping for grilled fish.

Lentils (Phases 3–4)
12g carbs per 50g cooked

Mung Beans (Phases 3–4)
14g carbs 50g cooked

Pinto Beans (Phases 3–4)
14.5g carbs per 50g cooked

Red Kidney Beans (Phases 3–4)
14.5g carbs per 50g cooked

Soya Beans (Phases 3–4)
6.2g carbs per 50g cooked

Split Peas (Phases 3–4)
12.5g carbs per 50g cooked

NOODLES

Ⓕ**Ⓨ**Ⓘ **Ken Hom Microwave Noodles (Phases 3–4)**
8.25g carbs per 25g uncooked
Contains wheat flour

Ⓕ**Ⓨ**Ⓘ **Sanchi Organic Ramen Noodles (Phases 3–4)**
⚠ 3.4g carbs per 25g uncooked
Contains wheat flour

Ⓕ**Ⓨ**Ⓘ **Yaki Soba Noodles (Phases 3–4)**
8.7g carbs per 25g uncooked
Contains wheat flour

Ⓕ**Ⓨ**Ⓘ **Yaki Udon Noodles (Phases 3–4)**
6.7g carbs per 25g uncooked
Contains wheat flour

PASTA

Ⓕ**Ⓨ**Ⓘ **Glutano Wheat Free Spirals (Phases 3–4)**
20.2g carbs per 25g uncooked
Contains maize starch

FYI ItalFresco Gnocchi di Patate (Phases 3–4)
8.5g carbs per 25g uncooked
Contains wheat flour

FYI Organico Fusilli (Phases 3–4)
18.5g carbs per 25g uncooked
Contains wheat flour

FYI Organico Whole Wheat Spaghetti (Phases 3–4)
18.5g carbs per 25g uncooked
Contains wheat flour

⚠ Orgran Rice and Corn Pasta
19.6g carbs per 25g uncooked
Contains white rice

Orgran Rice and Millet Pasta (Phases 3–4)
19.2g carbs per 25g uncooked

Orgran Vegetable Rice Pasta (Phases 3–4)
20g carbs per 25g uncooked

FYI Seeds of Change Organic Semi-Wholewheat
⚠ Tortiglioni (Phases 3–4)
18.7g carbs per 25g uncooked
Contains wheat flour

RICE

⚠ Merchant Gourmet Organic Basmati Rice
 19.5g carbs per 25g uncooked
Contains white rice

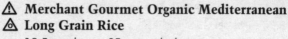

⚠ Merchant Gourmet Organic Mediterranean ⚠ Long Grain Rice
19.5g carbs per 25g uncooked
Contains white rice

⚠ Pataks Basmati Rice
18.5g carbs per 25g uncooked
Contains white rice

Rice, Brown (Phases 3–4)
20.5g carbs per 25g uncooked

DRIED VEGETABLES

Mushrooms

All mushrooms are acceptable on Induction. However, dried mushrooms can be high in carbs. In these instances, use them sparingly as a seasoning or your daily carb count will be too high.

Borde Girolles Mushrooms (Phases 1–4)
12.7g carbs per 25g

Borde Porcini Mushrooms (Phases 1–4)
7.8g carbs per 25g

Borde Shiitake Mushrooms (Phases 1–4)
14.1g carbs per 25g

Merchant Gourmet Mixed Mushrooms (Phases 1–4)
14.5g carbs per 25g

Merchant Gourmet Porcini Mushrooms (Phases 1–4)
1.25g carbs per 25g

 ### Unique Organic Porcini Mushrooms (Phases 1–4)
1.25g carbs per 25g

Whitworths Dried Sliced Mushrooms (Phases 1–4)
1.2g carbs per 25g

Onions

As with dried mushrooms, you need to pay attention to portion size. Because dried onions are high in carbs, it is easy to exceed your daily carb count unless you exercise caution.

Whitworths Dried Onions (Phases 3–4)
17.1g carbs per 25g

Peas

Batchelors Bigga Dried Peas (Phases 3–4)
9.4g carbs per 25g

Batchelors Quick Soak Dried Peas (Phases 3–4)
10.5g carbs per 25g

Whitworths Dried Marrowfat Peas (Phases 3–4)
12.5g carbs per 25g

Potatoes

⚠ **Smash Original Mashed Potatoes with Smoked Bacon/Cheddar & Onion/Fried Onion**

3.4–3.5 g carbs per 25g

Contains trans fats

Tomatoes

Merchant Gourmet Italian Sun Dried Tomatoes (Phases 2–4)

5.1g carbs per 25g

Merchant Gourmet Mi-Cuit Semi Dried Tomatoes Ready to Eat (Phases 2–4)

5.7g carbs per 25g

Mixed Vegetables

Whitworths Dried Mixed Country Vegetables (Phases 3–4)

22.1g carbs per 25g

ITALIAN SAUCES

Pasta is high in carbs and should be consumed in moderation when doing Atkins. Avoid white pasta and buy the whole-wheat variety instead; eat smaller portions, replacing some of the pasta you would have had in the past with appropriate vegetables and protein.

Be especially vigilant when checking ingredients labels on bottled and jarred sauces. Most contain added sugars and flour of some description.

BOLOGNESE SAUCE

 Dolmio Express Minced Beef Bolognese Original Sauce
7.1g carbs per 100g
Contains added sugars and modified maize starch

 Dolmio Extra Mushrooms Bolognese Sauce
8.4g carbs per 100g
Contains added sugars and modified maize starch

⚠ **Dolmio Extra Onion & Garlic Bolognese Sauce**
9g carbs per 100g
Contains added sugars and modified maize starch

⚠ **Dolmio Original Bolognese**
8.7g carbs per 100g
Contains added sugars and modified maize starch

⚠ **Dolmio Original Light Bolognese**
7.8g carbs per 100g
Contains added sugars and modified maize starch

⚠ **Knorr Ragu Traditional Bolognese Sauce**
5.8g carbs per 100g
Contains added sugars

⚠ **Loyd Grossman Bolognese Sauce**
10.2g carbs per 100g
Contains added sugars

OTHER PASTA SAUCES

⚠ **Bertolli Grilled Peppers & Chilli Oil Stir Through Pasta Sauce**
7.9g carbs per 100g
Contains added sugars

⚠ **Bertolli Grilled Vegetable Pasta Sauce (with Extra Virgin Olive Oil)**
8.7g carbs per 100g
Contains added sugars

⚠ **Bertolli Grilled Vegetables & Balsamic Vinegar Stir Through Pasta Sauce**
6.5g carbs per 100g
Contains added sugars

⚠ **Bertolli Sun Dried Tomato & Mascarpone Cheese Stir Through Pasta Sauce**
7.8g carbs per 100g
Contains added sugars

⚠ **Bertolli Tomato & Basil Pasta Sauce**
7.9g carbs per 100g
Contains added sugars

⚠ **Bertolli Tomato, Red Wine & Shallots Pasta Sauce with Extra Virgin Olive Oil**
7.2g carbs per 100g
Contains added sugars

⚠ **Bertolli Tomato, Romano & Garlic Pasta Sauce**
7.7g carbs per 100g
Contains added sugars

⚠ **Dolmio Express Rich Tomato with Basil Pesto Pasta Sauce**
6.2g carbs per 100g
Contains added sugars and modified maize starch

⚠ **Dolmio Express Spicy Italian Chilli Pasta Sauce**
7.5g carbs per 100g
Contains added sugars and modified maize starch

⚠ **Dolmio Express Tomato & Basil Pasta Sauce**
7.9g carbs per 100g
Contains added sugars and modified maize starch

⚠ **Dolmio Sun-Dried Tomato Pasta Bake Sauce**
10.4g carbs per 100g
Contains added sugars and modified maize starch

⚠ **Dolmio Tomato & Cheese Pasta Bake**
8.8g carbs per 100g
Contains added sugars and modified maize starch

⚠ **Go Organic Italian Tomato & Red Chilli Pasta**
⚠ **Sauce**
5g carbs per 100g
Contains added sugars

⚠ **Go Organic Italian Tomato & Sweet Basil**
⚠ **Pasta Sauce**
4.3g carbs per 100g
Contains added sugars

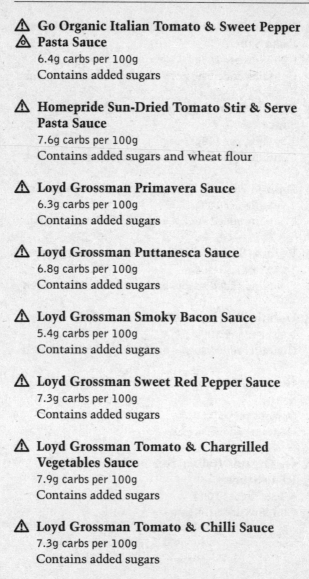

⚠ **Go Organic Italian Tomato & Sweet Pepper**
⚠ **Pasta Sauce**
   6.4g carbs per 100g
   Contains added sugars

⚠ **Homepride Sun-Dried Tomato Stir & Serve**
Pasta Sauce
   7.6g carbs per 100g
   Contains added sugars and wheat flour

⚠ **Loyd Grossman Primavera Sauce**
   6.3g carbs per 100g
   Contains added sugars

⚠ **Loyd Grossman Puttanesca Sauce**
   6.8g carbs per 100g
   Contains added sugars

⚠ **Loyd Grossman Smoky Bacon Sauce**
   5.4g carbs per 100g
   Contains added sugars

⚠ **Loyd Grossman Sweet Red Pepper Sauce**
   7.3g carbs per 100g
   Contains added sugars

⚠ **Loyd Grossman Tomato & Chargrilled**
Vegetables Sauce
   7.9g carbs per 100g
   Contains added sugars

⚠ **Loyd Grossman Tomato & Chilli Sauce**
   7.3g carbs per 100g
   Contains added sugars

Loyd Grossman Tomato & Spring Herbs Sauce
8.4 carbs per 100g
Contains added sugars

 Loyd Grossman Tomato & Wild Mushroom Sauce
7.4g carbs per 100g
Contains added sugars

 Sacla' Italia Olive & Tomato Stir Through
3.3g carbs per 100g
Contains added sugars

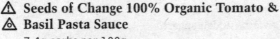 **Seeds of Change 100% Organic Tomato & Basil Pasta Sauce**
7.4g carbs per 100g
Contains added sugars

PESTO SAUCE

Bertolli Pesto (Phases 2–4)
4.4g carbs per 100g

Bertolli Pesto Rosso (Phases 2–4)
9.5g carbs per 100g

 Cirio Basilico
8.0g carbs per 100g
Contains added sugars

 Sacla' Italia Black Olive Pesto
1.9g carbs per 100g
Contains added sugars

Sacla' Italia Chargrilled Aubergine Pesto (Phases 1–4)
3.8g carbs per 100g

⚠ **Sacla' Italia Classic Pesto**
4.2g carbs per 100g
Contains added sugars

Sacla' Italia Sun-Dried Tomato Pesto (Phases 2–4)
5.2g carbs per 100g

⚠ **Sacla' Italia Organic Tomato Pesto**
 4.3g carbs per 100g
Contains added sugars

Sacla' Italia Wild Rocket Pesto (Phases 2–4)
3.2g carbs per 100g

BAKING

When you're doing Atkins, you should pay as much attention to the products you select as you do to how you cook them. In order to create delicious low-carb desserts and snacks, you'll have to look out for appropriate ingredients and low-carb products that can make the task easier and the result tastier. Some things, like unsweetened cocoa powder and soya flour, are naturally low in carbohydrate; others may be specially formulated items, such as Atkins™ Quick Quisine™ Bake Mix.

High in carbs, white flour is unacceptable on Atkins because the refining process strips it of virtually all its nutrients. Look for less processed whole-grain flours, but remember – whole grains are not low in carbs, and they must be saved for the maintenance phases of Atkins.

Sugar, whether it's white, brown, organic or in the form of a so-called healthy sweetener such as honey or molasses, should also be avoided no matter what phase of Atkins you are in. Sugar will do nothing but help you pile on the pounds and contribute to dental problems. Splenda®, a natural sugar substitute, is the Atkins sweetener of choice for baking with excellent results.

Splenda® Sweetener (Phases 1–4)
0.5g Net Carbs per teaspoon

EVAPORATED MILK

Evaporated milk has 60 per cent less water than regular milk. It can be used in recipes straight from the can, but if you're using it instead of regular milk it must be combined with an equal amount of water. There are two important things to remember when using evaporated milk. First, avoid low-fat and fat-free varieties; the evaporated milk made from whole milk has less naturally occurring sugar. Second, read the label *carefully* and be sure to choose evaporated – not sweetened condensed – milk. Still, milk is not acceptable until the maintenance phases of Atkins. A better bet is to use cream thinned with water, or a lactose-reduced dairy beverage.

Carnation Evaporated Milk (Phases 3–4)
1.8g carbs per 15ml

COOKING SPREADS

When you are baking while doing Atkins, you are
better avoiding the traditional cooking fats because
they contain trans fats. Use butter instead.

⚠ Cookeen Refined Vegetable Fat
0g carbs per 100g
Contains trans fats

⚠ Stork
0g carbs per 100g
Contains trans fats

⚠ Trex Pure Vegetable Fat
0g carbs per 100g
Contains trans fats

FLOUR

If you're looking for a flour to add crunch or stability to
a food before sautéing, substitute soya flour or Atkins
Quick Quisine™ Bake Mix. Note that these cannot be
used to replace regular flour in most baking recipes –
wheat flour contains gluten, which provides structure
to baked goods.

Gluten is a form of protein that is contained in
varying quantities and qualities in wheat, rye, barley
and oats. As rice and soya flour are gluten-free, strength
needs to be added when baking to prevent crumbling
and to improve the texture. You can use whey protein,
available in powder form from health food shops
(always look for unflavoured varieties), or xanthan.

Xanthan is a vegetable gum which is also useful for
thickening gravy, soups, sauces, etc. As it's classed as a

fibre rather than a starch, it has a minimal impact on blood sugar and is therefore ideal for use on any stage of Atkins.

Use the following quantities for best results:

- Bread – 1 teaspoon per 100g flour
- Cakes – ½ teaspoon per 100g flour
- Pizza bases – 2 teaspoons per 100g flour

Conventional cornflour, also referred to as cornstarch or maize starch, is off-limits on Atkins.

CAKE MIXES

Jenny Warden's CarboPhobia Luxury Coconut Cake Mix (Phases 2–4)
7g net carbs per 100g made as directed with eggs and butter

Jenny Warden's CarboPhobia Luxury Dark Chocolate Cake Mix (Phases 1–4)
3.6g net carbs per 100g made as directed with eggs and butter

Jenny Warden's CarboPhobia Luxury Lemon Cake Mix
3.8g net carbs per 100g made as directed with eggs and butter

FLOUR & BAKE MIXES

Atkins Quick Quisine™ Bake Mix
2.7g carbs per 25g

Biochem Ultimate Lo Carb Whey Powder (Phases 1–4)
1g carbs per 25g

⚠ **Dove's Farm Gluten Free Breadmachine Bread Flour (Phases 3–4)**
20g carbs per 25g

⚠ **Dove's Farm Organic Malthouse Flour (Phases 3–4)**
16g carbs per 25g

⚠ **Dove's Farm Organic Rice Flour (Phases 3–4)**
20g carbs per 25g

⚠ **Dove's Farm Organic Rye Flour (Phases 3–4)**
17g carbs per 25g

Nature's Store Soya Flour (Phases 1–4)
3.9g carbs per 25g

Powerhealth Wheyprotein (Phases 1–4)
Trace carbs per 25g

⚠ **Simple Chef Bake Mix**
4.75g carbs per 25g
Contains added sugars

RAISING AGENTS

Allinson's Active Dry Yeast (Phases 1–4)
0g carbs per ¼ teaspoon

Baking Powder, most brands (Phases 1–4)
0–1g carbs per teaspoon

COCOA POWDER

Cadbury's Cocoa (Phases 1–4)
10.5g carbs per 100g dry powder

⚠️ **Cadbury's Drinking Chocolate**
22.5g carbs per 18g serving (made with 200ml whole milk)
Contains added sugars

⚠️ **Green & Black's Organic Cocoa (Phases 1–4)**
1.7g carbs per teaspoon

⚠️ **Green & Black's Organic Hot Chocolate**
 16g carbs per 4 teaspoon serving
Contains added sugars

Flavouring Facts

Spices, extracts and seasonings are an excellent way to enhance flavour without adding a lot of carbs. Most spices and extracts provide 0 grams of carbs per serving. Cinnamon, for instance, has only 0.6 grams per teaspoon – the amount you often find per recipe, not per serving.

When it comes to extracts, opt for pure extracts, not artificial ones. You'll be astonished at the difference pure vanilla and pure almond extracts make, compared with their artificial counterparts.

DRIED FRUIT

If you think of dried fruit as a snack, it's time to change your attitude. When fruit is dried, the sugars become concentrated, so it's easy for the carbs to add up after just a few tablespoons of super-sweet morsels. Use dried fruit to add just a touch of fruity flavour to foods by sprinkling a few pieces on low-carb cereal, salads or main dishes. Despite its inherent sweetness, some brands of dried fruit also contain added sugars, which you want to avoid. Moreover, many major brands of dried fruits have been treated with sulphur dioxide, a preservative. Since some people experience an allergic reaction to it, look for those that don't list it in the ingredients.

When it comes to coconut, avoid sweetened flakes and look for the unsweetened variety, which has a fraction of the carbs and is acceptable in all four phases of Atkins. Health food shops or gourmet stores are a good source for finding unsweetened shredded or grated coconut – it's delicious when whirled into a low-carb shake.

Apricots

Humdinger Dried Chopped Apricots (Phases 3–4)
14.3g carbs per 25g serving

Sundora Mini Apricots (Phases 3–4)
9g carbs per 25g serving

Compotes & Jellies

⚠ Del Monte Fruitini, Strawberry Jelly with Peach Pieces
18.4g carbs per 120g pot
Contains added sugars

⚠ Hartley's Chunky Fruit Compote, Apple & Summer Fruit
14.7g carbs per 95g pot
Contains added sugars

⚠ Hartley's Smooth Fruit Compote
14g carbs per 90g pouch
Contains added sugars

Currants, Sultanas & Raisins

⚠ Crazy Jack Organic Sultanas (Phases 3–4)
17.3g carbs per 25g serving

⚠ Crazy Jack Organic Sun-Dried Raisins (Phases 3–4)
17.2g carbs per 25g serving

Mixed Raisins (Phases 3–4)
21.4g carbs per 30g bag

Own Brand Currants (Phases 3–4)
17g carbs per 25g serving

Own Brand Raisins (Phases 3–4)
16–18g carbs per 25g serving

Raisins & Apricots (Phases 3–4)
18.2g carbs per 30g bag

Whitworths Luxury Dried Mixed Fruit
16.3g carbs per 25g serving
Contains added sugars

Dates

Humdinger Dried Stone-out Dates (Phases 3–4)
18g carbs per 25g serving

 Whitworths Chopped Dates
17.2g carbs per 25g serving
Contains added sugars

 Whitworths Chopped Dates and Walnuts
14g carbs per 25g serving
Contains added sugars

Fruit Flakes

 Fruit Bowl Fruit Flakes, Blackcurrant
19.9g carbs per 25g serving
Contains added sugars

 Fruit Bowl Fruit Flakes, Strawberry
19.9g carbs per 25g serving
Contains added sugars

 **Fruit Bowl Fruit Flakes, Strawberry with
Yoghurt Coating**
18.2g carbs per 25g serving
Contains added sugars and trans fats

 Fruit Bowl Fruit Flakes, Tropical
20g carbs per 25g serving
Contains added sugars

Mixed

Del Monte Fruit Express No Added Sugar Peach & Pear Pieces in Fruit Juice (Phases 3–4)
20g carbs per 185g pot

Del Monte Fruit Express No Added Sugar Tropical Mixed Fruit in Juice (Phases 3–4)
20.7g carbs per 185g pot

Del Monte Fruit in Juice, Mixed Fruit Pieces in Fruit Juice (Phases 3–4)
14.4 carbs per 120g pot

Whitworths Dried Fruit Salad (Phases 3–4)
10g carbs per 25g serving

Others

⚠ **Fruit Bowl School Bars, Strawberry**
16.6g carbs per 20g serving
Contains added sugars

⚠ **Humdinger Stem Ginger**
21g carbs per 25g serving
Contains added sugar

Own Brand Desiccated Coconut (Phases 1–4)
1.6g carbs per 25g serving

⚠ **Sundora Apple Slices**
13.6g carbs per 25g serving
Contains added sugars

⚠ **Sundora Mini Pineapple Pieces**
22.2g carbs per 25g serving
Contains added sugars

Sundora Mini Prunes (Phases 3–4)
8.5g carbs per 25g serving

⚠ **Whitworths Honey Coated Banana Chips**
15g carbs per 25g serving
Contains added sugars

NUTS

⚠ **Crazy Jack Organic Brazil Nuts (Phases 2–4)**
1.8g carbs per 25g serving

Own Brand Flaked Almonds (Phases 2–4)
1.8g carbs per 25g serving

Own Brand Whole Almonds (Phases 2–4)
1.6g carbs per 25g serving

**Own Brand Whole Blanched Hazelnuts
(Phases 2–4)**
1.5g carbs per 25g serving

Own Brand Pine Nuts (Phases 2–4)
1g carbs per 25g serving

Own Brand Walnuts (Phases 2–4)
Trace carbs per 25g serving

PRESERVES, NUT BUTTERS & SPREADS

Even dedicated low-carb lifestylers want a little treat from time to time and a spoonful of fruit jam, marmalade or a nut butter can often do the trick. Fortunately there are some brands that are acceptable on Atkins, but even when a product is labelled 'sugar-free', you still need to scrutinize the ingredient label carefully. It may not have added *refined* sugar (sucrose) but it may well contain other forms of added sugar, such as fructose, which will make it unacceptable. A good guideline is to look for diabetic jams and marmalades. Marmite and Vegemite are acceptable from day one on Atkins.

When it comes to nut butters, natural is better. Nut butters are rich in protein, fibre and essential fatty acids, but many commercial brands may contain trans fats or fructose and other sweeteners. However, most of the organic brands contain none of these ingredients and are perfectly acceptable on Atkins.

JAMS

Apricot

⚠ **Meridian Apricot Spread**
5.4g carbs per 15g serving
Contains added sugars

⚠ **Own Brand Reduced Sugar Apricot Jam**
6.7–7.1g carbs per 15g serving
Contains added sugars

Streamline Reduced Sugar Apricot Jam with Extra Fruit
7.2g carbs per 15g serving
Contains added sugars

Black Cherry

 St Dalfour Black Cherry High Fruit Content Spread – No Added Sugar
8.4g carbs per 15g serving
Contains added sugars

Blackcurrant

 Own Brand Reduced Sugar Blackcurrant Jam
6.7g–7.1g carbs per 15g serving
Contains added sugars

 Streamline Reduced Sugar Blackcurrant Jam with Extra Fruit
7.2g carbs per 15g serving
Contains added sugars

FYI **Weight Watchers from Heinz Blackcurrant Spread (Phases 2–4)**
3.9g carbs per 15g serving
Contains aspartame

Morello Cherry

Stute Diabetic Morello Cherry Jam (Phases 3–4)
0.8g carbs per 15g serving

Raspberry

Stute Diabetic Raspberry Jelly (Phases 2–4)
0.3g carbs per 15g serving

(FYI) **Weight Watchers from Heinz Raspberry Spread (Phases 2–4)**
4.1g carbs per 15g serving
Contains aspartame

Rhubarb and Ginger
⚠ **Baxters Extra Fruit Reduced Sugar Rhubarb and Ginger Jam**
8g carbs per 15g serving
Contains added sugars

Strawberry
⚠ **Baxters Extra Fruit Reduced Sugar Strawberry Jam**
8g carbs per 15g serving
Contains added sugars

⚠ **Meridian Strawberry Spread – No Added Sugar**
5.5g carbs per 15g serving
Contains added sugars

⚠ **Own Brand Reduced Sugar Strawberry Jam**
6.7–7.1g carbs per 15g serving
Contains added sugars

⚠ **St Dalfour Strawberry High Fruit Content Spread – No Added Sugar**
8.4g carbs per 15g serving
Contains added sugars

⚠ **Streamline Reduced Sugar Strawberry Jam**
7.2g carbs per 15g serving
Contains added sugars

Stute Diabetic Strawberry Extra Jam (Phases 2–4)
8.5g carbs per 15g serving

⚠ Weight Watchers from Heinz Strawberry Spread
4.3g carbs per 15g serving
Contains added sugars and aspartame

Wild Blueberry

⚠ Meridian Wild Blueberry Spread
5.5g carbs per 15g serving
Contains added sugars

MARMALADE

⚠ Streamline Reduced Sugar Diced Cut Orange Marmalade
7.2g carbs per 15g serving
Contains added sugars

⚠ Streamline Reduced Sugar Thin Cut Orange Marmalade
7.2g carbs per 15g serving
Contains added sugars

Stute Fine Cut Diabetic Orange Extra Marmalade (Phases 3–4)
8.6g carbs per 15g serving

PEANUT BUTTER

Crunchy

⚠ **Sun-Pat Crunchy**
2.2g carbs per 15g serving
Contains added sugars

⚠ **Own Brand Crunchy Peanut Butter**
1.8g–1.9g carbs per 15g serving
Contains added sugars

⚠ **Whole Earth Organic Peanut Butter – Crunchy No Added Sugar (Phases 2–4)**
1.5g carbs per 15g serving

Smooth

⚠ **Sun-Pat Smooth**
2.2g carbs per 15g serving
Contains added sugars

Whole Earth Non-Organic Original Style Crunchy Peanut Butter – No Added Sugar (Phases 2–4)
1.5g carbs per 15g serving

⚠ **Whole Earth Organic Peanut Butter – Smooth No Added Sugar (Phases 2–4)**
1.5g carbs per 15g serving

OTHER NUT BUTTERS

Meridian Brazil Nut Butter (Phases 2–4)
3.4g carbs per 15g serving

Meridian Cashew Nut Butter (Phases 2–4)
2.6g carbs per 15g serving

Meridian Hazelnut Nut Butter (Phases 2–4)
0.8g carbs per 15g serving

Wallaby Natural Australian Macadamia Nut Spread (Phases 2–4)
1.5g carbs per 15g serving

SPREADS

Marmite (Phases 1–4)
0.8g carbs per 4g serving

Vegemite (Phases 1–4)
0.8g carbs per 4g serving

Chocolate Spread
⚠ Nutella
1g carbs per 15g serving
Contains added sugars

Drinks

NON-ALCOHOLIC DRINKS

When it comes to losing and later maintaining weight, what you drink can make a big difference to your success. Fluids can help curb your appetite by filling you up, and if what's in your glass is water, soda water or another non-caloric drink you won't add carbs. But if you consume sugary and sports drinks, sweetened elixirs or teas sweetened with some form of sugar, you could be heading for trouble. In addition to watching out for carbs, you should also limit your consumption of coffee, tea or other caffeinated soft drinks because they have a dehydrating effect and can impact blood sugars when consumed in excess. If you are not sensitive to the effects of caffeine, you can probably consume up to two cups a day.

When doing Atkins, you should drink at least eight (225ml) glasses of water per day. Water is vital for proper cell function and helps to prevent constipation, and, because you've probably increased your fibre intake since you began doing Atkins, drinking those eight glasses of water is even more critical. You can choose tap, mineral or spring water, but if you choose carbonated water be aware that the bubbles can fill you up and prevent you from getting all eight glasses. Try one of the new flavoured still waters – they're terrific for satisfying a juice craving – but make sure it's unsweetened or sweetened with Splenda® rather than sugar.

Hot drinks can also curb your appetite. Studies have shown that people who begin a meal with soup

eat less, so try a hot broth or drink a cup of unsweetened herbal tea as you prepare dinner. Just remember
to add whatever you drink to your daily carb count.

HOT DRINKS

Because many hot drink sachets contain milk they're
not permitted during Induction. (Many also contain
aspartame.) If you're craving something warm, have
decaffeinated coffee, tea or unsweetened cocoa made
with cream and sweetener. In the maintenance phases,
don't forget to add in carbs from the milk when making
cocoa.

Caffeinated or Decaffeinated Black Tea (Phases 1–4)
0g carbs per cup

Caffeinated or Decaffeinated Coffee (Phases 1–4)
0g carbs per cup

Cadbury's Cocoa (Phases 3–4)
9.9g carbs per 4g serving

⚠ Cadbury's Drinking Chocolate
22.5g carbs per 18g serving
Contains added sugars

⚠ Green & Black's Organic Cocoa (Phases 1–4)
1.7g carbs per teaspoon

⚠ Green & Black's Organic Hot Chocolate
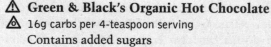
⚠ 16g carbs per 4-teaspoon serving
Contains added sugars

Herbal Tea (Phases 1–4)
0g carbs per cup

MILK & SOYA MILK

Only whole milk or controlled-carb is permitted when doing Atkins, and only after you have moved into the maintenance phases. If you prefer soya milk, you still need to exercise caution because a good deal of soya milk, even when not flavoured, is sweetened. Some sweetened soya milks have more than nine times the grams of carbs of unsweetened versions! Choose brands that have no added sugars and check the nutritional facts panels on products before you buy, since some are lower in carbs than others.

Cow's Milk

Gold Top Jersey & Guernsey (Phases 3–4)
4.7g carbs per 100ml

⚠ Organic Whole (Phases 3–4)
4.8g carbs per 100ml

Whole (Phases 3–4)
4.7g carbs per 100ml

UHT Milk

Whole (Phases 3–4)
4.8g carbs per 100ml

Goat's Milk

Whole (Phase 3–4)
4.3g carbs per 100ml

Low-Carb Milk

Atkins Low-Carb Semi-Skimmed Milk (Phases 1–4) (COMING SOON)
2g Net Carbs per 100ml

Oat & Rice Milk

⚠ Oat Supreme
3.3g carbs per 100ml
Contains added sugars

⚠ Oatly Organic Oat Drink
 6.5g carbs per 100ml
Contains added sugars

⚠ Provamel Alpro Rice Organic
⚠ 9.9g carbs per 100ml
Contains organic rice syrup

(FYI) Rice Dream Original (Phases 3–4)
9.4g carbs per 100ml
Contains partially milled brown rice

(FYI) Rice Dream Original with Added Calcium (Phases 3–4)
9.4g carbs per 100ml
Contains partially milled brown rice

Soya Milk

Holland & Barrett Unsweetened Soya (Phases 1–4)
0.6g carbs per 100ml

⚠ **Provamel Alpro Chilled Soya**
2.8g carbs per 100ml
Contains added sugars

⚠ **Provamel Alpro Soya Sweetened Organic UHT Soya**
2.8g carbs per 100ml
Contains added sugars

⚠ **Provamel Alpro Soya Unsweetened Organic UHT Soya (Phases 1–4)**
0.4g carbs per 100 ml

⚠ **Provamel Alpro Sweetened**
2.8g carbs per 100ml
Contains added sugars

Provamel Alpro Unsweetened (Phases 1–4)
2.8g carbs per 100ml

So Good Soya Chilled (Phases 2–4)
5.3g carbs per 100ml

So Good Soya Life (Phases 2–4)
5g carbs per 100ml

Flavoured Milks

Most flavoured milks are a no-go area while on Atkins
because, though they may come within acceptable carb
limits, they contain added sugars.

Atkins Advantage Ready-to-Drink Shake Chocolate Flavour (Phases 1–4)
2g Net Carbs per serving

**Atkins Advantage Ready-to-Drink Shake
Strawberry Flavour (Phases 1–4)**
2g Net Carbs per serving

**Atkins Advantage Ready-to-Drink Shake
Vanilla Flavour (Phases 1–4)**
2g Net Carbs per serving

⚠ **Café Met Choc'o'latte Milk Drink**
10g carbs per 100ml
Contains added sugars

⚠ **Café Met Mochalatte Milk Drink**
9g carbs per 100ml
Contains added sugars

⚠ **Campina Mild & Fruity Strawberry**
13.1g carbs per 100ml
Contains added sugars

⚠ **Campina Yazoo Chocolate Flavour Milkshake**
11.8g carbs per 100ml
Contains added sugars

⚠ **Campina Yazoo UHT Strawberry Flavour
Milk Drink**
10.3g carbs per 100ml
Contains added sugars

⚠ **Campina Yazoo UHT Strawberry Flavour
Milkshake**
10.3g carbs per 100ml
Contains added sugars

⚠ **Frijj Fresh Thick Banana Flavour Milkshake**
10.1g carbs per 100ml
Contains added sugars and modified maize starch

⚠ **Frijj Fresh Thick Strawberry Flavour Milkshake**
10.1g carbs per 100ml
Contains added sugars and modified maize starch

⚠ **Frijj Fresh Thick Vanilla Flavour Milkshake**
10.7g carbs per 100ml
Contains added sugars and modified maize starch

⚠ **Müller Froot**
14g carbs per 100ml
Contains added sugars and modified maize starch

⚠ **Provamel Alpro Soya Dairy Free Chocolate Flavour**
10.7g carbs per 100ml
Contains added sugars

⚠ **Rice Dream Vanilla Made from Partially Milled Brown Rice**
10.3g carbs per 100ml
Contains added sugars

⚠ **Yoplait Yop Strawberry Flavoured Yogurt Drink**
14g carbs per 100ml
Contains added sugars

Shake Mixes

Atkins Advantage Shake Mix Chocolate Flavour (Phases 1–4)
2g Net Carbs per serving

Atkins Advantage Shake Mix Strawberry Flavour (Phases 1–4)
3g Net Carbs per serving

Atkins Advantage Shake Mix Vanilla Flavour (Phases 1–4)
3g Net Carbs per serving

Biochem Ultimate Lo Carb Whey Powder Natural Flavour (Phases 1–4)
1g Net Carbs per serving

⚠ Carb Solutions High Protein Shake Mix Creamy Vanilla
3g Net Carbs per serving
Contains added sugars and trans fats

⚠ Carb Solutions High Protein Shake Mix Rich Chocolate
4g Net Carbs per serving
Contains added sugars and trans fats

Smoothies & Probiotic Drinks

Most regular smoothies and drinkable yogurts contain as many as 60 grams of carbs per 300ml bottle – a far cry from the healthy products they're touted to be. Instead, whip up smoothies at home with fresh fruit, tofu and Splenda®.

⚠ **Benecol Yogurt Drink**
9.9g carbs per 70g pot
Contains added sugars

⚠ **Danone Actimel 0% Fat Original**
6.8g carbs per 100ml
Contains added sugars and aspartame

⚠ **Danone Actimel 0% Fat Pineapple**
5.5g carbs per 100ml
Contains added sugars and aspartame

⚠ **Danone Actimel Multifruit**
16g carbs per 100ml
Contains added sugars and modified starch

⚠ **Danone Actimel Orange**
15.9g carbs per 100ml
Contains added sugars

⚠ **Danone Actimel Original**
14.3g carbs per 100ml
Contains added sugars

⚠ **Danone Actimel Strawberry**
15.9g carbs per 100ml
Contains added sugars and modified starch

⚠ **Müller Vitality Probiotic Low Fat Raspberry Yogurt Drink**
12.8g carbs per 100ml
Contains added sugars and modified starch

⚠ **Ocean Spray Plus Probiotic Cranberry & Raspberry Yogurt Drink**
15.2g carbs per 100ml
Contains added sugars

⚠ **PJ Smooothie Oranges, Mangoes & Bananas**
13.6g carbs per 100ml
Contains added sugars

⚠ **PJ Super Smooothie Daily Detox**
11.9g carbs per 100ml
Contains added sugars

⚠ **Yakult**
7.9g carbs per 65ml pot
Contains added sugars

⚠ **Yakult Light**
5.4g carbs per 65ml pot
Contains added sugars

⚠ **Yoplait Yop Strawberry Flavoured Yogurt Drink**
14g carbs per 100ml
Contains added sugars

JUICES

Juice contains all the carbohydrate of a fruit (sometimes more, if it has added sugars) but none of the fibre. Eat the whole fruit instead of pouring a glass of juice and you'll get the benefit of the fibre, which slows down the impact of the sugar on your bloodstream. If you must have a glass of juice, tomato and grapefruit are your best bets. Most other fruit juices – even

unsweetened ones – contain 30 grams of carbs or more
per 100ml serving. Instead, try using just a splash in
your water or dilute it with soda water for a refresh-
ingly light drink.

Atkins Apple & Cranberry Flavoured Drink (Phases 1–4)
1g Net Carbs per serving

Atkins Grapefruit & Lime Flavoured Drink (Phases 1–4)
1g Net Carbs per serving

Atkins Morning Shine™ Tropical Fruit Drink (Phases 3–4) (COMING SOON)
2g Net Carbs per serving

Copella Apple & Elderflower (Phases 3–4)
10.2g carbs per 100ml

Copella Apple & Mango (Phases 3–4)
10.1g carbs per 100ml

Copella Apple & Raspberry (Phases 3–4)
9.4g carbs per 100ml

Ocean Spray Cranberry & Blackcurrant Light (Phases 2–4)
5.7g carbs per 100ml

Ocean Spray Cranberry Classic Light (Phases 2–4)
5.5g carbs per 100ml

Ocean Spray Cranberry & Mango Light (Phases 3–4)
5.9g carbs per 100ml

⚠ **Ocean Spray Cranberry Select**
14.3g carbs per 100ml
Contains added sugars

Ocean Spray Orange & Cranberry (Phases 3–4)
11g carbs per 100ml

Tropicana Pure Premium Fibre – 4 Fruits & Carrot Juice (Phases 3–4)
15.8g carbs per 100ml

Tropicana Pure Premium Golden Grapefruit (Phases 3–4)
8g carbs per 100ml

Tropicana Pure Premium Original Orange (Phases 3–4)
9g carbs per 100ml

Tropicana Pure Premium Pink Grapefruit (Phases 3–4)
8g carbs per 100ml

Tropicana Pure Premium Purely Pineapple (Phases 3–4)
12.5g carbs per 100ml

FLAVOURED WATER

Watch out for carbs in innocuous-seeming waters.
Infused waters use non-caloric sweeteners and flavourings and can be incorporated into a low-carb eating
plan. However, some flavoured waters contain caloric
sweeteners, so if you choose such a brand you might as
well be drinking regular sweetened drinks.

Danone Activ (Phases 1–4)
0g carbs per 250ml serving

⚠ **Danone Activ Blackcurrant Still Water Drink**
12.4g carbs per 250ml serving
Contains added sugars

⚠ **Danone Activ Tropical Orange Still Water
Drink**
12.4g carbs per 250ml serving
Contains added sugars

Ⓕ **Own Brand Apple Flavoured Still Spring Water
Drink (Phases 1–4)**
0.1–0.5g carbs per 250ml serving
Contains aspartame

⚠ **Own Brand Berry (Blackberry, Blueberry,
Cranberry) Sparkling Spring Water Drink**
0.5–1.8g carbs per 250ml serving
Contains added sugars and aspartame

⚠ **Own Brand Elderflower Sparkling Spring
Water Drink**
0–3.3g carbs per 250ml serving
Contains added sugars and aspartame

⚠ **Own Brand Grapefruit Sparkling Spring Water Drink**
0.3g–0.5g carbs per 250ml serving
Contains added sugars and aspartame

⚠ **Own Brand Lemon and Lime Flavoured Sparkling Spring Water**
0.25–0.3g carbs per 250ml serving
Contains added sugars and aspartame

⚠ **Own Brand Lemon and Lime Still Spring Water Drink**
0–11.4g carbs per 250ml serving
Contains added sugars and aspartame

⚠ **Own Brand Peach Sparkling Spring Water Drink**
0.5–2.5g carbs per 250ml serving
Contains added sugars and aspartame

(FYI) **Own Brand Strawberry Still Spring Water Drink (Phases 1–4)**
0.5–12.8g carbs per 250ml serving
Some may contain added sugars and aspartame

(FYI) **Own Brand White Grape Still Spring Water Drink**
0.5–12.3g carbs per 250ml serving
Contains added sugars and aspartame

(FYI) **Perfectly Clear Sparkling Water, Peach Flavour (Phases 1–4)**
0g carbs per 250ml serving
Contains aspartame

FYI **Perfectly Clear Sparkling Water, Summer Fruits Flavour (Phases 1–4)**
0g carbs per 250ml serving
Contains aspartame

FYI **Perfectly Clear Still Spring Water, Citrus Fruits Flavour (Phases 1–4)**
0g carbs per 250ml serving
Contains aspartame

FYI **Perfectly Clear Still Spring Water, Summer Fruits Flavour (Phases 1–4)**
0g carbs per 250ml serving
Contains aspartame

⚠ **Volvic Touch of Fruit Lemon and Lime Still Water**
13.8g carbs per 250ml serving
Contains added sugars

⚠ **Volvic Touch of Fruit Orange and Peach Still Water**
13.8g carbs per 250ml serving
Contains added sugars

⚠ **Volvic Touch of Fruit Strawberry Still Water**
13.8g carbs per 250ml serving
Contains added sugars

SQUASHES & CORDIALS

If you think, because the bulk of these drinks is made up of water, that squashes and cordials don't contain carbs, you could not be more wrong. Take a look at the selection below if you need confirmation that you should stick to plain water or non-caloric flavoured water.

Squash – after dilution

Ocean Spray Dilutable Cranberry Juice Light (Phases 2–4)
7.1g carbs per 100ml

⚠ Own Brand No Added Sugar Apple and Blackcurrant Squash
0.5g carbs per 250ml serving
Contains added sugars and aspartame

⚠ Own Brand No Added Sugar Lemon Squash
0.1–0.2g carbs per 250ml serving
Contains added sugars and aspartame

⚠ Own Brand No Added Sugar Mixed Fruit/Summerfruit Squash
0.5g carbs per 250ml serving
Contains added sugars and aspartame

⚠ Own Brand No Added Sugar Orange Squash
0.3–0.5g carbs per 250ml serving
Contains added sugars and aspartame

⚠ Own Brand No Added Sugar Orange, Lemon and Pineapple Squash
0.3–0.4g carbs per 250ml serving
Contains added sugars and aspartame

⚠ Ribena Light
4.8 carbs per 250ml serving
Contains added sugars and aspartame

⚠ **Robinsons Classic Lemon Barley Water**
10.9g carbs per 250ml serving
Contains added sugars

⚠ **Robinsons Summer Fruits Smooth Fruit and Barley**
5.8g carbs per 250ml serving
Contains added sugars and aspartame

⚠ **Sunny Delight California Style No Added Sugar**
3.5g carbs per 250ml serving
Contains added sugars, aspartame and modified starch

⚠ **Sunny Delight California Style Original**
24.3g carbs per 250ml serving
Contains added sugars and modified starch

Cordials – after dilution

⚠ **Belvoir Organic Blackcurrant Cordial**
⚠ 14.5g carbs per 250ml serving
Contains added sugars

⚠ **Belvoir Organic Elderflower Cordial**
15g carbs per 250ml serving
Contains added sugars

⚠ **Belvoir Organic Ginger Cordial**
⚠ 11.8g carbs per 250ml serving
Contains added sugars

⚠ **Bottlegreen Elderflower Cordial**
14g carbs per 250ml serving
Contains added sugars

⚠ **Bottlegreen English Summer Cordial**
16.8g carbs per 250ml serving
Contains added sugars

⚠ **Bottlegreen Wellbeing Dandelion and Burdock Cordial**
16.5g carbs per 250ml serving
Contains added sugars

⚠ **Bottlegreen Wellbeing Raspberry and Lovage Cordial**
17g carbs per 250ml serving
Contains added sugars

⚠ **Vimto No Added Sugar**
0.7g carbs per 250ml serving
Contains added sugars and aspartame

FIZZY DRINKS

Nearly all diet soft drinks are sweetened with aspartame. Instead, look for brands that use sucralose (Splenda®) and where possible choose decaffeinated varieties. Too much caffeine can elevate blood sugar, and as caffeine is also a diuretic, it is a good idea to have one glass of water for every 250ml of caffeinated drink you consume.

Fruit-flavoured Fizzy Drinks
FYI **Diet Tango Orange (Phases 1–4)**
1.8g carbs per 250ml serving
Contains aspartame

⚠ **Duchy Originals Organic Apple Refresher**
 25g carbs per 250ml serving
Contains added sugars

⚠ **Fanta Light, Icy Lemon**
1g carbs per 250ml serving
Contains added sugars and aspartame

FYI **Fanta Light, Orange (Phases 1–4)**
1.3g carbs per 250ml serving
Contains aspartame

⚠ **Fanta Low Sugar Apple Splash**
11.8g carbs per 250ml serving
Contains added sugars and aspartame

FYI **Irn-Bru, Diet (Phases 1–4)**
Trace carbs per 250ml serving
Contains aspartame

⚠ **Lilt Fruit Crush**
11.5g carbs per 250ml serving
Contains added sugars and aspartame

⚠ **Lilt Fruit Crush Light**
1g carbs per 250ml serving
Contains added sugars and aspartame

FYI **Own Brand Cherryade, No Added Sugar/Sugar-Free (Phases 1–4)**
Trace carbs per 250ml serving
Contains aspartame

ⓕⓨⓘ Own Brand Diet/Light Ginger Beer (Phases 1–4)
Trace carbs per 250ml serving
Contains aspartame

**ⓕⓨⓘ Own Brand Diet/Sugar-Free Lemonade
(Phases 1–4)**
Trace carbs per 250ml serving
Contains aspartame

**⚠ Own Brand No Added Sugar/Diet Orange
Crush/Orangeade**
0.5–2g carbs per 250ml serving
Contains added sugars and aspartame

**ⓕⓨⓘ Own Brand No Added Sugar/Sugar-Free
Limeade (Phases 1–4)**
Trace carbs per 250ml serving
Contains aspartame

ⓕⓨⓘ Sprite Lite (Phases 1–4)
0g carbs per 250ml serving
Contains aspartame

Other Fruit-flavoured Drinks

⚠ Amé Crisp Dry Fruit Drink
10.5g carbs per 250ml serving
Contains added sugars

⚠ Amé Delicate White Fruit Drink
17g carbs per 250ml serving
Contains added sugars

⚠ Amé Radiant Red Fruit Drink
14.3g carbs per 250ml serving
Contains added sugars

⚠ **Amé Refreshing Rosé Fruit Drink**
14.8g carbs per 250ml serving
Contains added sugars

⚠ **AquaLibra Berry**
16.3g carbs per 250ml serving
Contains added sugars

⚠ **AquaLibra Dry**
11.3g carbs per 250ml serving
Contains added sugars

⚠ **AquaLibra Original**
12.8g carbs per 250ml serving
Contains added sugars

Atkins Apple and Cranberry Flavoured Drink
Trace Net Carbs per 500ml serving

Atkins Grapefruit and Lime Flavoured Drink
Trace Net Carbs per 500ml serving

⚠ **Belvoir Organic Elderflower Pressé**
⚠ 25g carbs per 250ml serving
Contains added sugars

⚠ **Bottlegreen Blueberry Pressé**
18.5g carbs per 250ml serving
Contains added sugars

⚠ **Bottlegreen Cranberry Pressé**
18.5g carbs per 250ml serving
Contains added sugars

⚠ **Bottlegreen Elderflower Pressé**
22.3g carbs per 250ml serving
Contains added sugars

⚠ **Bottlegreen Elderlight Pressé**
7.8g carbs per 250ml serving
Contains added sugars and aspartame

⚠ **Bottlegreen Ginger and Lemongrass Pressé**
17g carbs per 250ml serving
Contains added sugars

⚠ **Carpe Diem Kombucha**
21.3g carbs per 250ml serving
Contains added sugars

Mixers

Ⓕ**Ⓨ**Ⓘ **Own Brand Diet/Low Calorie American Ginger Ale (Phases 1–4)**
0–0.1g carbs per 250ml serving
Contains aspartame

⚠ **Own Brand Diet/Low Calorie Bitter Lemon**
0.3–0.5g carbs per 250ml serving
Contains added sugars and aspartame

Ⓕ**Ⓨ**Ⓘ **Own Brand Diet/Low Calorie Indian Tonic Water (Phases 1–4)**
Trace carbs per 250ml serving
Contains aspartame

Own Brand Soda Water (Phases 1–4)
0g carbs per 250ml serving

FYI Schweppes Original Slimline Bitter Lemon (Phases 1–4)

0.3g carbs per 250ml serving

Contains aspartame

Schweppes Original Soda Water (Phases 1–4)

0g carbs per 250ml serving

FYI Schweppes Slimline Indian Tonic Water (Phases 1–4)

0g carbs per 250ml serving

Contains aspartame

ALCOHOL

Although alcohol is not permitted during Induction, you may enjoy the occasional tipple once you've moved on to Ongoing Weight Loss. But it's important to exercise discretion – some alcoholic drinks have higher carb counts than others. Additionally, the body burns alcohol as a fuel before fat, so imbibing can slow down the fat-burning process, which then postpones weight loss. Alcohol does not act as a carbohydrate, so it will not interfere with burning fat in the same way that sugars and other carbohydrates do. However, if you add alcohol to your regime and suddenly stop losing weight, reduce or discontinue your alcohol intake.

If you drink spirits, use only mixers that contain no added sugars or fruit juices. In the later phases of Atkins, you may use vegetable-based mixers.

Even if you choose alcohol that is relatively low in carbs, it should be consumed in moderation. That means, at most, one drink a day.

BEER

If you choose to drink beer, light and low-carb beers are your best bet. Some light beers are nearly as high in carbs as regular beers, however, so be sure to check labels.

Michelob Ultra (Phases 2–4)
2.5g carbs per 275ml

Sleeman Breweries Extra Light Beer (Phases 2–4)
Trace carbs per 275ml

Weissbier Alcohol-free Beer (Phases 2–4)
2.9g carbs per 275ml

SPIRITS, CHAMPAGNE & WINE

Bourbon, Gin, Rum, Vodka, Whisky (Phases 2–4)
0g carbs per 100ml

Sherry, Dry (Phases 1–4)
3.6g carbs per 100ml

Champagne (Phases 2–4)
1.8–3.6g carbs per 100 ml

White Wine (Phases 2–4)
1g carbs per 100ml

Red Wine (Phases 2–4)
2g carbs per 100ml

Dessert Wine, Dry (Phases 2–4)
4g carbs per 100ml

Dessert Wine, Sweet (Phases 3–4)
12g carbs per 100ml

Fish

Fish is a wonderful source of protein and provides essential vitamins, minerals and omega oils. With the exception of some shellfish, which have a higher carb count, fish contains virtually no carbs, which makes it an ideal food while doing Atkins. Fresh fish is remarkably easy to prepare. Whether baked, poached, barbecued, grilled or cooked in a stew, it doesn't take long to put a nutritious, protein-rich meal on the table. Tinned fish offers a handy alternative when you want to create a quick salad. And as long as you steer clear of products swimming in sauces, deli and smoked fish are a perfect way to get your protein without having to cook.

Note that we have used the FYI symbol **FYI** to draw your attention to products in which you would not normally expect to find carbohydrates. While most of these fish products should have a zero carb rating, because of the rules that dictate the way in which we report naturally occurring carbs we have to indicate the possible carb content. For further information, see Naturally Occurring Carbs on page 126 of the Listings Section introduction.

FRESH FISH

Just as we now prefer to shop for fresh meat at the supermarket instead of specialist butchers' shops, so too have we eschewed the fishmonger in favour of the supermarket fish counter. The fresh fish department is an amazing sight to behold, with its wonderful selection of international seafood: succulent tuna from tropical oceans, arctic cod, Scottish salmon and Mediterranean langoustines.

Fresh fish should smell of the ocean. If it smells unpleasant and its eyes have a milky look, it's not at its best, so pass it over in favour of a fresher specimen. If you buy a whole fish, the counter assistant will gut it and remove scales, fins, tail and head if you ask. Ideally, you should cook fresh fish within a day of buying it.

Anchovies (Phases 1–4)
0g carbs per 100g

Bream (Phases 1–4)
0g carbs per 100g

Catfish (Phases 1–4)
0g carbs per 100g

Cod (Phases 1–4)
0g carbs per 100g

Coley (Phases 1–4)
0g carbs per 100g

Dab (Phases 1–4)
0g carbs per 100g

Dover Sole (Phases 1–4)
0g carbs per 100g

Eel (Phases 1–4)
0g carbs per 100g

Haddock (Phases 1–4)
0g carbs per 100g

Hake (Phases 1–4)
0g carbs per 100g

Halibut (Phases 1–4)
0g carbs per 100g

Herring (Phases 1–4)
0g carbs per 100g

John Dory (Phases 1–4)
0g carbs per 100g

Lemon Sole (Phases 1–4)
0g carbs per 100g

Ling (Phases 1–4)
0g carbs per 100g

Mackerel (Phases 1–4)
0g carbs per 100g

Mahi Mahi (Dolphin Fish) (Phases 1–4)
0g carbs per 100g

Marlin (Phases 1–4)
0g carbs per 100g

Monkfish (Phases 1–4)
0g carbs per 100g

Mullet, Grey or Red (Phases 1–4)
0g carbs per 100g

Plaice (Phases 1–4)
0g carbs per 100g

Salmon (Phases 1–4)
0g carbs per 100g

Sardines (Phases 1–4)
0g carbs per 100g

Sea Bass (Phases 1–4)
0g carbs per 100g

Skate (Phases 1–4)
0g carbs per 100g

Snapper (Phases 1–4)
0g carbs per 100g

Swordfish (Phases 1–4)
0g carbs per 100g

Tilapia (Phases 1–4)
0g carbs per 100g

Trout (Phases 1–4)
0g carbs per 100g

Tuna (Phases 1–4)
0g carbs per 100g

Whitebait (Phases 1–4)
0g carbs per 100g

Whiting (Phases 1–4)
0g carbs per 100g

FRESH SHELLFISH

Clams (Phases 1–4)
5.3g carbs per 100g

Cockles (Phases 1–4)
Trace carbs per 100g

Crab (Phases 1–4)
0g carbs per 100g

Dublin Bay Prawns (Phases 1–4)
0g per 100g

Lobster (Phases 1–4)
1.3g carbs per 100g

Mussels (Phases 1–4)
2.5g carbs per 100g

Oysters (Phases 1–4)
4.5g carbs per 100g

Prawns (Phases 1–4)
0g carbs per 150g

Scallops (Phases 1–4)
2.6g carbs per 100g

Squid (Phases 1–4)
4g carbs per 100g

Whelks (Phases 1–4)
Trace carbs per 100g

PREPARED FISH AND SHELLFISH

Worst Bites

It takes about two minutes to bread haddock or prawns, and five minutes to whip up crab cakes or fish cakes, so prepared foods aren't huge timesavers. What they are, however, is laden with empty carbs, making them unacceptable on Atkins. So steer clear of prepared breaded fish and do it yourself. When you make your own breading, use Atkins™ Quick Quisine Bake Mix or crumbs made from low-carb bread to ensure you keep within your daily carb count. Once you are in Ongoing Weight Loss, you can also use a blend of soya flour and ground nuts as a coating. Beware of sweet and sour sauces as they are full of sugar and other empty carbs.

Breaded Prawns
22g carbs per 7 prawns

Crab Cakes
18g carbs per cake

Fish Cakes
29g carbs per 2 cakes

Stuffed Clams
16g carbs per clam

Sweet & Sour Prawns
28g carbs per 6 prawns

Pickled Herring, Boneless (Phases 1–4)
4g carbs per 50g

Salt Cod (Phases 1–4)
0g carbs per 75g

Scampi (Phases 1–4)
5g carbs per 100g serving (8–10 pieces)

DELI FISH

Poached salmon, smoked mackerel and marinated anchovies are just some of the deli fish options that make a convenient low-carb base for a delicious protein-rich salad. Deli fish is not without its drawbacks, however; be sure to avoid fish in sauce, which might contain added sugars and other unacceptable ingredients. Checking whether deli food is acceptable can present a bit of a challenge: while you can check nutrition labels on pre-packed deli fish, it's more of a tall order when you're shopping at the deli counter. When in doubt, ask the counter assistant!

MACKEREL

**(FYI) Own Brand Peppered Mackerel Fillets
(Phases 1–4)**
0.6–1.6g carbs per 100g

**(FYI) Own Brand Smoked Mackerel Fillets
(Phases 1–4)**
0.3–0.7g carbs per 100g

SALMON

**John West Mild Oak Smoked Salmon
(Phases 1–4)**
0.5g carbs per 100g

(FYI) **Own Brand Poached Salmon (Phases 3–4)**
Trace carbs per 100g
Some may contain maize starch

(FYI) **Own Brand Smoked Salmon (Phases 1–4)**
0.1–0.8g carbs per 100g
Some may contain trace added sugars

(FYI) **Own Brand Smoked Salmon Parcels
(Phases 3–4)**
1.2–3.5g carbs per 100g
Some may contain trace added sugars and
modified maize starch

TROUT

**Own Brand Smoked Rainbow Trout Fillets
(Phases 1–4)**
0.1g carbs per 100g

(FYI) **Own Brand Smoked Rainbow Trout Slices
(Phases 1–4)**
0.1g carbs per 100g
Some may contain trace added sugars

⚠ **RR Spink Arbroath Smoked Trout**
0.1g carbs per 100g
Contains trace added sugars

OTHER DELI FISH

**Own Brand Marinated Anchovy Fillets
(Phases 1–4)**
2g carbs per 100g

⚠ **Own Brand Marinated Seafood Salad**
5.5g carbs per 100g
Contains added sugars

⚠ **Own Brand Rollmop Herrings**
17.3g carbs per 100g
Contains added sugars

⚠ **Own Brand Sushi Fish Selection Pack**
25.8–27.9g carbs per 100g
Contains added sugars, maize starch and wheat
flour

PATÉ

 Own Brand Crab Paté (Phases 3–4)
5.5–5.9g carbs per 100g
Contains modified maize starch and wheat flour

⚠ **Own Brand Mackerel Paté**
0.6–1g carbs per 100g
Contains added sugars

⚠ **Own Brand Smoked Salmon Paté**
0.2–3.4g carbs per 100g
Contains added sugars and modified maize starch

⚠ **Own Brand Tuna Paté**
Trace–0.9g carbs per 100g
Contains added sugars and modified maize starch

TINNED FISH

ANCHOVIES

FYI **Admiral Anchovy Paste with Olive Oil
(Phases 1–4)**
1.8g carbs per 100g

FYI **Gia Anchovy Paste (Phases 1–4)**
2.1g carbs per 100g

FYI **John West Flat Fillets of Anchovies in Olive
Oil (Phases 1–4)**
Trace carbs per 10g serving

FYI **Own Brand Anchovies in Olive Oil with
Garlic and Parsley (Phases 1–4)**
Trace carbs per 100g

FYI **Own Brand Anchovy Fillets in Olive Oil,
Jarred (Phases 1–4)**
Trace carbs per 100g

FYI **Own Brand Anchovy Fillets in Olive Oil,
Tinned (Phases 1–4)**
Trace carbs per 100g

CAVIAR

FYI **Marina Lumpfish Caviar (Phases 1–4)**
2g carbs per 100g

CLAMS

⚠ **John West Baby Clams in Brine**
3g carbs per 100g
Contains added sugars

COCKLES

⚠ **Van Smirren Seafoods Cockles Cooked and Pickled**
9g carbs per 100g
Contains added sugars

COD & HERRING ROE

FYI **John West Pressed Cod Roe (Phases 1–4)**
2.3g carbs per 100g

FYI **John West Soft Cod Roes (Phases 1–4)**
Trace carbs per 100g

FYI **John West Soft Herring Roes (Phases 1–4)**
Trace carbs per 100g

CRAB

FYI **John West Dressed Crab (Phases 3–4)**
2g carbs per 100g
Contains added wheat flour

⚠ **Kingfisher Crabmeat in Brine**
1.7g carbs per 100g
Contains added sugars and MSG

⚠ **Kingfisher De-Luxe Lump Crabmeat in Brine**
1.7g carbs per 100g
Contains added sugars and MSG

Shippam's Crab Spread (Phases 2–4)
5.4g carbs per 100g

HERRINGS

⚠ **John West Herring Fillets in Tomato Sauce**
4.8g carbs per 95g serving
Contains added sugars and modified cornflour

⚠ **Princes Marinated Herring**
1.6g carbs per 100g
Contains added sugars

KIPPERS

ⓕⓨⓘ **John West Kipper Fillets in Brine (Phases 1–4)**
Trace carbs per 100g

ⓕⓨⓘ **John West Kipper Fillets in Sunflower Oil (Phases 1–4)**
Trace carbs per 100g

ⓕⓨⓘ **Princes Kippers in Lightly Salted Water (Phases 1–4)**
Trace carbs per 100g
Contains MSG

Princes Kippers in Sunflower Oil (Phases 1–4)
0g carbs per 100g

LOBSTER

(FYI) John West Dressed Lobster (Phases 3–4)
2g carbs per 100g
Contains added wheat flour

MACKEREL

⚠ **John West Mackerel Fillets in Curry Sauce**
3.5g carbs per 100g
Contains added sugars and modified cornflour

⚠ **John West Mackerel Fillets in Green Peppercorn Sauce**
2.6g carbs per 100g
Contains added sugars and modified cornflour

⚠ **John West Mackerel Fillets in Mustard Sauce**
4.7g carbs per 100g
Contains added sugars and modified cornflour

(FYI) John West Traditional Wood Smoked Peppered Mackerel Fillets in Sunflower Oil (Phases 1–4)
0.5g carbs per 100g

(FYI) Princes Mackerel Fillets in a Hot Chilli Dressing (Phases 1–4)
Trace carbs per 100g

Princes Mackerel Fillets in Lightly Salted Water (Phases 1–4)
0g carbs per 100g

⚠ **Princes Mackerel Fillets in Mustard Sauce**
6g carbs per 100g
Contains added sugars, trans fats, modified maize
starch and wheat flour

**Princes Mackerel Fillets in Olive Oil
(Phases 1–4)**
0g carbs per 100g

⚠ **Princes Mackerel Fillets in a Rich Spicy
Tomato Sauce**
4.7g carbs per 100g
Contains added sugars

**Princes Mackerel Fillets in a Rich Tomato
Sauce (Phases 1–4)**
3.3g carbs per 100g

MUSSELS

**John West Smoked Mussels in Sunflower Oil
(Phases 1–4)**
10g carbs per 100g

**Palacio de Oriente Mussels in Galician Sauce
(Phases 1–4)**
5.5g carbs per 100g

**Van Smirren Seafoods Mussels in Brine
(Phases 1–4)**
1g carbs per 100g

⚠ **Van Smirren Seafoods Mussels Cooked and Pickled**
1g carbs per 100g
Contains added sugars

OYSTERS

John West Smoked Oysters in Sunflower Oil (Phases 1–4)
10g carbs per 100g

PILCHARDS

Glenryck Atlantic Pilchards in Brine (Phases 1–4)
0g carbs per 100g

⚠ **Glenryck South Atlantic Pilchard Fillets in Spicy Tomato Sauce**
3.5g carbs per 100g
Contains added sugars

🅕🅨🅘 **Glenryck South Atlantic Pilchards in Tomato Sauce (Phases 3–4)**
2.3g carbs per 100g
Contains modified maize starch

PRAWNS

⚠ **John West Prawns in Brine**
1g carbs per 100g
Contains added sugars and MSG

⚠ **Kingfisher Prawns in Brine**
0.5g carbs per 100g
Contains added sugars and MSG

SALMON

(FYI) **Glenryck Medium Red Salmon in Brine
(Phases 1–4)**
0g carbs per 100g

(FYI) **Glenryck Medium Red Salmon, Skinless and
Boneless (Phases 1–4)**
0.3g carbs per 100g

(FYI) **John West Pink Salmon (Phases 1–4)**
Trace carbs per 100g

(FYI) **John West Red Salmon (Phases 1–4)**
Trace carbs per 100g

La Piara Smoked Salmon Paté (Phases 1–4)
1.5g carbs per 100g

**Princes Wild Medium Red Salmon
(Phases 1–4)**
0g carbs per 100g

Princes Wild Pink Salmon (Phases 1–4)
0g carbs per 100g

⚠ **Shippam's Finest Potted Salmon**
1g carbs per 100g
Contains added sugars

Shippam's Salmon Spread (Phases 1–4)
4.2g carbs per 100g

⚠ **Weight Watchers from Heinz Salmon in Lemon Mayonnaise Dressing Made with John West Salmon**
6.4g carbs per 100g
Contains added sugars and modified cornflour

SARDINES

Bela Sardines in Hot Sauce (Phases 1–4)
0g carbs per 100g

Bela Sardines in Lemon Sauce (Phases 1–4)
0g carbs per 100g

(FYI) **John West Boneless Sardines in Sunflower Oil (Phases 1–4)**
Trace carbs per 100g

John West Boneless Sardines in Tomato Sauce (Phases 1–4)
1.5g carbs per 100g

⚠ **Princes Sardine and Tomato Paste**
3.1g carbs per 100g
Contains added sugars

Princes Sardines in a Rich Tomato Sauce (Phases 1–4)
1.6g carbs per 100g

SHRIMPS

⚠ **John West Shrimps in Brine**
1g carbs per 100g
Contains added sugars

SILD

🔲 **John West Sild in Sunflower Oil (Phases 1–4)**
Trace carbs per 100g

⚠ **John West Sild in Tomato Sauce**
2.5g carbs per 100g
Contains added sugars and cornflour

SKIPPERS

⚠ **John West Traditional Smoked Skippers Brisling in Tomato Sauce**
3g carbs per 100g
Contains added sugars and cornflour

🔲 **John West Traditional Wood Smoked Skippers Brisling in Sunflower Oil (Phases 1–4)**
Trace carbs per 100g

TROUT

⚠ **Shippam's Trout and Lemon Paté**
6.2g carbs per 100g
Contains added sugars

TUNA

⚠ **John West Everything But the Salad Leaves Tuna French Style**
4.6g per 100g
Contains added sugars

⚠ **John West Everything But the Salad Leaves Tuna Italian Style**
4.3g per 100g
Contains added sugars

⚠ **John West Everything But the Salad Leaves Tuna, Lemon and Chive**
4.6g per 100g
Contains added sugars

⚠ **John West Skipjack Tuna in Mayonnaise with Sweet Corn**
4.5g carbs per 100g
Contains added sugars

⚠ **John West Skipjack Tuna Salad with Three Bean Mix in Vinaigrette Dressing**
9.6g carbs per 100g
Contains added sugars

⚠ **John West Skipjack Tuna in Thousand Island Dressing**
5.1g carbs per 100g
Contains added sugars and modified cornflour

(FYI) **John West Tuna Light Lunch French Style (Phases 3–4)**
7.6g carbs per 100g
Contains modified cornflour

⚠ **John West Tuna Light Lunch Mediterranean**
6.4g carbs 100g
Contains added sugars and modified cornflour

⚠ **John West Tuna Light Lunch Niçoise Style**
8.9g carbs per 100g
Contains added sugars and modified cornflour

⚠ **John West Tuna Light Lunch Tomato Salsa**
7.5g carbs per 100g
Contains added sugars

(FYI) **John West Yellowfin Tuna Steak in Olive Oil (Phases 1–4)**
Trace carbs per 100g

(FYI) **John West Yellowfin Tuna Steak in Springwater (Phases 1–4)**
Trace carbs per 100g

La Piara Tuna with Olive Oil Paté (Phases 2–4)
5.1g carbs per 100g

⚠ **Princes Slimming World Tuna in a Light Lemon Mayonnaise**
3.5g carbs per 100g
Contains added sugars

⚠ **Princes Slimming World Tuna in a Lime and Black Pepper Dressing**
3.5g carbs per 100g
Contains added sugars

⚠ **Princes Slimming World Tuna in a Red Chilli and Lime Dressing**
1g carbs per 100g
Contains added sugars

Princes Tuna & Mayonnaise Paste (Phases 1–4)
1g carbs per 100g

⚠ **Princes Tuna & Red Onion Paste**
5.4g carbs per 100g
Contains added sugars

⚠ **Weight Watchers from Heinz Tuna in Coronation Style Dressing Made with John West Tuna**
6.5g carbs per 100g
Contains added sugars

⚠ **Weight Watchers from Heinz Tuna in Mayonnaise Style Dressing with Sweet Corn Made with John West Tuna**
6.1g carbs per 100g
Contains added sugars

⚠ **Weight Watchers from Heinz Tuna in Tomato and Herb Dressing Made with John West Tuna**
5.1g carbs per 100g
Contains added sugars and modified cornflour

FROZEN FISH

Fish freezes well. You can either buy it fresh and freeze it yourself – in which case, make sure that it hasn't been previously frozen – or buy it already frozen. Raw frozen fish, when thawed, contains the same number of carbs as fresh fish. You might enter a minefield, however, when you buy pre-cooked fish in sauces, as these more often than not will contain trans fats, flour and other unacceptable ingredients, as you can see from the examples below.

COD

(FYI) **Birds Eye Cod Steaks in Butter Sauce (Phases 3–4)**
5g carbs per 100g
Contains maize starch and wheat flour

(FYI) **Birds Eye Cod Steaks in Parsley Sauce (Phases 3–4)**
5.6g carbs per 100g uncooked
Contains maize starch and wheat flour

(FYI) **Birds Eye Simply Cod Fillets in a Light Breadcrumb (Phases 3–4)**
15g carbs per 100g uncooked
Contains wheat flour

⚠ **Own Brand Cod Portions in Butter Sauce**
2.9–5g carbs per 100g
Contains added sugars, modified maize starch and wheat flour

⚠ **Own Brand Cod Portions in Parsley Sauce**
2.4–5g carbs per 100g
Contains added sugars, trans fats, modified maize starch and wheat flour

FISH CAKES

FYI **Birds Eye Cod Fish Cakes in Crunch Crumb (Phases 3–4)**
15.9g carbs per 100g uncooked
Contains wheat flour

FYI **Own Brand Economy Fish Cakes (Phases 3–4)**
21.2–22g carbs per 100g
Contains wheat flour

FISH FILLETS IN SAUCE

⚠ **Birds Eye SteamFresh Fish 100% Pink Salmon Fillets in a Dill Sauce**
2.9 carbs per 100g
Contains added sugars and maize starch

⚠ **Ross Fish Steaks in Parsley Sauce**
3.1g carbs per 100g
Contains added sugars, trans fats, modified starch and wheat flour

FYI **Young's Garlic & Herb Fish Fillets (Phases 3–4)**
16.2g carbs per 100g uncooked
Contains wheat flour

⚠ **Young's Lemon & Pepper Fish Fillets**
15.3g carbs per 100g uncooked
Contains added sugars and wheat flour

FISH FINGERS

(FYI) Birds Eye 100% Cod Fillet Fish Fingers (Phases 3–4)
15.6g carbs per 100g uncooked
Contains wheat flour

(FYI) Own Brand Cod Fillet Fish Fingers (Phases 3–4)
16.8–18g carbs per 100g
Some may contain wheat flour

(FYI) Own Brand Economy Fish Fingers (Phases 3–4)
11.9–16g carbs per 100g
Can contain added sugars and wheat flour

(FYI) Own Brand Freefrom Cod Fillet Fish Fingers (Phases 3–4)
15.6–18g carbs per 100g
Contains maize flour, maize starch and modified maize starch

HADDOCK

⚠ Birds Eye SteamFresh Fish 100% Haddock Fillets in Cheese & Leek Sauce
2.5 carbs per 100g
Contains added sugars and maize starch

⚠ Own Brand Breaded Haddock Portions
17.8–20g carbs per 100g
Contains added sugars, trans fats and wheat flour

KIPPERS

Own Brand Smoked Kippers with Butter (Phases 1–4)
0g–trace carbs per 100g

MEDITERRANEAN-STYLE FISH

FYI **Birds Eye Italiano Fish Bake (Phases 3–4)**
3.9g carbs per 100g
Contains maize starch

FYI **Birds Eye Vegetable Tuscany Fish Bake (Phases 3–4)**
4.3g carbs per 100g
Contains maize starch

⚠ **Own Brand Mediterranean Style Cod Fillets**
0.1–2.5g carbs per 100g
Contains added sugars, trans fats and modified maize starch

PRAWNS

⚠ **Tahay Prawn Ring**
4.7g carbs per 100g
Contains added sugars

TUNA

Own Brand Tuna Steaks (Phases 1–4)
Trace–0.3g carbs per 100g

Frozen Food

Sometimes, if it's been a long day or you've been too busy to get to the supermarket, all you want to do is reach into the freezer and find something you can pop in the oven or the microwave. There's nothing wrong with that notion – after all, why was the freezer invented? – but if you want to ensure that you still eat healthily, you must pay attention to how you stock your freezer. Frozen vegetables pose little problem and nor does frozen fruit as long as you are careful to avoid those with added sugars, but you will have to exercise caution when buying meals made with fish and meat.

DESSERTS & ICE CREAM

Until low-carb ice creams and desserts are manufactured in the UK, the frozen desserts aisle is a no-go area. While some of the ice creams we reviewed came within acceptable carb limits, all of them contained added sugars, which means they are unacceptable on any phase of Atkins. Once you are past Induction, if you cannot live without ice cream, consider making your own using natural yogurt, fromage frais and berries, and sweetening it with Splenda®.

DESSERTS

 Slim-Fast Chocolate and Caramel Stick Bars
14.5g carbs per stick
Contains added sugars

Slim-Fast Vanilla and Strawberry Mini Tubs
18g carbs per 60g tub
Contains added sugars

⚠ Viennetta Vanilla
22.9g carbs per 100g
Contains added sugars

⚠ Weight Watchers Chocolate with Honeycomb Pieces
15.2g carbs per 100ml pot
Contains added sugars and modified maize starch

⚠ Weight Watchers Vanilla with Raspberry Swirl
13.3g carbs per 100ml pot
Contains added sugars and modified cornflour

⚠ Weight Watchers Vanilla with Strawberry Swirl
13.3g carbs per 100ml pot
Contains added sugars and modified cornflour

ICE CREAM

⚠ Duchy Originals Organic Vanilla Ice Cream
 15.8g carbs per 100g
Contains added sugars

⚠ Green & Black's Organic Chocolate Ice Cream
18.6 carbs per 100g
Contains added sugars

⚠ Green & Black's Vanilla Ice Cream
15.2g carbs per 100g
Contains added sugars

⚠ **Hill Station Dark Roast Coffee Ice Cream**
17.3g carbs per 100g
Contains added sugars

⚠ **Hill Station Mango and Lime Ice Cream**
19.9g carbs per 100g
Contains added sugars

⚠ **Hill Station Stem Ginger Ice Cream**
20.2g carbs per 100g
Contains added sugars

⚠ **Hill Station Vanilla Bean Ice Cream**
17.8g carbs per 100g
Contains added sugars

⚠ **Mackie's of Scotland Traditional Luxury Dairy**
⚠ **Ice Cream**
18g carbs per 100g
Contains added sugars

⚠ **Minghella Dolce Vita Real Vanilla Ice Cream**
17g carbs per 100g
Contains added sugars

⚠ **Yeo Valley Organic Vanilla Dairy Ice Cream**
⚠ 21.3 carbs per 100g
Contains added sugars

⚠ **Yorkshire Dales Natural Flavour Old**
Fashioned Luxury Dairy Ice Cream
18.6g carbs per 100g
Contains added sugars

⚠ **Yorkshire Dales Old English Sticky Toffee Crunch Luxury Dairy Ice Cream**
10.9g carbs per 100g
Contains added sugars

⚠ **Yorkshire Dales Triple Chocolate Chunk Luxury Dairy Ice Cream**
12.5g carbs per 100g
Contains added sugars and modified maize starch

FISH

Portions of fish that have simply been frozen – for example, a haddock fillet or a tuna steak – will have the same carb content that fresh fish has. The same cannot be said for most of the other fish products you'll find in supermarket freezers. Even seemingly simple dishes such as cod in butter sauce are swimming in added sugars and wheat flours, while many other fish dishes contain manufactured trans fats and modified maize starch.

Stick to plain frozen fillets and steaks, or buy fresh and freeze them yourself.

Cod

(FYI) Birds Eye Cod Steaks in Butter Sauce (Phases 3–4)
5g carbs per 100g
Contains maize starch and wheat flour

(FYI) Birds Eye Cod Steaks in Parsley Sauce (Phases 3–4)
5.6g carbs per 100g uncooked
Contains maize starch and wheat flour

Ⓕ⒴⒤ **Birds Eye Simply Cod Fillets in a Light Breadcrumb (Phases 3–4)**
15g carbs per 100g uncooked
Contains wheat flour

Ⓕ⒴⒤ **Own Brand Cod Portions in Butter Sauce**
2.9–5g carbs per 100g
Contains added sugars, modified maize starch and wheat flour

⚠ **Own Brand Cod Portions in Parsley Sauce**
2.4–5g carbs per 100g
Contains added sugars, trans fats, modified maize starch and wheat flour

Fish Cakes

Ⓕ⒴⒤ **Birds Eye Cod Fish Cakes in Crunch Crumb (Phases 3–4)**
15.9g carbs per 100g uncooked
Contains wheat flour

Ⓕ⒴⒤ **Own Brand Economy Fish Cakes (Phases 3–4)**
21.2–22g carbs per 100g
Contains wheat flour

Fish Fillets in Sauce

⚠ **Birds Eye SteamFresh Fish 100% Pink Salmon Fillets in a Dill Sauce**
2.9 carbs per 100g
Contains added sugars and maize starch

⚠ **Ross Fish Steaks in Parsley Sauce**
3.1g carbs per 100g
Contains added sugars, trans fats, modified starch and wheat flour

Ⓕ🅨 **Young's Garlic & Herb Fish Fillets (Phases 3–4)**
16.2g carbs per 100g uncooked
Contains wheat flour

⚠ **Young's Lemon & Pepper Fish Fillets**
15.3g carbs per 100g uncooked
Contains added sugars and wheat flour

Fish Fingers

Ⓕ🅨 **Birds Eye 100% Cod Fillet Fish Fingers (Phases 3–4)**
15.6g carbs per 100g uncooked
Contains wheat flour

Ⓕ🅨 **Own Brand Cod Fillet Fish Fingers (Phases 3–4)**
16.8–18g carbs per 100g
Contains wheat flour

Ⓕ🅨 **Own Brand Economy Fish Fingers (Phases 3–4)**
11.9–16g carbs per 100g
Some may contain added sugars and wheat flour

Ⓕ🅨 **Own Brand Freefrom Cod Fillet Fish Fingers (Phases 3–4)**
15.6–18g carbs per 100g
Contains maize flour, maize starch and modified maize starch

Haddock

⚠ **Birds Eye SteamFresh Fish 100% Haddock Fillets in Cheese & Leek Sauce**
2.5 carbs per 100g
Contains added sugars and maize starch

⚠ **Own Brand Breaded Haddock Portions**
17.8–20g carbs per 100g
Contains added sugars, trans fats and wheat flour

Kippers

**Own Brand Smoked Kippers with Butter
(Phases 1–4)**
0g–trace carbs per 100g

Mediterranean-Style Fish

ⒻⓎⒾ **Birds Eye Italiano Fish Bake (Phases 3–4)**
3.9g carbs per 100g
Contains maize starch

ⒻⓎⒾ **Birds Eye Vegetable Tuscany Fish Bake
(Phases 3–4)**
4.3g carbs per 100g
Contains maize starch

⚠ **Own Brand Mediterranean Style Cod Fillets**
0.1–2.5g carbs per 100g
Contains added sugars, trans fats and modified
maize starch

Prawns

⚠ **Tahay Prawn Ring**
4.7g carbs per 100g
Contains added sugars

Tuna

Own Brand Tuna Steaks (Phases 1–4)
Trace–0.3g carbs per 100g

FRUIT

Just as with frozen vegetables, frozen fruit is higher in carbs than fresh. When frozen foods thaw, ice crystals rupture the cell walls, so water escapes and other nutrients, including carbohydrates, are concentrated. There isn't a wide range of choice in this category, largely because, apart from summer berries, most other fruit is available fresh all year round. Make sure that any frozen fruit you buy is unsweetened. Look out for the words 'unsweetened', 'sugar-free' or 'no-added-sugar' on the label and check the ingredient list for all forms of sugar, including fruit juice concentrate.

Blackberries (Phases 2–4)
10.6g carbs per 100g

Blueberries (Phases 2–4)
9.4g carbs per 100g

Cranberries (Phases 2–4)
7.6g carbs per 100g

Raspberries (Phases 2–4)
10g carbs per 100g

Shearway Black Forest Fruits (Phases 3–4)
10.9g carbs per 100g

Shearway Luxury Fruit Salad with Camarosa Strawberries (Phases 3–4)
10g carbs per 100g

⚠ **Shearway Organic Raspberries (Phases 2–4)**
4.6g carbs per 100g

Shearway Raspberries (Phases 2–4)
4.6g carbs per 100g

Shearway Summer Fruits (Phases 3–4)
6.9g carbs per 100g

Strawberries, Whole (Phases 2–4)
7g carbs per 100g

MEAT & POULTRY

As with frozen fish, frozen meat and poultry need to be
carefully scanned when it comes to counting carbs.
Frozen cuts, such as lamb chops or chicken breasts, are
handy stand-bys to keep in your freezer, with the same
carb counts as their fresh counterparts. You might
think that frozen burgers or frozen whole chickens
would be no different either, but you would be wrong.
Burgers often contain added sugars and wheat flour,
while frozen roasts may contain manufactured trans
fats. Not every item in the freezer case is off limits, but
pay close attention to nutritional labelling.

Be aware also that some frozen meat, such as
burgers, might seem to contain carbs, even when there
are no other ingredients. This is due to naturally occurring carbs (see Naturally Occurring Carbs on page 126
of the introduction to the Listings Section). In these
cases we have drawn your attention to the fact with an
FYI symbol **FYI** .

BEEF

Burgers

FYI **Birds Eye 100% Beef Burgers (Phases 3–4)**
0g carbs per 100g
Contains wheat flour

Birds Eye 100% Beef Mega Burgers (Phases 1–4)
0g carbs per 100g

FYI **Birds Eye Captain's Beef Burgers (Phases 3–4)**
3.9g carbs per 100g
Contains wheat flour

FYI **Birds Eye Mexican Chilli Beef Quarter Pounders (Phases 3–4)**
6.5g carbs per 100g
Contains wheat flour

FYI **Birds Eye Original & Best Beef Burgers (Phases 3–4)**
5.1g carbs per 100g
Contains wheat flour

⚠ **Own Brand Beef Burgers with Onion**
3.8–6.9g carbs per 100g
Contains added sugars and wheat flour

⚠ **Own Brand Economy Burgers**
11–12g carbs per 100g
Contains added sugars, MSG and wheat flour

⚠ **Own Brand Prime Beef Quarter Pounders**
1.3–6g carbs per 100g
Contains added sugars and wheat flour

ⓕ **Planet Hollywood Beef Burgers (Phases 1–4)**
1.4g carbs per 100g

⚠ **Ross 100% Beef Burgers**
1.1g carbs per 100g
Contains added sugars and wheat flour

⚠ **Ross Chilli Beef Quarter Pounders**
2.8g carbs per 100g
Contains added sugars and wheat flour

⚠ **Ross Quarter Pounders**
2.8g carbs per 100g
Contains added sugars and wheat flour

Grills

⚠ **Dalepak Cracked Black Pepper Marinade Style Beef Grills**
6.2g carbs per 100g
Contains added sugars, modified maize starch and wheat

⚠ **Dalepak Peppered Beef Marine Style Grillsteaks**
5.5g carbs per 100g
Contains added sugars, modified maize starch and wheat flour

ⓕ **Own Brand Beef Grillsteaks (Phases 1–4)**
1.6g carbs per 100g
Some may contain added sugars

⚠ Own Brand Peppered Beef Grillsteaks
8.6–12.8g carbs per 100g
Contains added sugars, modified maize starch and
wheat flour

⚠ Ross Beef Grillsteaks
3.7g carbs per 100g
Contains added sugars and wheat flour

⚠ Ross 100% Beef Grillsteaks
1.1g carbs per 100g uncooked
Contains added sugars and wheat flour

Miscellaneous
Ⓕ Aria Beef Strips (Phases 1–4)
1.1g carbs per 100g

⚠ Birds Eye Roast Beef in Gravy
3.2g carbs per 100g
Contains added sugars, maize starch and wheat
flour

⚠ Own Brand Sliced Beef in Gravy
2.6–2.7g carbs per 100g
Contains added sugars, trans fats, modified maize
starch and wheat flour

PORK
Ribs
⚠ Dalepak Chinese Style Ribsteaks
10.4g carbs per 100g
Contains added sugars

⚠ **Dalepak Smokey Barbecue Style Ribsteaks**
8.8g carbs per 100g uncooked
Contains added sugars, aspartame, modified maize
starch and wheat flour

⚠ **Farmers Table Chinese Style Pork Ribs**
5.4g carbs per 100g
Contains added sugars, modified maize starch and
wheat flour

Sausages

⚠ **Own Brand Cocktail Sausages**
11–15.8g carbs per 100g
Contains added sugars and wheat flour

⚠ **Own Brand Thick Pork Sausages**
11–12.9g carbs per 100g
Contains added sugars and wheat flour

⚠ **Own Brand Thick Pork & Beef Sausages**
10.6–15.4g carbs per 100g
Contains added sugars and wheat flour

⚠ **Own Brand Thin Pork Sausages**
8.7–13g carbs per 100g
Contains added sugars and wheat flour

(FYI) **Richmond Thick Sausages (Phases 3–4)**
12.8g carbs per 100g
Contains wheat flour

⚠ **Wall's Jumbo Pork Sausages**
10.2g carbs per 100g
Contains added sugars and wheat flour

(FYI) Wall's Skinless Pork Sausages (Phases 3–4)
9g carbs per 100g
Contains wheat flour

POULTRY

Burgers

(FYI) Birds Eye Captain's Chicken Burgers (Phases 3–4)
16.6g carbs per 100g
Contains wheat flour

⚠ Birds Eye Captain's Roasted Chicken Bites
3.4g carbs per 100g
Contains added sugars, maize starch and wheat flour

⚠ Birds Eye 100% Chicken Fillet Burgers Cajun
2.6g carbs per 100g
Contains added sugars, maize starch and wheat flour

⚠ Birds Eye 100% Chicken Fillet Burgers Original
3g carbs per 100g
Contains added sugars, maize starch and wheat flour

Grills

⚠ Birds Eye Captain's Mini BBQ Chicken Griddlers
6.7g carbs per 100g
Contains added sugars, maize starch and wheat flour

⚠ **Birds Eye Chicken Chargrills Garlic**
3.1g carbs per 100g
Contains added sugars, maize starch and wheat
flour

⚠ **Birds Eye Chicken Chargrills Original**
2.5g carbs per 100g
Contains added sugars, maize starch and wheat
flour

🅵🆈🅸 **Birds Eye Chicken Quarter Pounders
(Phases 3–4)**
19.2g carbs per 100g
Contains maize flour and wheat flour

Miscellaneous

🅵🆈🅸 **Aria Chicken Strips (Phases 1–4)**
0.9g carbs per 100g

🅵🆈🅸 **Bernard Matthews Mini Cheese & Herb Kievs
(Phases 3–4)**
12.1g carbs per 100g
Contains wheat flour

⚠ **Bernard Matthews Original Turkey Sausages**
13.5g carbs per 100g
Contains added sugars and wheat flour

⚠ **Birds Eye Chicken Tikka**
3.5g carbs per 100g
Contains added sugars, maize starch and wheat
flour

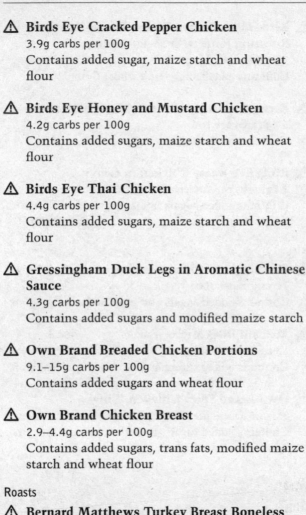 Birds Eye Cracked Pepper Chicken
3.9g carbs per 100g
Contains added sugar, maize starch and wheat
flour

Birds Eye Honey and Mustard Chicken
4.2g carbs per 100g
Contains added sugars, maize starch and wheat
flour

Birds Eye Thai Chicken
4.4g carbs per 100g
Contains added sugars, maize starch and wheat
flour

Gressingham Duck Legs in Aromatic Chinese Sauce
4.3g carbs per 100g
Contains added sugars and modified maize starch

Own Brand Breaded Chicken Portions
9.1–15g carbs per 100g
Contains added sugars and wheat flour

Own Brand Chicken Breast
2.9–4.4g carbs per 100g
Contains added sugars, trans fats, modified maize
starch and wheat flour

Roasts

Bernard Matthews Turkey Breast Boneless Roasting Joint
2.7g carbs per 100g
Contains added sugars

⚠ **Bernard Matthews Turkey Breast Boneless Roasting Joint with Sage & Onion**
3.2g carbs per 100g
Contains added sugars and wheat flour

⚠ **Bernard Matthews Turkey Breast Roast**
3.4g carbs per 100g
Contains added sugars

⚠ **Birds Eye Roast Chicken in Gravy**
2.7g carbs per 100g uncooked
Contains added sugars, maize starch and wheat flour

Wings

⚠ **Gressingham Chinese Barbeque Duck Wings**
11g carbs per 100g
Contains added sugars and modified maize starch

⚠ **McCain BBQ Micro Wings**
6g carbs per serving, 4.4g carbs per 100g
Contains added sugars and modified maize starch

⚠ **Own Brand Spicy Chicken Wings**
3.2–3.5g carbs per 100g
Contains added sugars, modified maize starch and wheat flour

LAMB

Grills

⚠ **Dalepak Lamb Dalesteaks**
1.9g carbs per 100g
Contains added sugars and wheat flour

⚠ **Dalepak Minted Lamb Marinade Style Grills**
4.4g carbs per 100g
Contains added sugars, modified maize starch and
wheat flour

FYI **Own Brand Lamb Grillsteaks (Phases 3–4)**
2.2–5.2g carbs per 100g
Contains wheat flour

Miscellaneous
FYI **Aria Lamb Strips (Phases 1–4)**
1.3g carbs per 100g

Roasts
⚠ **Bernard Matthews Boneless Leg Joint in
Rosemary & Garlic Marinade**
6.6g carbs per 100g
Contains added sugars and modified maize starch

Bernard Matthews Lamb Roast (Phases 1–4)
0.1g carbs per 100g

VEGETABLES

As with fresh vegetables, most frozen vegetables are
acceptable on Atkins – as long as what you're buying
is *just* vegetables. Avoid frozen vegetables swimming
in sauces made with starches; also, butter-flavoured
and cheese-flavoured sauces usually contain partially
hydrogenated vegetable oils as the first ingredient.
Choose plain vegetables and cook them in stock for
added flavour, then dress them with butter or olive
oil.

You may find that frozen vegetables are higher in
carbs than fresh ones. This is because frozen vegetables

are always cooked, which frequently concentrates their nutrients.

Asparagus Spears (Phases 1–4)
2.2g carbs per 100g

Broccoli (Phases 1–4)
2g carbs per 100g

Brussels Sprouts (Phases 1–4)
4g carbs per 100g

Butternut Squash (Phases 3–4)
13g carbs per 100g

Carrots (Phases 3–4)
5g carbs per 100g

Cauliflower (Phases 1–4)
2.3g carbs per 100g

Courgettes (Phases 1–4)
2.2g carbs per 100g

Green Beans (Phases 1–4)
4.8g carbs per 100g

Kale (Phases 1–4)
2.9g carbs per 100g

Okra (Phases 1–4)
4.4g carbs per 100g

Onions (Phases 1–4)
5g carbs per 100g

Peas (Phases 3–4)
9.5g carbs per 100g

Peppers, Red & Yellow (Phases 1–4)
2.8g carbs per 100g

Petits Pois (Phases 3–4)
7g carbs per 100g

Spinach, Creamed (Phases 1–4)
5.4g carbs per 100g

Spinach, Leaf (Phases 1–4)
1.2g carbs per 100g

Sweetcorn (Phases 3–4)
20g carbs per 100g

VEGETARIAN ALTERNATIVES

You need to approach meat alternatives carefully when doing Atkins, as they do not always equate with low carbs. Many of the products will be bulked up with breadcrumbs, beans, potatoes or rice. Be aware that a low carb count doesn't necessarily mean that a product is suitable for all phases.

Importantly, no matter how healthy some of these products purport to be, many of the most popular brands contain added sugars and added trans fats, which should be avoided on all phases of Atkins.

BEEF, POULTRY & BACON SUBSTITUTES

⚠ **Morningstar Farms Meat-free Streaky Strips**
13.4g carbs per 100g
Contains added sugars and modified cornflour

Quorn Chicken Style Roast (Phases 1–4)
4g carbs per 100g

⚠ **Quorn Crispy Fillets**
14.2g carbs per 100g
Contains added sugars, trans fats and wheat flour

Quorn Fillets (Phases 1–4)
5.9g carbs per 100g

⚠ **Quorn Garlic & Herb Fillets**
16.7g per 100g
Contains wheat flour

⚠ **Quorn Pork Style Ribsters**
4.8g carbs per 100g
Contains trans fats

Quorn Swedish Style Balls (Phases 1–4)
5.4g carbs per 100g

Realeat Vege Mince (Phases 1–4)
6g carbs per 100g

SAUSAGES

⚠ **Linda McCartney Sausages**
8.6g carbs per 100g
Contains added sugars and trans fats

ⒻⓎ **Own Brand Vegetarian/Meatfree Hot Dog Sausages (Phases 1–4)**
6g carbs per 100g
Some may contain added sugars

ⒻⓎ **Own Brand Vegetarian Sausages (Phases 1–4)**
2–20.5g carbs per 100g
Some may contain added sugars and wheat

BURGERS

ⒻⓎ **Birds Eye Captain's Vegetable Burgers (Phases 3–4)**
25.5g carbs per 100g
Contains wheat flour

ⒻⓎ **Birds Eye Crunchy Vegetable Quarter Pounders (Phases 3–4)**
24.9g carbs per 100g
Contains wheat flour

⚠ **Dalepak Vegetable Quarter Pounders**
20.8g carbs per 100g
Contains added sugars, trans fats and wheat flour

⚠ **Goodlife Organic Vegetable Burgers (Phases 3–4)**
26.3g carbs per 100g

⚠ **Linda McCartney Flame Grilled Burgers**
2.9g carbs per 100g
Contains trans fats

⚠ **Own Brand Vegetable & Spicy Bean Quarter Pounders**
28–35g carbs per 100g
Contains added sugars, trans fats and wheat flour

Ⓕ **Own Brand Vegetarian/Meatfree Burgers (Phases 1–4)**
3.9–7g carbs per 100g
Some may contain added sugars

Ⓕ **Own Brand Vegetarian/Meatfree Quarterpounders (Phases 1–4)**
0.3–7g carbs per 100g
Some may contain added sugars and trans fats

Ⓕ **Quorn Burgers (Phases 3–4)**
8.8g carbs per 100g
Contains starch

⚠ **Quorn Premium Burgers**
5.5g carbs per 100g
Contains trans fats

⚠ **Quorn Southern Style Burgers**
17g carbs per 100g
Contains trans fats and wheat flour

NUT PRODUCTS

Ⓕ **Goodlife Nut Cutlets (Phases 3–4)**
21.8g carbs per 100g
Contains wheat flour

Own Brand Vegetable and Nut Cutlets
22g carbs per 100g
Some may contain added sugars, trans fats and
wheat flour

Own Brand Vegetarian Nuggets
10.5–14.7g carbs per 100g
Contains added sugars, breadcrumbs and wheat
flour

FYI Quorn Southern Style Nuggets (Phases 3–4)
18.8g carbs per 100g
Contains wheat flour

FALAFEL

Goodlife Falafel with Yogurt and Mint Dip (Phases 3–4)
22.4g carbs per 100g

READY MEALS

⚠ Linda McCartney Lasagne
14.6g carbs per 100g
Contains added sugars, modified maize starch and
wheat flour

PASTA & RICE

⚠ Own Brand Spinach & Ricotta Cannelloni
12.5–17.3g carbs per 100g
Contains added sugars, trans fats, modified maize
starch and wheat flour

(FYI) **Ross Spinach and Ricotta Cannelloni
(Phases 3–4)**
13.2g carbs per 100g
Contains modified maize starch and wheat flour

VEGETABLE PRODUCTS

(FYI) **Birds Eye Captain's Vegetable Fingers
(Phases 3–4)**
23.8g carbs per 100g
Contains wheat flour

(FYI) **Dalepak Cauliflower Cheese Grills
(Phases 3–4)**
20.1g carbs per 100g
Some may contain added sugars, trans fats, maize
starch and wheat flour

⚠ **Dalepak Vegetable Fingers**
26.7g carbs per 100g
Contains added sugars, trans fats and wheat flour

⚠ **Dalepak Vegetable Grills**
22.5g carbs per 100g
Contains added sugars and wheat flour

⚠ **Own Brand Potato & Cheese Bakes**
22.4–24.5g carbs per 100g
Contains trans fats, modified maize starch and
wheat flour

Fruit

FRESH FRUIT

Once you have completed Induction and moved on to
Ongoing Weight Loss, you may start to add fruit other
than avocados, tomatoes and olives back into your diet.
Berries are relatively low in carbohydrates and thus are
among the first foods you'll be able to reintroduce into
your eating plan. Fresh fruit is always best, but pay
attention to portion size and buy small specimens
because a large apple or pear, for example, counts as
more than one serving.

When you start to add berries back into your diet, be
aware that you should do so cautiously. Keep your
portions small – you should be looking at a serving size
of 5 grams of carbs – to avoid loading up on carbs. Some
berries will be more appropriate for OWL than others, as
you will see from the listing below. If in doubt, always
weigh out a portion of fruit. Eventually you will become
accustomed to an appropriate visual serving size.

BERRIES

Blackberries (Phases 2–4)
5.1g carbs per 100 grams

Blueberries (Phases 2–4)
5g carbs per 100g

Cranberries (Phases 2–4)
7.6g carbs per 100g – raw

Gooseberries (Phases 2–4)
3g carbs per 100g

Loganberries (Phases 2–4)
5.1g carbs per 100g

Raspberries (Phases 2–4)
4.6g carbs per 100g

Redcurrants (Phases 2–4)
4.4g carbs per 100g

Strawberries (Phases 2–4)
6g carbs per 100g

CITRUS FRUITS

Clementines (Phases 3–4)
13.8g carbs per 100g

Grapefruit (Phases 3–4)
6.8g carbs per 100g

Grapefruit, Pink (Phases 3–4)
9.2g carbs per 100g

Kumquats (Phases 3–4)
15.9g carbs per100g

Lemon Juice (Phases 3–4)
2.5g carbs per 2 tablespoons

Lime Juice (Phases 3–4)
2.9g carbs per 2 tablespoons

Oranges (Phases 3–4)
8.5g carbs per 100g

Tangerines (Phases 3–4)
8g carbs per 100g

MELONS

Cantaloupe (Phases 3–4)
4.2g carbs per 100g

Galia (Phases 3–4)
5.6g carbs per 100g

Honeydew (Phases 3–4)
6.6g carbs per 100g

Watermelon (Phases 3–4)
7.1g carbs per 100g

TROPICAL FRUITS

Avocado, Haas (Phases 1–4)
0.5g carbs per 100g

Bananas (Phases 3–4)
20.9g carbs per 100g

Carambola (Star Fruit) (Phases 3–4)
7.8g carbs per 100g

Cherimoya (Phases 3–4)
17.7g carbs per 100g

Guava (Phases 3–4)
4.9g carbs per 100g

Kiwi (Phases 3–4)
10.3g carbs per 100g

Mango (Phases 3–4)
13.8g carbs per 100g

Papaya (Phases 3–4)
8.8g carbs per 100g

Passion fruit (Phases 3–4)
5.8g carbs per 100g

Pineapple (Phases 3–4)
10.1g carbs per 100g

Plantains (Phases 3–4)
31.9g carbs per 100g

STONE FRUITS

Apricots (Phases 3–4)
7.2g carbs per 100g

Cherries (Phases 3–4)
11.5g carbs per 100g

Nectarines (Phases 3–4)
9g carbs per 100g

Peaches (Phases 3–4)
7.6g carbs per 100g

Plums (Phases 3–4)
8.8g carbs per 100g

OTHER FRUITS

Apples, Cooking (Phases 3–4)
8.9g carbs per 100g

Apples, Eating (Phases 3–4)
11.8g carbs per 100g

Dates (Phases 3–4)
31.3g carbs per 100g

Figs (Phases 3–4)
48.6g carbs per 100g

Grapes, Green (Phases 3–4)
15.4g carbs per 100g

Grapes, Red (Phases 3–4)
15.4 g carbs per 100g

Loquats (Phases 3–4)
12.2g carbs per 100g

Lychees (Phases 3–4)
14.3g carbs per 100g

Pears (Phases 3–4)
15.1g carbs per 100g

Pears, Bosc (Phases 3–4)
12.9g carbs per 100g

Physalis (Cape Gooseberry) (Phases 3–4)
11g carbs per 100g

Pomegranate (Phases 3–4)
17.2g carbs per 100g

Quince (Phases 3–4)
15.3g carbs per 100g

Rhubarb (Phases 1–4)
0.8g carbs per 100g

TINNED & JARRED FRUIT

Thanks to advances in canning technology, tinned and jarred fruit can be as fresh as newly-picked fruit, but because it has been preserved in liquid it will lack bite. Avoid varieties that have been packed in syrup.

APPLES

John West Apple Slices (Phases 3–4)
5g carbs per 100g

⚠ **Morton Fruit Fillings Apple & Blackberry**
22.2g carbs per 100g
Contains added sugars and modified maize starch

⚠ **Morton Fruit Fillings Bramley Apple**
21.1g carbs per 100g
Contains added sugars and modified maize starch

Own Brand Apple Slices No Added Sugar (Phases 3–4)
7.8–9g carbs per 100g

APRICOTS

(FYI) Own Brand Apricot Halves in Fruit Juice (Phases 3–4)
8–10g carbs per 100g
Some may contain added sugars

BLACKBERRIES

⚠ Hartley's Blackberries in Apple Juice
8.2g carbs per 100g
Contains added sugars

⚠ John West Blackberries in Fruit Juice (Phases 2–4)
7.1g carbs per 100g
Contains added sugars

⚠ Own Brand Blackberries in Fruit Juice (Phases 2–4)
7–8.6g carbs per 100g
Contains added sugars

BLACKCURRANTS

⚠ Hartley's Blackcurrants in Apple Juice
9g carbs per 100g
Contains added sugars

(FYI) Own Brand Blackcurrants in Fruit Juice (Phases 3–4)
8–9.2g carbs per 100g
Some may contain added sugars

CHERRIES

⚠ **Hartley's Black Cherries in Apple Juice**
11.4g carbs per 100g
Contains added sugars

⚠ **Morton Red Cherry Fruit Fillings**
23.9g carbs per 100g
Contains added sugars and modified maize starch

⚠ **Own Brand Black Cherry Pie Filling**
17.7g carbs per 100g
Contains added sugars and modified maize starch

CITRUS FRUITS

Del Monte Mandarin Oranges Whole Segments in Own Juice (Phases 3–4)
10g carbs per 100g

Opies Sliced Lemons in Lemon Juice (Phases 3–4)
7.8g carbs per 100g

Own Brand Mandarin Segments in Fruit/Orange/Natural Juice (Phases 3–4)
7.7–10g carbs per 100g

FRUIT COCKTAIL

Del Monte Fruit Cocktail in Juice (Phases 3–4)
11.2g carbs per 100g

⚠ **Own Brand Fruit Cocktail in Fruit/Apple Juice**
10–12g carbs per 100g
Contains added sugars

GOOSEBERRIES

⚠ **Hartley's Gooseberries in Apple Juice**
9.4g carbs per 100g
Contains added sugars

GRAPEFRUIT

Del Monte Grapefruit Segments in Juice (Phases 3–4)
10.5g carbs per 100g

Own Brand Grapefruit Segments in Fruit/Natural Juice (Phases 3–4)
8.7–10g carbs per 100g

OLIVES, JARRED

Belazu Black Olives with Herbs (Phases 1–4)
5.8g carbs per 100g

Belazu Green Olives with Basil and Garlic (Phases 1–4)
1.6g carbs per 100g

Fora Domat Turkish Olives (Phases 1–4)
0.7g carbs per 100g

Karyatis Garlic Stuffed Olives in Extra Virgin Oil (Phases 1–4)
1g carbs per 100g

Karyatis Kalamata Olives in Extra Virgin Oil (Phases 1–4)
0.8g carbs per 100g

Karyatis Mixed Olives in Extra Virgin Oil (Phases 1–4)
0.8g carbs per 100g

FYI **McIlhenny Tabasco Spiced Spanish Olives (Phases 1–4)**
0.5g carbs per 100g
Contains MSG

Own Brand Black Olives (Phases 1–4)
3.3–6g carbs per 100g

Own Brand Green Olives (Phases 1–4)
3.6g carbs per 100g

Own Brand Green Olives Stuffed with Jalapeño Paste (Phases 1–4)
3.5g carbs per 100g

Own Brand Green Olives Stuffed with Pimento Paste (Phases 1–4)
3.5g carbs per 100g

OLIVES, TINNED

FYI **Own Brand Green Tinned Olives (Phases 1–4)**
Trace–0.6g carbs per 100g
Contains MSG

Own Brand Pitted Black Tinned Olives in Brine (Phases 1–4)
Trace–7g carbs per 100g

PEACHES

Del Monte Peach Slices in Juice (Phases 3–4)
11.2g carbs per 100g

⚠ Own Brand Peach Slices in Fruit/Grape Juice (Phases 3–4)
10–12g carbs per 100g
Contains added sugars

PEARS

Del Monte Pear Halves in Juice (Phases 3–4)
10.5g carbs per 100g

Own Brand Pear Halves/Quarters in Fruit/Natural/Pear Juice (Phases 3–4)
9–11g carbs per 100g

PINEAPPLE

Own Brand Pineapple Slices/Chunks in Natural/Pineapple Juice (Phases 3–4)
12–12.2g carbs per 100g

Princes Pineapple Crushed in Juice (Phases 3–4)
12.2g carbs per 100g

PRUNES

⚠ **Del Monte Prunes in Juice**
25g carbs per 100g
Contains added sugars

Own Brand Prunes in Fruit Juice (Phases 3–4)
19–25.7g carbs per 100g

RASPBERRIES

⚠ **Hartley's Raspberries in Apple Juice**
8.1g carbs per 100g
Contains added sugars

⚠ **John West Raspberries in Fruit Juice**
6.7g carbs per 100g
Contains added sugars

RHUBARB

Own Brand Rhubarb (Phases 1–4)
1–7g carbs per 100g

SUMMER FRUITS

⚠ **Hartley's Summer Fruits in Apple Juice**
8.6g carbs per 100g
Contains added sugars

⚠ **Morton Fruit Fillings Summer Fruits**
19g carbs per 100g
Contains added sugars and modified maize starch

DRIED FRUIT

Dried fruit should be regarded as an extra-special treat, as it only takes a few pieces to dramatically increase your carb count. Scatter a few pieces over yoghurt, cereal or a salad, but never be tempted to nibble dried fruit out of the packet!

APRICOTS

Humdinger Dried Chopped Apricots (Phases 3–4)
14.3g carbs per 25g serving

Sundora Mini Apricots (Phases 3–4)
9g carbs per 25g serving

COMPOTES & JELLIES

⚠ **Del Monte Fruitini, Strawberry Jelly with Peach Pieces**
18.4g carbs per 120g pot
Contains added sugars

⚠ **Hartley's Chunky Fruit Compote, Apple & Summer Fruit**
14.7g carbs per 95g pot
Contains added sugars

⚠ **Hartley's Smooth Fruit Compote**
14g carbs per 90g pouch
Contains added sugars

CURRANTS, SULTANAS & RAISINS

⚠ **Crazy Jack Organic Sultanas (Phases 3–4)**
17.3g carbs per 25g serving

⚠ **Crazy Jack Organic Sun-Dried Raisins
(Phases 3–4)**
17.2g carbs per 25g serving

Mixed Raisins (Phases 3–4)
21.4g carbs per 30g bag

Own Brand Currants (Phases 3–4)
17g carbs per 25g serving

Own Brand Raisins (Phases 3–4)
16–18g carbs per 25g serving

Raisins & Apricots (Phases 3–4)
18.2g carbs per 30g bag

⚠ **Whitworths Luxury Dried Mixed Fruit**
16.3g carbs per 25g serving
Contains added sugars

DATES

Humdinger Dried Stone-out Dates (Phases 3–4)
18g carbs per 25g serving

⚠ **Whitworths Chopped Dates**
17.2g carbs per 25g serving
Contains added sugars

Whitworths Chopped Dates and Walnuts
14g carbs per 25g serving
Contains added sugars

FRUIT FLAKES

 Fruit Bowl Fruit Flakes, Blackcurrant
19.9g carbs per 25g serving
Contains added sugars

 Fruit Bowl Fruit Flakes, Strawberry
19.9g carbs per 25g serving
Contains added sugars

 Fruit Bowl Fruit Flakes, Strawberry with Yoghurt Coating
18.2g carbs per 25g serving
Contains added sugars and trans fats

 Fruit Bowl Fruit Flakes, Tropical
20g carbs per 25g serving
Contains added sugars

MIXED

Del Monte Fruit Express No Added Sugar Peach & Pear Pieces in Fruit Juice (Phases 3–4)
20g carbs per 185g pot

Del Monte Fruit Express No Added Sugar Tropical Mixed Fruit in Juice (Phases 3–4)
20.7g carbs per 185g pot

Del Monte Fruit in Juice, Mixed Fruit Pieces in Fruit Juice (Phases 3–4)
14.4 carbs per 120g pot

Whitworths Dried Fruit Salad (Phases 3–4)
10g carbs per 25g serving

OTHERS

 Fruit Bowl School Bars, Strawberry
16.6g carbs per 20g serving
Contains added sugars

 Humdinger Stem Ginger
21g carbs per 25g serving
Contains added sugars

Own Brand Desiccated Coconut (Phases 1–4)
1.6g carbs per 25g serving

 Sundora Apple Slices
13.6g carbs per 25g serving
Contains added sugars

 Sundora Mini Pineapple pieces
22.2g carbs per 25g serving
Contains added sugars

Sundora Mini Prunes (Phases 3–4)
8.5g carbs per 25g serving

 Whitworths Honey Coated Banana Chips
15g carbs per 25g serving
Contains added sugars

FROZEN FRUIT

Frozen fruit is higher in carbohydrates than fresh fruit. When frozen foods thaw, ice crystals rupture the cell walls, so water escapes. With less water, other nutrients, including carbohydrates, are concentrated.

As frozen fruits may be sweetened, make sure the product you purchase is unsweetened. Look for the words 'unsweetened', 'sugar-free' or 'no-added-sugar' on the label, and examine the ingredients list for sugar in all its forms, including fruit juice concentrate.

Blackberries (Phases 2–4)
10.6g carbs per 100g

Blueberries (Phases 2–4)
9.4g carbs per 100g

Cranberries (Phases 2–4)
7.6g carbs per 100g

Raspberries (Phases 2–4)
10g carbs per 100g

Shearway Black Forest Fruits (Phases 2–4)
10.9g carbs per 100g

Shearway Luxury Fruit Salad with Camarosa Strawberries (Phases 2–4)
10g carbs per 100g

Shearway Raspberries (Phases 2–4)
4.6g carbs per 100g

⚠ **Shearway Organic Raspberries (Phases 2–4)**
4.6g carbs per 100g

Shearway Summer Fruits (Phases 3–4)
6.9g carbs per 100g

Strawberries, whole (Phases 2–4)
7g carbs per 100g

International Foods

A wonderful feature of the modern supermarket is the sheer variety of food available to choose from. Nowhere is this better reflected than in the international aisles: Asian, Indian, Caribbean, Tex-Mex and Mexican ... the list goes on. Every element you need to create an authentic meal is on hand, as well as the snacks and condiments to add the final touches to a delicious dinner.

While some of these products are acceptable when you're doing Atkins, in general you need to approach them with caution. Many contain added sugars that make them unacceptable no matter which phase you're in. Others are full of trans fats, refined white flour and cornflour. Examine the nutritional information on the packaging carefully to ensure that you aren't consuming forbidden ingredients.

To make it as easy as possible to gather together everything you need for a delicious international dinner, we have divided this section first into cuisines and then further into the following categories:

Ingredients	Components you use when you are cooking from scratch, such as fish sauce or coconut milk
Cooking sauces	Ready-made sauces in which you cook the main ingredient (such as meat, poultry, fish or seafood) to transform it into an international meal

Condiments   Things you put on the side of
                          your plate to enhance the meal,
                          as you would with mustard or
                          mayonnaise

Accompaniments   All the things that go together
                          with a main dish – for example,
                          soup, seaweed, taco shells or
                          chapattis

It's worth noting that fresh sauces often contain more
acceptable ingredients than jarred ones. Or why not
consider making your own? It's not as time-consuming
or complicated as you might imagine!

- Roast peppers in the oven (or, if you are in a hurry,
  open a jar instead) then blend in a food processor
  with a tin of chopped tomatoes to produce a
  delicious sauce. This freezes very well, so prepare a
  large batch to make it worth your while.
- Mix whole-milk Greek yogurt with a handful of
  finely chopped fresh mint, coriander and parsley, a
  finely chopped clove of garlic and a teaspoon of
  korma spice mix for a delicious quick mild curry
  cooking sauce that contains very few carbs.
- Quickly blend a teaspoon of pesto in a food
  processor with 125g butter, a clove of garlic, a small
  handful of flat-leaf parsley and freshly ground black
  pepper. Place in the refrigerator for 30 minutes. A
  teaspoon of this tasty herb butter on top of a piece
  of grilled steak, chicken or fish makes a delicious
  quick sauce. Place any leftover herb butter into ice-
  cube trays and freeze.
- A few ready-made curry pastes are acceptable on
  Atkins and make delicious sauces when added to

whole-milk natural yogurt or coconut milk. Curry pastes can also be used sparingly on meat or fish before grilling.

- For a delicious Thai marinade for meat or fish, place a small handful of finely chopped coriander, 1 teaspoon of grated fresh ginger, 1 tablespoon of lime juice, a finely chopped red chilli and 250ml vegetable oil in a screw-top jar. Shake well to mix together and leave to stand for 30 minutes. A few tablespoons of the marinade can also be poured over chopped peppers before roasting to give them a delicious Thai flavour.

In this chapter, we have deviated from our usual 100g/100ml-only listings to give carb counts for portion sizes in certain cases.

ASIAN (CHINESE, JAPANESE, THAI)

Fish sauce is common in Thailand (where it's called *nam pla*) and Vietnam (where it's called *nuoc nam*). It is a pungent, salty condiment made from fermented fish. Major brands contain added sugars.

INGREDIENTS

Bart Coconut Cream (Phases 2–4)
3.4g carbs per 100ml

FYI **Bart Coconut Milk (Phases 3–4)**
1.6g carbs per 100ml
Contains cornflour

Bart Creamed Coconut (Phases 2–4)
22.6g carbs per 100g

(FYI) **Bart Organic Coconut Milk (Phases 3–4)**
⚠ 1.5g carbs per 100ml
Contains cornflour

(FYI) **Bart Reduced Fat Coconut Milk (Phases 3–4)**
3.6g carbs per 100ml
Contains cornflour

⚠ **Blue Dragon Fish Sauce Nam Pla**
1.5g carbs per 5ml serving, 30.9g carbs per 100ml
Contains added sugars

Blue Dragon Silken Tofu (Phases 1–4)
2.4g carbs per 100g

⚠ **Legend Organics Desiccated Coconut (Phases 2–4)**
11.1g carbs per 100g

⚠ **Sharwood's Oyster Sauce**
3.4g carbs per 25g serving, 13.6g carbs per 100g
Contains added sugars and wheat flour

⚠ **Sharwood's Plum Sauce**
14.8g carbs per 25g serving, 59.4g carbs per 100g
Contains added sugars and modified cornflour

⚠ **Tom Yum Soup Paste**
1g carbs per 15g serving, 6.6g carbs per 100g
Contains trans fats and MSG

⚠ **Wing Yip Super Grade Oyster Sauce**
4g carbs per 17g serving, 23.8g carbs per 100g
Contains added sugars, modified starch, MSG and wheat flour

World Harbors Maui Mountain Hawaiian Style Teriyaki Sauce & Marinade
5.2g carbs per 10g serving, 52g carbs per 100g
Contains added sugars

COOKING SAUCES

 Blue Dragon Stir Fry Teriyaki Sauce
28.6g carbs per 100g
Contains added sugars, modified maize starch and wheat flour

 Go Organic Mild Thai Curry Sauce with Lime & Coconut
6.2g carbs per 100g
Contains added sugars

 Go Organic Thai Green Curry Sauce with Coriander & Lime
6.3g carbs per 100g
Contains added sugars

Go Organic Thai Red Curry Sauce with Galangal and Red Chilli (Phases 2–4)
5.5g carbs per 100g

Loyd Grossman Red Thai Curry Sauce
13.7g carbs per 100g
Contains added sugars and modified maize starch

Sharwoods Black Bean Stir Fry Base
16.8g carbs per 100g
Contains added sugars, modified cornflour and wheat flour

⚠ **Sharwoods Spicy Tomato Szechuan Stir Fry Base**
17.4g carbs per 100g
Contains added sugars, modified cornflour and wheat flour

⚠ **Sharwood's Wok Soy**
5.6g carbs per 25g serving, 22.4g carbs per 100g
Contains added sugars and modified starch

⚠ **Wing Yip Vegetarian Mushroom Sauce**
4.2g carbs per 17g serving, 24.7g carbs per 100g
Contains added sugars, modified starch and wheat flour

CONDIMENTS
Chilli Sauce

 Amoy Chilli Sauce (Phases 3–4)
1.3g carbs per 25g serving, 5.2g carbs per 100g
Contains modified starch

⚠ **Lemon Myrtle Chilli Sauce**
8g carbs per 30g serving, 27g carbs per 100g
Contains added sugars and modified starch

⚠ **Namjai Dipping Chilli Sauce**
12g carbs per 25g serving, 48g carbs per 100g
Contains added sugars

Nando's Hot Peri-Peri Sauce (Phases 1–4)
1.7g carbs per 25g serving, 6.7g carbs per 100g

⚠ Sharwood's Sweet Chilli Sauce
10.9g carbs per 25g serving, 43.7g carbs per 100g
Contains added sugars

⚠ Sharwood's Thai Chilli Sauce
9.7g carbs per 25g serving, 39.1g carbs per 100g
Contains added sugars and modified cornflour

⚠ Wing Yip Sweet Chilli Sauce
7.9g carbs per 17g serving, 46.5g carbs per 100g
Contains added sugars

Soy Sauce

Soy sauce can be made with soya beans, wheat or barley. The key to choosing a top-quality product is to look for the word 'fermented' on the label. Other soy sauces are chemically processed and have an unpleasant, harsh taste. Soy sauce is extremely high in sodium, so we recommend using reduced-sodium soy sauce. Tamari is a Japanese soy sauce similar to Chinese sauces. Be wary of added sweeteners, such as molasses, in soy sauce.

⚠ Amoy Dark Soy Sauce
2g carbs per 10g serving, 20g carbs per 100g
Contains added sugars and wheat flour

⚠ Amoy Light Soy Sauce
0.7g carbs per 10g serving, 7.5g carbs per 100g
Contains added sugars and wheat flour

⚠ Amoy Reduced Salt Soy Sauce
1g carbs per 10g serving, 10g carbs per 100g
Contains added sugars and wheat flour

ⓕⓨⓘ Sanchi Organic Shoyu Soy Sauce (Phases 3–4)
⚠ 0.7g carbs per 10g serving, 7.1g carbs per 100g
Contains wheat flour

Others

Wasabi paste (the green condiment served alongside pickled ginger with sushi) is a fiery Japanese condiment made from horseradish.

Hoisin is a thick, tangy sauce made of fermented soya beans. Check the ingredients list carefully. Most brands have sugar, syrup or water as the first ingredient but keep looking until you find a brand with soya beans first and no added sugar.

⚠ **Hot Oz Green Devil Wasabi Sauce**
4.3g carbs per 30g serving, 14.3g carbs per 100g
Contains added sugars and modified starch

⚠ **Sharwood's Hoi-Sin Sauce**
12.3g carbs per 25g serving, 49.5g carbs per 100g
Contains added sugars

ACCOMPANIMENTS

⚠ **Blue Dragon Crispy Seaweed**
19.2g carbs per 100g
Contains added sugars

⚠ **Blue Dragon Wonton Soup**
2g carbs per 100g
Contains added sugars, MSG and wheat flour

INDIAN

INGREDIENTS

FYI **Discovery Soured Cream (Phases 3–4)**
5.4g carbs per 100g
Contains modified maize starch

Namjai Green Curry Paste (Phases 2–4)
20g carbs per 100g

Namjai Red Curry Paste (Phases 2–4)
20g carbs per 100g

⚠ **Patak's Original Balti Curry Paste Tomato &
Coriander**
17.2g carbs per 100g
Contains added sugars, gram flour and maize flour

⚠ **Patak's Original Jalfrezi Curry Paste**
13.5g carbs per 100g
Contains added sugars and maize starch

⚠ **Patak's Original Korma Curry Paste Coconut
& Coriander**
11.6g carbs per 100g serving
Contains added sugars and maize flour

FYI **Patak's Original Madras Curry Paste Cumin &
Chilli (Phases 3–4)**
21.6g carbs per 100g
Contains maize flour

⚠ **Patak's Original Rogan Josh Curry Paste Tomato & Paprika**
12.7g carbs per 100g
Contains added sugars

Patak's Original Tandoori Curry Paste Tamarind & Ginger (Phases 2–4)
23.1g carbs per 100g

⚠ **Patak's Original Tikka Masala Curry Paste Coriander & Lemon**
16.7g carbs per 100g
Contains added sugars and maize starch

🆗 **Patak's Original Vindaloo Curry Paste Tamarind & Chilli (Phases 3–4)**
16g carbs per 100g
Contains maize flour

⚠ **Patak's Raita Spicy Tomato & Onion**
13.3g carbs per 100g
Contains added sugars, trans fats and modified maize starch

⚠ **Patak's Raita Yoghurt, Cucumber and Mint**
8.4g carbs per 100g
Contains added sugars

Sharwood's Vegetable Ghee (Phases 1–4)
Trace carbs per 100g

COOKING SAUCES

⚠ **Go Organic Jalfrezi Curry Sauce with Bell Pepper, Tomato & Coriander (Phases 2–4)**
4.3g carbs per 100g

⚠ **Homepride 97% Fat Free Balti**
9.1g carbs per 100g
Contains added sugars and cornflour

⚠ **Homepride 98% Fat Free Curry**
10g carbs per 100g
Contains added sugars and cornflour

⚠ **Homepride 95% Fat Free Korma**
10.6g carbs per 100g
Contains added sugars and cornflour

⚠ **Homepride 95% Fat Free Tikka Masala**
10g carbs per 100g
Contains added sugars and cornflour

⚠ **Loyd Grossman Jalfrezi Curry Sauce**
8.2g carbs per 100g
Contains added sugars and modified maize starch

⚠ **Loyd Grossman Madras Curry Sauce**
6.8g carbs per 100g
Contains added sugars

⚠ **Loyd Grossman Rogan Josh Curry Sauce**
10.5g carbs per 100g
Contains added sugars

⚠ **Patak's Original Madras Cumin & Chilli Sauce**
7.6g carbs per 100g
Contains added sugars and modified maize starch

⚠ **Patak's Original Rogan Josh Curry Paste with Tomato & Paprika**
12.7g carbs per 100g
Contains added sugars

⚠ **Patak's Original Rogan Josh Tomato & Cardamom Sauce**
9.4g carbs per 100g
Contains added sugars and modified maize starch

⚠ **Patak's Original Tikka Masala Lemon & Coriander Sauce**
6.2g carbs per 100g
Contains added sugars and modified maize starch

Ⓕ**Ⓨ**Ⓘ **Patak's Original Vindaloo Curry Paste with Tamarind & Chilli (Phases 3–4)**
3.5g carbs per 100g
Contains maize flour

⚠ **Sharwoods Bundh Pasanda Oven Sauce**
12.4g carbs per 100g
Contains added sugars and modified cornflour

⚠ **Sharwoods Dhansak Cooking Sauce**
11.1g carbs per 100g
Contains added sugars and modified cornflour

⚠ **Sharwoods Jalfrezi Cooking Sauce**
8.1g carbs per 100g
Contains added sugars and modified cornflour

Sharwoods Madras Cooking Sauce
9.7g carbs per 100g
Contains added sugars and modified cornflour

 Sharwoods Tikka Masala Cooking Sauce
10.4g carbs per 100g
Contains added sugars and modified cornflour

**Shere Khan Restaurant Balti Sauce
(Phases 2–4)**
3.9g carbs per 100g

**Shere Khan Restaurant Karahi Sauce
(Phases 2–4)**
3.9g carbs per 100g

**Shere Khan Restaurant Madras Sauce
(Phases 2–4)**
3.8g carbs per 100g

CONDIMENTS

△ Patak's Original Brinjal Aubergine Pickle
10.4g carbs per 30g serving, 34.6g carbs per 100g
Contains added sugars

Patak's Original Lime Pickle (Phases 1–4)
1.2g carbs per 30g serving, 4g carbs per 100g

△ Patak's Premium Mango Chutney Mild
22g carbs per 35g serving, 62.8g carbs per 100g
Contains added sugars

⚠ **Sharwood's Bengal Spice Mango Chutney**
14.5g carbs per 25g serving, 58g carbs per 100g
Contains added sugars and modified cornflour

⚠ **Sharwood's Green Label Mango Chutney**
14.4g carbs per 25g serving, 57.8g carbs per 100g
Contains added sugars

⚠ **Sharwood's Green Label Spreadable Chutney**
12.4g carbs per 25g serving, 49.8g carbs per 100g
Contains added sugars

⚠ **Sharwood's Lime Pickle**
3.7g carbs per 25g serving, 15g carbs per 100g
Contains added sugars

⚠ **Sharwood's Sweet Major Grey Mango Chutney**
13.2g carbs per 25g serving, 52.9g carbs per 100g
Contains added sugars

⚠ **Sharwood's Tropical Lime Mango Chutney**
12.6g carbs per 25g serving, 50.5g carbs per 100g
Contains added sugars

ACCOMPANIMENTS

Chapattis

Patak's Original Chapatti Wraps (Phases 3–4)
17.9g carbs per chapatti

Poppadoms (Ready-to-Eat)

**Sharwoods Indian Garlic and Coriander
Puppodums (Phases 2–4)**
4.7g carbs per poppadom

Sharwoods Indian Mildly Spiced Puppodums (Phases 2–4)
4.4g carbs per poppadom

Sharwoods Indian Plain Puppodums (Phases 2–4)
4.9g carbs per poppadom

Poppadoms (Require Cooking)

Patak's Original Pappadums Garlic (Phases 2–4)
4.4g carbs per poppadom

Patak's Original Pappadums Plain (Phases 2–4)
4.32g carbs per poppadom

Sharwoods Indian Garlic and Green Chilli Pappads (Phases 2–4)
5.41g carbs per poppadom

Sharwoods Indian Plain Puppodums (Phases 2–4)
5.25g carbs per poppadom

CARIBBEAN

COOKING SAUCES

⚠ Encona Jamaican Jerk Sauce
1.3g carbs per 5ml serving, 27.1g carbs per 100ml
Contains added sugars and cornflour

⚠ **English Provender Co More Than a Marinade, Cajun Spice**
15.3g carbs per 100g
Contains added sugars

⚠ **Uncle Ben's Cajun Sauce**
8.4g carbs per 100g
Contains added sugars and modified maize starch

CONDIMENTS

Discovery Jalapeños Chillies (Phases 1–4)
0.8g carbs per 25g serving, 3.4g carbs per 100g

⚠ **Discovery Red Jalapeños**
4.1g carbs per 25g serving, 16.4g carbs per 100g
Contains added sugars

Encona Cajun Hot Pepper Sauce (Phases 1–4)
Trace carbs per 5ml serving, 0.4g carbs per 100ml

FYI **Encona West Indian Original Hot Pepper Sauce – Scotch Bonnet Peppers (Phases 3–4)**
0.5g carbs per 5ml serving, 10g carbs per 100ml
Contains cornflour

FYI **Encona West Indian Smooth Hot Pepper Sauce with Papaya (Phases 3–4)**
0.3g carbs per 5ml serving, 6g carbs per 100ml
Contains cornflour

⚠ **Old El Paso Original Salsa Hot**
6g carbs per 100g
Contains added sugars

Old El Paso Original Salsa Mild
6g carbs per 100g
Contains added sugars

Old El Paso Sliced Jalapeños (Phases 1–4)
0.8g carbs per 25g serving, 3.4g carbs per 100g

 Peppadew Piquante Pepper Ketchup
9.3g carbs per 25g serving, 37.4g carbs per 100g
Contains added sugars and modified starch

ACCOMPANIMENTS

Grace Green Pigeon Peas (Phases 3–4)
21.2g carbs per 100g

Sea Isle Gunga Peas (Phases 3–4)
19.3g carbs per 100g

TEX-MEX & MEXICAN

INGREDIENTS

 Discovery Jalapeño & Lime Instant Marinade
15.4g carbs per 100g
Contains added sugars

 **Discovery Roasted Cumin & Coriander
Instant Marinade**
32.3g carbs per 100g
Contains added sugars

 Newman's Own Creamy Cajun Marinade
6.3g carbs per 100g
Contains added sugars and modified maize starch

⚠ **Newman's Own Mustard & Honey Marinade**
23.9g carbs per 100g
Contains added sugars

⚠ **Newman's Own Sticky BBQ Marinade**
32.6g carbs per 100g
Contains added sugars and modified maize starch

⚠ **Old El Paso Spice Mix for Chilli**
57g carbs per 100g
Contains added sugars and wheat flour

⚠ **Old El Paso Spice Mix for Fajitas**
54g carbs per 100g
Contains added sugars

⚠ **Old El Paso Spice Mix for Tacos**
69g carbs per 100g
Contains added sugars and wheat flour

COOKING SAUCES

⚠ **Discovery Buffalo Wings Sauce**
8.8g carbs per 100g
Contains added sugars and modified maize starch

⚠ **Discovery Hot & Smoky BBQ Sauce**
8.5g carbs per 100g
Contains added sugars and modified maize starch

⚠ **Discovery Louisiana Cajun Chicken Seasoning & Sauce**
14.7g carbs per 100g
Contains added sugars and modified maize starch

⚠ **Discovery Mexican Chilli Con Carne Seasoning & Sauce**
17.6g carbs per 100g
Contains added sugars and modified maize starch

⚠ **Discovery Rio Grande Mexican Recipe Sauce**
12.3g carbs per 100g
Contains added sugars and modified maize starch

⚠ **Discovery Stir Fry Californian Creamy Cajun Sauce**
12.2g carbs per 100g
Contains added sugars and modified maize starch

⚠ **Discovery Texan Fajitas Seasoning & Sauce**
13.2g carbs per 100g
Contains added sugars and modified maize starch

⚠ **Homepride Medium Chilli Sauce**
10.4g carbs per 100g
Contains added sugars and cornflour

⚠ **Hot Oz Three Cs Hot Sauce**
61.3g carbs per 100g
Contains added sugars and modified maize starch

⚠ **Nando's Hot Peri-Peri Marinade**
12.84g carbs per 100g
Contains added sugars and modified cornflour

ACCOMPANIMENTS

⚠ **Discovery Gluten Free Corn Tortillas**
8.6g carbs per tortilla
Contains added sugars

Discovery Spicy Refried Beans (Phases 3–4)
11.9g carbs per 100g

(FYI) **Old El Paso Crunchy Taco Shells (Phases 3–4)**
6.86g carbs per shell
Contains cornflour

Old El Paso Refried Beans
16.1g carbs per 100g

(FYI) **Old El Paso Taco Nachips (Phases 3–4)**
61g carbs per 100g
Contains cornflour

(FYI) **Old El Paso Taco Shells (Phases 3–4)**
6.7g carbs per 11g shell, 61g carbs per 100g
Contains cornflour

AFRICAN

COOKING SAUCES

⚠ **Ukuva iAfrica Malawi Gold African Curry Sauce**
12.5g carbs per 100g
Contains added sugars

⚠ **Zulu Spicy BBQ Fire Sauce with Sweet Potato & Fire Roasted Tomato**
7.4g carbs per 100g
Contains added sugars

Meat and Poultry

Meat and poultry are two of the most important sources of protein when you're doing Atkins. Whether you choose fresh, tinned or cured meat, it's important to pay attention to portion sizes because if you fill up on meat, you won't be hungry enough to eat vegetables, which are an equally important source of vitamins and minerals.

Few of us have the time to use an independent butcher, preferring instead to buy meat and poultry from the supermarket. This development has, in turn, heralded the demise of the traditional butcher's shop, which is no longer a fixture of every high street. Because of the increase in demand, the quality of supermarket meat has improved greatly over the past few years, with traceability becoming an important issue. Fresh meat can be bought either from the butcher's counter or from chilled cabinets, where prepacked cuts are available.

Fresh meat is expensive in the UK, but a little can go a long way. Don't ignore cheaper cuts, which can be cooked slowly to produce mouth-wateringly tender casseroles and stews. Cold and cured meats – the sugar-free varieties of course – make ideal and portable lunches or snacks.

In the case of products that contain naturally occurring carbs where you would expect to see a zero rating, we have drawn your attention to them with a FYI icon **FYI**. For further information turn to page 126 in the Listings Section introduction.

FRESH MEAT AND POULTRY

MEAT
Beef

Blade Bone (Phases 1–4)
0g carbs per 100g

Brisket (Phases 1–4)
0g carbs per 100g

Chuck Steak (Phases 1–4)
0g carbs per 100g

Fillet (Phases 1–4)
0g carbs per 100g

Flank (Phases 1–4)
0g carbs per 100g

Forerib (Phases 1–4)
0g carbs per 100g

Ground or Minced (Phases 1–4)
0g carbs per 100g

Neck, Clod or Sticking (Phases 1–4)
0g carbs per 100g

Rump (Phases 1–4)
0g carbs per 100g

Shin (Phases 1–4)
0g carbs per 100g

Silverside (Phases 1–4)
0g carbs per 100g

Sirloin (Phases 1–4)
0g carbs per 100g

Skirt (Phases 1–4)
0g carbs per 100g

Top Rump (Phases 1–4)
0g carbs per 100g

Topside (Phases 1–4)
0g carbs per 100g

Veal

Belly (Phases 1–4)
0g carbs per 100g

Loin (Phases 1–4)
0g carbs per 100g

Neck (Phases 1–4)
0g carbs per 100g

Rump (Phases 1–4)
0g carbs per 100g

Shin (Phases 1–4)
0g carbs per 100g

Shoulder (Phases 1–4)
0g carbs per 100g

Silverside (Phases 1–4)
0g carbs per 100g

Top Rump (Phases 1–4)
0g carbs per 100g

Topside (Phases 1–4)
0g carbs per 100g

Lamb

Best End (Phases 1–4)
0g carbs per 100g

Breast (Phases 1–4)
0g carbs per 100g

Chump (Phases 1–4)
0g carbs per 100g

Chump Chops (Phases 1–4)
0g carbs per 100g

Fillet (Phases 1–4)
0g carbs per 100g

Leg (Phases 1–4)
0g carbs per 100g

Leg Steaks (Phases 1–4)
0g carbs per 100g

Loin (Phases 1–4)
0g carbs per 100g

Middle End (Phases 1–4)
0g carbs per 100g

Saddle (Phases 1–4
0g carbs per 100g

Scrag End (Phases 1–4)
0g carbs per 100g

Shoulder (Phases 1–4)
0g carbs per 100g

Shoulder Chops (Phases 1–4)
0g carbs per 100g

Pork

Bath Chaps (Phases 1–4)
0g carbs per 100g

Blade (Phases 1–4)
0g carbs per 100g

Knuckle (Phases 1–4)
0g carbs per 100g

Leg (Phases 1–4)
0g carbs per 100g

Loin Best End (Phases 1–4)
0g carbs per 100g

Loin Chops (Phases 1–4)
0g carbs per 100g

Neck (Phases 1–4)
0g carbs per 100g

Shoulder (Phases 1–4)
0g carbs per 100g

Spare Rib Chops (Phases 1–4)
0g carbs per 100g

Spare Rib Joint (Phases 1–4)
0g carbs per 100g

Spare Ribs (Phases 1–4)
0g carbs per 100g

Steaks (Phases 1–4)
0g carbs per 100g

Tenderloin (Phases 1–4)
0g carbs per 100g

Offal

Calves' Kidney (Phases 1–4)
0g carbs per 100g

Calves' Liver (Phases 1–4)
0g carbs per 100g

Lambs' Heart (Phases 1–4)
0g carbs per 100g

Lambs' Kidney (Phases 1–4)
0g carbs per 100g

Lambs' Liver (Phases 1–4)
0g carbs per 100g

Lambs' Sweetbreads (Phases 1–4)
0g carbs per 100g

Marrow Bones (Phases 1–4)
0g carbs per 100g

Ox Kidney (Phases 1–4)
0g carbs per 100g

Ox Liver (Phases 1–4)
0g carbs per 100g

Ox Tongue (Phases 1–4)
0g carbs per 100g

Oxtail (Phases 1–4)
0g carbs per 100g

Pigs' Head (Phases 1–4)
0g carbs per 100g

Pigs' Kidneys (Phases 1–4)
0g carbs per 100g

Pigs' Liver (Phases 1–4)
0g carbs per 100g

Pigs' Trotters (Phases 1–4)
0g carbs per 100g

Pork Belly (Phases 1–4)
0g carbs per 100g

Tripe (Phases 1–4)
2g carbs per 100g

Veal Sweetbreads (Phases 1–4)
0g carbs per 100g

Game

Goat (Phases 1–4)
0g carbs per 100g

Hare (Phases 1–4)
0g carbs per 100g

Rabbit (Phases 1–4)
0g carbs per 100g

Venison (Phases 1–4)
0g carbs per 100g

POULTRY

Chicken

Breasts (Phases 1–4)
0g carbs per 100g

Drumsticks (Phases 1–4)
0g carbs per 100g

Thighs (Phases 1–4)
0g carbs per 100g

Wings (Phases 1–4)
0g carbs per 100g

Turkey

Breasts (Phases 1–4)
0g carbs per 100g

Drumsticks (Phases 1–4)
0g carbs per 100g

Minced (Phases 1–4)
0g carbs per 100g

Wings (Phases 1–4)
0g carbs per 100g

Whole (Phases 1–4)
0g carbs per 100g

Duck

Breasts (Phases 1–4)
0g carbs per 100g

Whole (Phases 1–4)
0g carbs per 100g

Game

Goose (Phases 1–4)
0g carbs per 100g

Guinea Fowl (Phases 1–4)
0g carbs per 100g

Ostrich (Phases 1–4)
0g carbs per 100g

Pheasant (Phases 1–4)
0g carbs per 100g

TINNED MEAT & POULTRY

Your Atkins storecupboard should always include tinned meat, so that you are never caught short. Many tinned meats are ideal while on Atkins, but don't be lulled into a false sense of security: be on the lookout for added sugars and nitrates, trans fats, MSG and other unsavoury ingredients lurking in tinned stews and casseroles.

BEEF

Corned Beef

⚠ **Fray Bentos Corned Beef**
0.8g carbs per 100g
Contains added sugars and nitrates

⚠ **Own Brand Corned Beef**
1g carbs per 100g
Contains added sugars and nitrates

(FYI) **Princes Corned Beef and Onion Paste (Phases 1–4)**
2.8g carbs per 100g
Contains nitrates

⚠ **Princes Delicious Corned Beef Hash**
5.1g carbs per 100g
Contains added sugars and nitrates

⚠ **Princes Lean Corned Beef**
1g carbs per 100g
Contains added sugars and nitrates

Shippam's Corned Beef and Onion (Phases 1–4)
2.8g carbs per 100g

Beef & Stews

⚠ **Own Brand Irish Stew**
5.9–7g carbs per 100g
Contains added sugars, trans fats, modified maize starch and wheat flour

⚠ **Own Brand Minced Beef & Onions**
2.8–3.1g carbs per 100g
Contains added sugars, trans fats, cornflour and wheat flour

⚠ **Own Brand Stewed Steak**
1.6–4.5g carbs per 100g
Contains added sugars, cornflour and wheat flour

⚠ **Princes Chunky Premium Lean Steak**
3g carbs per 100g
Contains added sugars and wheat flour

(FYI) **Princes Full Flavour Beef 'n' Beer (Phases 3–4)**
5.5g carbs per 100g
Contains cornflour and wheat flour

⚠ **Princes Goulash**
5g carbs per 100g
Contains added sugars, modified cornflour and wheat flour

⚠ **Princes Minced Beef with Onions in Gravy**
5.5g carbs per 100g
Contains added sugars, modified flour and wheat
flour

⚠ **Princes Premium Lean Steak**
3g carbs per 100g
Contains added sugars and wheat flour

⚠ **Princes Rich & Tasty Beef in Red Wine**
5g carbs per 100g
Contains added sugars, modified cornflour and
wheat flour

FYI **Princes Slices of Beef in Gravy (Phases 3–4)**
2g carbs per 100g
Contains wheat flour

FYI **Princes Succulent Steak and Kidney
(Phases 3–4)**
4g carbs per 100g
Contains cornflour, MSG and wheat flour

FYI **Princes Tender Stewed Steak (Phases 3–4)**
3.1g carbs per 100g
Contains cornflour and wheat flour

⚠ **Stagg Classic Chili Con Carne**
8.6g carbs per 100g
Contains added sugars and cornflour

⚠ **Stagg Dynamite Hot Chili Con Carne**
9.6g carbs per 100g
Contains added sugars and cornflour

⚠ **Stagg Silverado Beef Chili Con Carne**
10.9g carbs per 100g
Contains added sugars, cornflour and modified starch

Hamburgers

⚠ **Goblin Hamburgers**
4.6g carbs per 100g
Contains added sugars and wheat flour

Meat Balls

⚠ **Campbell's Meat Balls in 'Brilliant' Bolognese Sauce**
12.1g carbs per 100g
Contains added sugars, cornflour and wheat flour

⚠ **Campbell's Meat Balls in 'Gorgeous' Gravy**
9.6g carbs per 100g
Contains added sugars, cornflour, MSG and wheat flour

⚠ **Campbell's Meat Balls in 'Tasty' Tomato Sauce**
11.6g carbs per 100g
Contains added sugars, cornflour and wheat flour

CHICKEN

John West Chicken Light Lunch French Style (Phases 2–4)
6.7g carbs per 100g

⚠ **John West Chicken Light Lunch Italian Style**
9.6g carbs per 100g
Contains added sugars

🄵🄸 **Princes Chicken Roll (Phases 3–4)**
12.5g carbs per 100g
Contains MSG

🄵🄸 **Princes Chicken Roll with Sage & Onion (Phases 3–4)**
12.5g carbs per 100g
Contains MSG

Shippam's Chicken Spread (Phases 1–4)
2.2g carbs per 100g

⚠ **Stagg Less Than 3% Fat Chicken Grande**
10.2g carbs per 100g
Contains added sugars, modified starch and wheat flour

HAM

⚠ **Own Brand Ham**
0.2g carbs per 100g
Contains added sugars and nitrates

🄵🄸 **Princes Bacon Grill (Phases 3–4)**
11g carbs per 100g
Contains nitrates and wheat starch

⚠ **Princes Ham**
2g carbs per 100g
Contains added sugars and nitrates

PASTES & SPREADS

(FYI) La Piara Paté with Provence Herbs (Phases 1–4)
1g carbs per 100g
Contains MSG and nitrates

⚠ Princes Chicken and Ham Paste
4.5g carbs per 100g
Contains trans fats and nitrates

(FYI) Princes Ham and Beef Paste (Phases 2–4)
3.7g carbs per 100g
Contains nitrates

Shippam's Beef Spread (Phases 1–4)
3g carbs per 100g

Shippam's Chicken Spread (Phases 1–4)
2.2g carbs per 100g

⚠ Shippam's Classic Lamb and Mint Paté
2.9g carbs per 100g
Contains added sugars

PORK

⚠ Own Brand Pork and Ham
2.2g carbs per 100g
Contains added sugars and nitrates

(FYI) PEK Braised Pork Kidneys in Gravy (Phases 3–4)
4g carbs per 100g
Contains modified starch and wheat flour

(FYI) **PEK Chopped Pork (Phases 1–4)**
1.8g carbs per 100g
Contains nitrates

⚠ **Princes Pork Luncheon Meat**
7.4g carbs per 100g
Contains added sugars, nitrates and wheat starch

⚠ **Spam Lite**
2.1g carbs per 100g
Contains added sugars, nitrates and starch

SAUSAGES

(FYI) **Princes American Style Hot Dogs (Phases 2–4)**
4.5g carbs per 100g
Contains nitrates

⚠ **Princes Authentic Bockwurst German Sausages**
1.5g carbs per 100g
Contains added sugars and nitrates

⚠ **Princes Hot Dogs in Brine**
4.5g carbs per 100g
Contains added sugars, nitrates and wheat starch

TONGUE

⚠ **Princes Finest Hand Packed Ox Tongue**
0.3g carbs per 100g
Contains added sugars and nitrates

FYI **Princes Lunch Tongue (Phases 1–4)**
0.3g carbs per 100g
Contains nitrates

COLD & CURED MEATS

BACON & HAM

Back Bacon (Phases 1–4)
0g carbs

Ham, Boneless (Phases 1–4)
0g carbs

Luncheon Meat (Phases 1–4)
1g carbs per 100g serving

Middle Cut Bacon (Phases 1–4)
0g carbs

Pork Roll (Phases 1–4)
0.4g carbs per 100g serving

Smoked Bacon (Phases 1–4)
0g carbs

Streaky Bacon (Phases 1–4)
0g carbs

Unsmoked Bacon (Phases 1–4)
0g carbs

COLD CUTS

COOKED MEAT PRODUCTS

Atkins Gourmet Chargrilled Chicken Strips (Phases 1–4)
1g Net Carbs per serving

Own Brand Carved Roast Beef (Phases 1–4)
0–0.4g carbs per 100g

(FYI) Own Brand Chicken Slices (Phases 3–4)
2.1g carbs per 100g
Some may contain added sugars and maize starch

Own Brand Ham, Boneless (Phases 1–4)
0g carbs per 100g

Own Brand Luncheon Meat (Phases 1–4)
1g carbs per 100g serving

(FYI) Own Brand Roast Chicken Fillet (Phases 1–4)
Trace–0.7g carbs per 100g
Some may contain trace added sugars

(FYI) Own Brand Roast Pork (Phases 1–4)
0.1–0.7g carbs per 100g
Some may contain nitrates

(FYI) Own Brand Sliced Chicken Breast (Phases 1–4)
0.1–0.5g carbs per 100g
Some may contain trace added sugars and nitrates

(FYI) Own Brand Sliced Corned Beef (Phases 1–4)
Trace carbs per 100g
Some may contain trace added sugars

(FYI) Own Brand Sliced Gammon (Phases 1–4)
0.1–0.2g carbs per 100g
Contains nitrates

(FYI) Own Brand Sliced Turkey Breast (Phases 1–4)
Trace–0.2g carbs per 100g
Some may contain trace added sugars

(FYI) Own Brand Turkey Slices (Phases 3–4)
Trace–1.3g carbs per 100g
Some may contain maize starch and MSG

INTERNATIONAL MEATS

⚠ Own Brand Bresaola
0.1g carbs per 100g
Contains added sugars and nitrates

⚠ Own Brand Garlic Sausage
0.7–1.4g carbs per 100g
Contains added sugars, nitrates and wheat flour

⚠ Own Brand Mortadella
0.1–1g carbs per 100g
Contains added sugars and nitrates

⚠ Own Brand Pancetta
Trace–0.1g carbs per 100g
Contains added sugars and nitrates

⚠ **Own Brand Pepperoni**
0.1–2.4g carbs per 100g
Contains added sugars and nitrates

⚠ **Own Brand Prosciutto di Parma/di Speck –**
Parma Ham
Trace–1g carbs per 100g
Contains added sugars and nitrates

⚠ **Own Brand Salt Beef**
0.1–2.2g carbs per 100g
Contains added sugars and nitrates

⚠ **Peperami Grab the HOT Meat Snack**
0.6g carbs per 25g stick, 2.5g carbs per 100g
Contains added sugars, MSG and nitrates

⚠ **Peperami Grab the SPICY Meat Snack**
0.4g carbs per 25g stick, 1.7g carbs per 100g
Contains added sugars, MSG and nitrates

⚠ **Rocking JC Original Flavour Beef Jerky**
5.5g carbs per 28g serving, 19.4g carbs per 100g
Contains added sugars, MSG and nitrates

SAUSAGES
British Sausages

FYI **Black Pudding (Phases 3–4)**
14.6–17.8g carbs per 100g
Contains nitrates and wheat flour

Flavoured Sausages (Phases 1–4)
0–2g carbs per 100g

Pork Sausages (Phases 1–4)
1g carbs per link

International Sausages

Andouille (Phases 1–4)
1g carbs per 100g

Beef Frankfurters (Phases 1–4)
1.2g carbs per frankfurter

Beef-Pork Frankfurters (Phases 1–4)
1.5g carbs per 100g

Bratwurst (Phases 1–4)
2.1g carbs per link

Chorizo Sausage (Phases 1–4)
1g carbs per 100g

⚠ **Garlic Sausage**
0.7–1.4g carbs per 100g
Contains added sugars, nitrates and wheat flour

Italian Sausage, Pork (Phases 1–4)
0.9g carbs per 100g

Knockwurst (Phases 1–4)
2.3g carbs per link

Linguiça Sausage (Phases 1–4)
1g carbs per 100g

⚠ **Liverwurst**
2g carbs per 100g
Contains added sugars

⚠ **Peperami, Green Hot Pork**
1.7–2.5g carbs per 100g
Contains added sugars, MSG and nitrates

⚠ **Peperami, Red Spicy Pork**
1.7–2.5g carbs per 100g
Contains added sugars, MSG and nitrates

⚠ **Pepperoni**
0.1–2.4g carbs per 100g
Contains added sugars and nitrates

Polish Sausage (Phases 1–4)
0.8g carbs per 100g

Salami, Danish (Phases 1–4)
0.5g per 100g

Salami, French (Phases 1–4)
0.5g per 100g

Salami, Italian (Phases 1–4)
0.5g per 100g

Salami, Pork (Phases 1–4)
0.5g carbs per 100g

Smoked Sausages, Beef (Phases 1–4)
1g carbs per link

Smoked Sausages, Hot (Phases 1–4)
2g carbs per link

Smoked Sausages, Sweet (Phases 1–4)
3g carbs per link

PATÉ

⚠ Ardennes Paté
0.5–2.4g carbs per 100g
Contains added sugars, nitrates and wheat flour

⚠ Brussels Paté
2.8–8.4g carbs per 100g
Contains added sugars and nitrates

⚠ Chicken Liver Paté
1.9–6.4g carbs per 100g
Contains added sugars, nitrates and wheat flour

⚠ Duck Paté
1.7–9.3g carbs per 100g
Contains added sugars and nitrates

⚠ Duck & Orange Paté
3–3.9g carbs per 100g
Contains added sugars and nitrates

FROZEN BEEF & POULTRY

BEEF
Burgers

FYI Birds Eye 100% Beef Burgers (Phases 3–4)
0g carbs per 100g
Contains wheat flour

Birds Eye 100% Beef Mega Burgers (Phases 1–4)
0g carbs per 100g

Ⓕ Birds Eye Captain's Beef Burgers (Phases 3–4)
3.9g carbs per 100g
Contains wheat flour

Ⓕ Birds Eye Mexican Chilli Beef Quarter
Pounders (Phases 3–4)
6.5g carbs per 100g
Contains wheat flour

Ⓕ Birds Eye Original & Best Beef Burgers
(Phases 3–4)
5.1g carbs per 100g
Contains wheat flour

⚠ Own Brand Beef Burgers with Onion
3.8–6.9g carbs per 100g
Contains added sugars and wheat flour

⚠ Own Brand Economy Burgers
11–12g carbs per 100g
Contains added sugars, MSG and wheat flour

⚠ Own Brand Prime Beef Quarter Pounders
1.3–6g carbs per 100g
Contains added sugars and wheat flour

Ⓕ Planet Hollywood Beef Burgers (Phases 1–4)
1.4g carbs per 100g

⚠ Ross 100% Beef Burgers
1.1g carbs per 100g
Contains added sugars and wheat flour

⚠ Ross Chilli Beef Quarter Pounders
2.8g carbs per 100g
Contains added sugars and wheat flour

⚠ Ross Quarter Pounders
2.8g carbs per 100g
Contains added sugars and wheat flour

Grills

⚠ Dalepak Cracked Black Pepper Marinade Style Beef Grills
6.2g carbs per 100g
Contains added sugars, modified maize starch and wheat flour

⚠ Dalepak Peppered Beef Marine Style Grillsteaks
5.5g carbs per 100g
Contains added sugars, modified maize starch and wheat flour

ⓕⓥⓘ Own Brand Beef Grillsteaks (Phases 1–4)
1.6g carbs per 100g
Some may contain added sugars

⚠ Own Brand Peppered Beef Grillsteaks
8.6–12.8g carbs per 100g
Contains added sugars, modified maize starch and wheat flour

⚠ Ross Beef Grillsteaks
3.7g carbs per 100g
Contains added sugars and wheat flour

⚠ **Ross 100% Beef Grillsteaks**
1.1g carbs per 100g uncooked
Contains added sugars and wheat flour

Miscellaneous

ⒻⓎⒾ **Aria Beef Strips (Phases 1–4)**
1.1g carbs per 100g

⚠ **Birds Eye Roast Beef in Gravy**
3.2g carbs per 100g
Contains added sugars, maize starch and wheat
flour

⚠ **Own Brand Sliced Beef in Gravy**
2.6–2.7g carbs per 100g
Contains added sugars, trans fats, modified maize
starch and wheat flour

PORK

Ribs

⚠ **Dalepak Chinese Style Ribsteaks**
10.4g carbs per 100g
Contains added sugars

⚠ **Dalepak Smokey Barbecue Style Ribsteaks**
8.8g carbs per 100g uncooked
Contains added sugars, aspartame, modified maize
starch and wheat flour

⚠ **Farmers Table Chinese Style Pork Ribs**
5.4g carbs per 100g
Contains added sugars, modified maize starch and
wheat flour

Sausages

⚠ **Own Brand Cocktail Sausages**
11–15.8g carbs per 100g
Contains added sugars and wheat flour

⚠ **Own Brand Thick Pork Sausages**
11–12.9g carbs per 100g
Contains added sugars and wheat flour

⚠ **Own Brand Thick Pork & Beef Sausages**
10.6–15.4g carbs per 100g
Contains added sugars and wheat flour

⚠ **Own Brand Thin Pork Sausages**
8.7–13g carbs per 100g
Contains added sugars and wheat flour

ⒻⓎⒾ **Richmond Thick Sausages (Phases 3–4)**
12.8g carbs per 100g
Contains wheat flour

⚠ **Wall's Jumbo Pork Sausages**
10.2g carbs per 100g
Contains added sugars and wheat flour

ⒻⓎⒾ **Wall's Skinless Pork Sausages (Phases 3–4)**
9g carbs per 100g
Contains wheat flour

POULTRY

Burgers

(FYI) **Birds Eye Captain's Chicken Burgers (Phases 3–4)**
16.6g carbs per 100g
Contains wheat flour

⚠ **Birds Eye Captain's Roasted Chicken Bites**
3.4g carbs per 100g
Contains added sugars, maize starch and wheat flour

⚠ **Birds Eye 100% Chicken Fillet Burgers Cajun**
2.6g carbs per 100g
Contains added sugars, maize starch and wheat flour

⚠ **Birds Eye 100% Chicken Fillet Burgers Original**
3g carbs per 100g
Contains added sugars, maize starch and wheat flour

Grills

⚠ **Birds Eye Captain's Mini BBQ Chicken Griddlers**
6.7g carbs per 100g
Contains added sugars, maize starch and wheat flour

⚠ **Birds Eye Chicken Chargrills Garlic**
3.1g carbs per 100g
Contains added sugars, maize starch and wheat flour

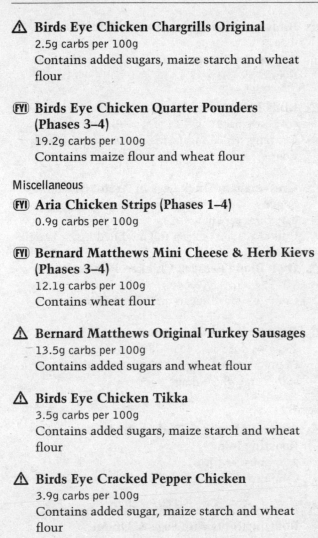

⚠️ **Birds Eye Chicken Chargrills Original**
2.5g carbs per 100g
Contains added sugars, maize starch and wheat
flour

FYI **Birds Eye Chicken Quarter Pounders
(Phases 3–4)**
19.2g carbs per 100g
Contains maize flour and wheat flour

Miscellaneous

FYI **Aria Chicken Strips (Phases 1–4)**
0.9g carbs per 100g

FYI **Bernard Matthews Mini Cheese & Herb Kievs
(Phases 3–4)**
12.1g carbs per 100g
Contains wheat flour

⚠️ **Bernard Matthews Original Turkey Sausages**
13.5g carbs per 100g
Contains added sugars and wheat flour

⚠️ **Birds Eye Chicken Tikka**
3.5g carbs per 100g
Contains added sugars, maize starch and wheat
flour

⚠️ **Birds Eye Cracked Pepper Chicken**
3.9g carbs per 100g
Contains added sugar, maize starch and wheat
flour

⚠ **Birds Eye Honey and Mustard Chicken**
4.2g carbs per 100g
Contains added sugars, maize starch and wheat
flour

⚠ **Birds Eye Thai Chicken**
4.4g carbs per 100g
Contains added sugars, maize starch and wheat
flour

⚠ **Gressingham Duck Legs in Aromatic Chinese
Sauce**
4.3g carbs per 100g
Contains added sugars and modified maize starch

⚠ **Own Brand Breaded Chicken Portions**
9.1–15g carbs per 100g
Contains added sugars and wheat flour

⚠ **Own Brand Chicken Breast**
2.9–4.4g carbs per 100g
Contains added sugars, trans fats, modified maize
starch and wheat flour

Roasts

⚠ **Bernard Matthews Turkey Breast Boneless
Roasting Joint**
2.7g carbs per 100g
Contains added sugars

⚠ **Bernard Matthews Turkey Breast Boneless
Roasting Joint with Sage & Onion**
3.2g carbs per 100g
Contains added sugars and wheat flour

⚠ Bernard Matthews Turkey Breast Roast
3.4g carbs per 100g
Contains added sugars

⚠ Birds Eye Roast Chicken in Gravy
2.7g carbs per 100g uncooked
Contains added sugars, maize starch and wheat flour

Wings

⚠ Gressingham Chinese Barbeque Duck Wings
11g carbs per 100g
Contains added sugars and modified maize starch

⚠ McCain BBQ Micro Wings
6g carbs per serving, 4.4g carbs per 100g
Contains added sugars and modified maize starch

⚠ Own Brand Spicy Chicken Wings
3.2–3.5g carbs per 100g
Contains added sugars, modified maize starch and wheat flour

LAMB
Grills

⚠ Dalepak Lamb Dalesteaks
1.9g carbs per 100g
Contains added sugars and wheat flour

⚠ Dalepak Minted Lamb Marinade Style Grills
4.4g carbs per 100g
Contains added sugars, modified maize starch and wheat flour

🔲 **Own Brand Lamb Grillsteaks (Phases 3–4)**
2.2–5.2g carbs per 100g
Contains wheat flour

Miscellaneous

⚠ **Aria Lamb Strips (Phases 1–4)**
1.3g carbs per 100g

Roasts

⚠ **Bernard Matthews Boneless Leg Joint in Rosemary & Garlic Marinade**
6.6g carbs per 100g
Contains added sugars and modified maize starch

Bernard Matthews Lamb Roast (Phases 1–4)
0.1g carbs per 100g

Ready Meals

Apart from Scandinavia, the British consume more ready meals than anyone in the world and, as such, the ready meals market in the UK cannot be ignored.

With our increasingly busy lives, we are all occasionally tempted to reach for ready meals, and with miles of supermarket aisles dedicated to these products, making an acceptable choice can be especially tricky for Atkins followers. Even when carb counts fall within acceptable limits, the most basic meals can contain problematic ingredients at best and unacceptable ingredients at worst. So, although ready meals are a godsend at certain times, you may wish to reconsider how you use them if you want to do Atkins successfully:

1   Avoid meals where pasta, rice or potato is the main component, as these will nearly always contain too many carbs.
2   Buy ready meals where the rice, potato or pasta is packaged separately – these will often be take-away ethnic meals in the chilled section. This way, you can remove the high-carb element and still enjoy the convenience of a dinner that has been prepared for you.
3   Look for main-meal components such as meat or fish to which a salad or cooked vegetables can be added, thereby keeping the overall carb count under control.
4   Be on the lookout for added sugars in the ingredients list as they are used frequently to enhance the flavour. Added sugars are unacceptable on any phase of Atkins.

In this section of the book we have changed the format slightly to make it even easier for you to choose ready meals. As own-label products dominate the ready meals market in the UK, with Marks & Spencer, Tesco, Sainsbury's and Asda leading the way, we have named the supermarkets in the product listing. The four market leaders we have chosen are nationwide, but you may have a favourite local supermarket selling its own brands.

INDIAN

⚠ **Asda Extra Special Tandoori Chicken Dil Pasanda**
16g carbs per 350g serving, 5g carbs per 100g
Contains added sugars and modified maize starch

⚠ **Asda Good for You! Bombay Style Chicken**
7g carbs per 370g serving, 2.1g carbs per 100g
Contains added sugars and modified maize starch

⚠ **Asda Indian Chicken Pasanda**
24g carbs per 350g serving, 7g carbs per 100g
Contains added sugars and modified maize starch

⚠ **Asda Indian Vegetable Curry**
26g carbs per 350g serving, 8g carbs per 100g
Contains added sugars and modified maize starch

⚠ **Marks & Spencer Chicken Kashmiri**
23.8g carbs per 350g serving, 6.8g carbs per 100g
Contains added sugars and modified maize starch

⚠ **Marks & Spencer Chicken Korma**
13.3g carbs per 350g serving, 3.8g carbs per 100g
Contains added sugars

⚠ **Marks & Spencer Chicken Piri Piri**
15.4g carbs per 350g serving, 8.8g carbs per 100g
Contains added sugars

(FYI) **Marks & Spencer King Prawn Makhani (Phases 3–4)**
10.2g carbs per 350g serving, 2.9g carbs per 100g
Contains maize starch

Marks & Spencer Matar Paneer (Phases 3–4)
13.8g carbs per 225g serving, 6.2g carbs per 100g

Marks & Spencer Mushroom Bhaji (Phases 2–4)
11.5g carbs per 225g serving, 5.1g carbs per 100g

Marks & Spencer Tarka Dal (Phases 3–4)
27.9g carbs per 225g serving, 12.4g carbs per 100g

Sainsbury's Butter Chicken (Phases 2–4)
8.8g carbs per 200g serving, 4.4g carbs per 100g

⚠ **Sainsbury's Chicken Balti**
7.4g carbs per 200g serving, 3.7g carbs per 100g
Contains added sugars

Sainsbury's Chicken Dopiaza (Phases 1–4)
6.2g carbs per 200g serving, 3.1g carbs per 100g

⚠ **Sainsbury's Chicken Tikka Masala**
14g carbs per 200g serving, 7g carbs per 100g
Contains added sugars and modified maize starch

⚠ **Sainsbury's Lamb Rogan Josh**
6g carbs per 200g serving, 3g carbs per 100g
Contains added sugars

Sainsbury's Tandoori King Prawn Masala (Phases 2–4)
10.2g carbs per 200g serving, 5.1g carbs per 100g

⚠ **Sainsbury's Taste the Difference Bengal Style Mustard & Honey Chicken Brochettes**
23.6g carbs per 400g serving, 5.9g carbs per 100g
Contains added sugars

Sainsbury's Vegetable Masala (Phases 2–4)
10.4g carbs per 200g serving, 5.2g carbs per 100g

FYI **Tesco Indian Chicken Jalfrezi (Phases 3–4)**
17.5g carbs per 350g serving, 5g carbs per 100g
Contains cornflour

⚠ **Tesco Indian Chicken Madras**
19.6g carbs per 350g serving, 5.6g carbs per 100g
Contains added sugars and modified maize starch

⚠ **Tesco Indian Chicken Tikka Masala**
7g carbs per 350g serving, 2g carbs per 100g
Contains added sugars and modified maize starch

FYI **Tesco Indian Mushroom Dopiaza (Phases 3–4)**
23.6g carbs per 350g serving, 6.7g carbs per 100g
Contains modified maize starch

BRITISH

(FYI) **Asda Cauliflower Cheese (Phases 3–4)**
9g carbs per 225g serving, 4g carbs per 100g
Contains modified maize starch and wheat flour

⚠ **Asda Chicken Escalopes with Hawaiian Pizza Style Topping**
12g carbs per 320g serving, 4.2g carbs per 100g
Contains added sugars, modified maize starch and nitrates

⚠ **Asda Extra Special Pork Fillets in a Creamy Cider Sauce with Apple**
25g carbs per 500g serving, 5g carbs per 100g
Contains added sugars, modified maize starch and wheat flour

⚠ **Asda Extra Special Pork Medallions with Mushrooms & Madeira Sauce**
3.7g carbs per 210g serving, 2.2g carbs per 100g
Contains added sugars and modified maize starch

⚠ **Asda Good for You! Cod in Parsley Sauce**
3.6g carbs per 180g serving, 2g carbs per 100g
Contains added sugars and modified maize starch

⚠ **Asda Plaice Fillets with Prawns in a White Wine & Mushroom Sauce**
0.7g carbs per 180g serving, 0.4g carbs per 100g
Contains added sugars and modified maize starch

(FYI) **Asda Regional Recipe Bacon Loin Steaks (Phases 3–4)**
2.9g carbs per 170g serving, 1.7g carbs per 100g
Contains nitrates, modified maize starch and wheat flour

⚠ **Asda Salmon Fillets Stuffed with Mozzarella & Sundried Tomatoes**
1g carbs per 240g serving, 0.4g carbs per 100g
Contains added sugars

⚠ **Asda Steak & Mushroom Casserole**
13g carbs per 300g serving, 4.2g carbs per 100g
Contains added sugars and modified maize starch

(FYI) **Marks & Spencer Cauliflower Cheese (Phases 3–4)**
11.1g carbs per 300g serving, 3.7g carbs per 100g
Contains wheat flour

(FYI) **Marks & Spencer Classic Salmon Parcels in Lemon Sauce (Phases 3–4)**
2.6g carbs per 185g serving, 1.4g carbs per 100g
Contains maize starch and wheat flour

⚠ **Marks & Spencer Favourites Chicken Breast Roast**
15.1g carbs per 265g serving, 5.7g carbs per 100g
Contains added sugars, maize starch and wheat flour

(FYI) **Marks & Spencer Favourites Chicken, Mushroom & Bacon (Phases 3–4)**
1.6g carbs per 198g serving, 0.8g carbs per 100g
Contains maize starch, nitrates and wheat flour

FYI **Marks & Spencer Favourites Liver & Bacon (Phases 3–4)**
6.1g carbs per 210g serving, 2.9g carbs per 100g
Contains maize starch, nitrates and wheat flour

FYI **Marks & Spencer Favourites Smoked Haddock in Cheese Sauce (Phases 3–4)**
22.8g carbs per 400g serving, 5.7g carbs per 100g
Contains maize starch and wheat flour

⚠ **Marks & Spencer Mini Favourites Beef Casserole**
18.4g carbs per 200g serving, 9.2g carbs per 100g
Contains trans fats, maize starch and wheat flour

FYI **Marks & Spencer Salmon with Watercress Sauce (Phases 3–4)**
6.6g carbs per 200g serving, 3.3g carbs per 100g
Contains maize starch and wheat flour

⚠ **Sainsbury's Gammon Steaks with Mature Cheddar Cheese and Pineapple Topping**
14.8g carbs per 200g serving, 7.4g carbs per 100g
Contains added sugars, modified maize starch, nitrates and wheat flour

⚠ **Sainsbury's Taste the Difference Beef Stroganoff**
10.4g carbs per 200g serving, 5.2g carbs per 100g
Contains added sugars, trans fats, modified maize starch and wheat flour

⚠ **Sainsbury's Taste the Difference Pork in a Somerset Cider Brandy Sauce with Apple**
10.3g carbs per 240g serving, 4.3g per 100g
Contains added sugars, modified maize starch and wheat flour

⚠ **Tesco British Classics Liver & Bacon**
11g carbs per 200g serving, 5.5g carbs per 100g
Contains added sugars, modified maize starch, nitrates and wheat flour

ⒻⓎⒾ **Tesco Cauliflower Cheese (Phases 3–4)**
19.3g carbs per 350g serving, 5.5g carbs per 100g
Contains wheat flour

⚠ **Tesco Finest Chicken & Asparagus with a Creamy White Wine & Basil Sauce**
4g carbs per 200g serving, 2g carbs per 100g
Contains added sugars and modified maize starch

ⒻⓎⒾ **Tesco Finest Chicken & Bacon Parcels (Phases 3–4)**
8.6g carbs per 232g serving, 3.7g carbs per 100g
Contains nitrates and wheat flour

⚠ **Tesco Finest Chicken Breasts with Cranberry Stuffing**
19.1g carbs per 200g serving, 9.6g carbs per 100g
Contains added sugars, modified maize starch and wheat flour

Tesco Finest Salmon Parcels with Garlic Butter (Phases 1–4)
0.9g carbs per 164g serving, 0.6g carbs per 100g

FYI Tesco Healthy Living British Classics Haddock in a Cheese and Chive Sauce (Phases 3–4)
4.4g carbs per 200g serving, 2.2g carbs per 100g
Contains modified maize starch and wheat flour

MEDITERRANEAN

⚠ Asda Broccoli Mornay
10g carbs per 225g, 4.3g carbs per 100g serving
Contains added sugars, trans fats, modified maize starch and wheat flour

⚠ Asda Good for You! Beef Moussaka
26g carbs per 400g, 7g carbs per 100g serving
Contains added sugars, modified maize starch and wheat flour

⚠ Asda Good for You! Duck with Apple & Calvados Sauce
7g carbs per 160g, 4.2g carbs per 100g serving
Contains added sugars and modified maize starch

⚠ Marks & Spencer Café Culture Aubergine Parmigiana
25.8g carbs per 350g serving, 7.6g carbs per 100g
Contains added sugars and maize starch

⚠ Marks & Spencer Café Culture Leek, Lentil and Spinach Fritatta
19.2g carbs per 350g serving, 5.5g carbs per 100g
Contains added sugars and modified maize starch

(FYI) Marks & Spencer Classic Chicken in White Wine Sauce (Phases 3–4)
2.5g carbs per 228g serving, 1.1g carbs per 100g
Contains maize starch

(FYI) Marks & Spencer Classic Haddock Mornay (Phases 3–4)
1.5g carbs per 190g serving, 0.8g carbs per 100g
Contains maize starch and wheat flour

⚠ Sainsbury's Taste the Difference Beef Stifado
23.2g carbs per 400g serving, 5.8g carbs per 100g
Contains added sugars, trans fats and modified maize starch

⚠ Tesco Finest Chicken Chasseur
5.4g carbs per 200g serving, 2.7g carbs per 100g
Contains added sugars and modified maize starch

(FYI) Tesco Finest Chicken Florentine (Phases 3–4)
21.8g carbs per 225g serving, 9.7g carbs per 100g
Contains maize starch and wheat flour

⚠ Tesco Finest Mediterranean Style Vegetables
22g carbs per 300g serving, 7.3g carbs per 100g
Contains added sugars

(FYI) Tesco Finest Steak au Poivre (Phases 3–4)
11.7g carbs per 450g serving, 2.6g carbs per 100g
Contains modified maize starch and wheat flour

(FYI) Tesco Finest Steak Diane (Phases 3–4)
8.8g carbs per 225g serving, 3.9g carbs per 100g
Contains maize starch and wheat flour

ORIENTAL

⚠ Asda Chicken Peanut Curry
5g carbs per 170g serving, 3.8g carbs per 100g
Contains added sugars, modified maize starch and wheat flour

⚠ Asda Good for You! Sweet & Sour Prawn Stir Fry
19g carbs per 175g serving, 11g carbs per 100g
Contains added sugars and maize starch

⚠ Marks & Spencer Beef in Black Bean Sauce
20g carbs per 350g serving, 5.7g carbs per 100g
Contains added sugars, maize starch and wheat flour

⚠ Sainsbury's Beef with Chilli Black Bean Sauce
25.8g carbs per 300g serving, 8.6g carbs per 100g
Contains added sugars, cornflour, modified maize starch and wheat flour

⚠ Sainsbury's Cantonese Mini Sticky Ribs
22.2g carbs per 150g serving, 14.8g carbs per 100g
Contains added sugars, modified maize starch and wheat flour

⚠ Sainsbury's Cantonese Roasted Duck in Plum Sauce
21.2g carbs per 150g serving, 14.1g carbs per 100g
Contains added sugars, modified maize starch and wheat flour

⚠ **Sainsbury's Thai Mango Chicken Curry**
9.6g carbs per 200g serving, 4.8g carbs per 100g
Contains added sugars and modified maize starch

⚠ **Sainsbury's Thai Red Chicken Curry**
11g carbs per 200g serving, 5.5g carbs per 100g
Contains added sugars

⚠ **Sainsbury's Thai Red Prawn Curry**
28.2g carbs per 300g serving, 9.4g carbs per 100g
Contains added sugars and modified maize starch

⚠ **Sainsbury's Thai Yellow Vegetable Curry**
14.2g carbs per 200g serving, 7.1g carbs per 100g
Contains added sugars, modified maize starch and
wheat flour

⚠ **Tesco Cantonese Chicken**
16.5g carbs per 175g, 9.4g carbs per 100g
Contains added sugars and modified maize starch

⚠ **Tesco Chinese Style Spare Ribs**
15.7g carbs per 175g serving, 9g carbs per 100g
Contains added sugars and modified maize starch

⚠ **Tesco Finest Aromatic Duck with a Plum
Sauce**
16.8g carbs per 250g serving, 6.7g carbs per 100g
Contains added sugars, modified maize starch and
wheat flour

⚠ **Tesco Finest Malaysian Chicken Breasts with
Thai Green Curry**
3.9g carbs per 200g serving, 2g carbs per 100g
Contains added sugars and modified maize starch

TEX/MEX

⚠ **Asda Spanish Style Chicken with Chorizo**
11g carbs per 310g, 4.1g carbs per 100g serving
Contains added sugars, modified maize starch and
nitrates

⚠ **Marks & Spencer Southern Style Barbecue Ribs**
19.1g carbs per 180g serving, 10.6g carbs per 100g
Contains added sugars and modified maize starch

CARIBBEAN

⚠ **Asda Caribbean Jamaican Jerk Style Chicken Breasts in a Sweet BBQ Flavour Sauce**
21g carbs per 180g, 13g carbs per 100g serving
Contains added sugars

Snacks

Whichever aisle you find them in, most prepackaged snacks are off-limits on Atkins, no matter what the phase – and that includes Lifetime Maintenance. Snacks are an important consideration when it comes to doing Atkins properly. While it's good to build snacks into your menu, not all snacks are acceptable. Not only are many processed snacks high in carbohydrates, thanks to flour and added sugars, but more often than not you will also find trans fats – often referred to as hydrogenated oils – lurking in the ingredients list. You should also be aware that even many so-called healthy snacks – protein bars, for example – often have astronomically high carb counts and can contain unacceptable ingredients, such as added sugars.

The protein- and nutrition-bar shelf can be one of the most confusing areas of the supermarket. It seems that every company has a line of bars in a never-ending variety of flavours and textures. When evaluating bars, look for carb counts of no more than 3 grams per bar, and make sure there are no added sugars or trans fats. Keep in mind too that a bar labelled 'high-protein' is not necessarily low in carbs.

Savoury snacks are another minefield. Crunchy, salty snacks can pack a double wallop: they're typically high in carbs because they're made with refined white flour and they almost always contain hydrogenated oils, meaning they are high in trans fats.

It's no surprise, then, that your best snack bets are those foods that are minimally processed – particularly nuts and cheese. They make much smarter choices than cheese puffs with that nuclear orange glow or vegetable snacks that look more like polystyrene than anything that came from the earth. When it comes to popcorn, pop it yourself! Of the 11 ready-made brands we reviewed, not one was suitable as they each contained added sugars and astronomical carb levels.

NUTS & SEEDS

Nuts and seeds are among the first foods you add back to your eating plan as you climb the carbohydrate ladder. In addition to being relatively low in carbs, they are also rich sources of protein, beneficial fats, fibre and a wide range of other nutrients: almonds are a good source of calcium, walnuts are high in omega-3 fats, pecans in thiamin and hazelnuts in vitamin E.

There's very little difference between dry-roasted and oil-roasted nuts, except in calories, but skip the honey-roasted or seasoned varieties. Nuts are also pretty consistent in carbs from one brand to another.

You should, however, limit your portions to 25g. To learn what a serving size looks like, measure that amount into the palm of your hand. That way, the next time you are helping yourself to a bowl of nuts at a party, you'll know your limit. If you find it too difficult to *stop* eating nuts once you get started, you should buy individual-size portions.

Contrary to popular belief, neither soy nuts nor peanuts are real nuts. Peanuts belong to the legumes food group, while soy nuts are made by roasting whole, water-soaked dried soya beans.

False Friends: Unexpected Carbs and Trans-fat Alert

Healthy snacks are often touted as being much more nutritious than the regular versions. Don't be fooled: if something sounds too good to be true, it probably is.

Baked crisps, for example: these are lower in fat than regular fried potato and corn crisps, but weigh in with significantly higher carb counts of 22 grams per serving (on average). In addition, many are loaded with sugar and hydrogenated oils.

SHOP SMART

You'll be a smart snack shopper if you remember two rules:

1 There can be tremendous variation within one food type. Be vigilant when reading ingredients labels!
2 Practise label logic. Fat-free isn't relevant when you are doing Atkins, so don't automatically be impressed with products labelled as such. 'Fat-free' is often a tip-off for added sugars.

BOMBAY MIX

FYI **Imperial Organic Bombay Mix (Phases 3–4)**
⚠ 9.6g carbs per 25g serving
  May contain maize starch

FYI **Imperial Original Karachi Crunch (Phases 3–4)**
9.6g carbs per 25g serving
Contains maize flour and MSG

FYI **Own Brand Bombay Mix (Phases 3–4)**
2.5–12.3g carbs per 25g serving
May contain maize starch

CEREAL BARS & FRUIT ROLLS

⚠ **Lyme Regis Foods, Fruit 4 U, Cherry**
20.6g carbs per 28g bar
Contains added sugars

⚠ **Lyme Regis Foods, Fruit 4 U, Raspberry**
20.6g carbs per 28g bar
Contains added sugars

⚠ **Lyme Regis Foods, Kidz Organic Fruit Bar, Blackcurrant Buzz (Phases 3–4)**
13.5g carbs per 20g bar

Lyme Regis Foods, La Fruit, Blackcurrant (Phases 3–4)
19.9g carbs per 25g serving

Lyme Regis Foods, La Fruit, Raspberry (Phases 3–4)
18.8g carbs per 25g serving

⚠ **Lyme Regis Foods, Organic Fruitus Bar, Apricot (Phases 3–4)**
21.4g carbs per 35g bar

⚠ **Lyme Regis Foods, Organic Fruitus Bar, Mixed**
⚠ **Berry**
22.3g carbs per 35g bar
Contains added sugars

⚠ **Lyme Regis Foods, Organic Seven Seeds and Nut Bar (Phases 3–4)**
17.4g carbs per 40g bar

Lyme Regis Foods, Zaps Apricot Fruit Bar (Phases 3–4)
16.6g carbs per 25g bar

Lyme Regis Foods, Zaps Orange Fruit Bar (Phases 3–4)
17.4g carbs per 25g bar

⚠ **The Village Bakery Fruit, Nut & Seed Bar**
18.4g carbs per 25g bar
Contains added sugars

SNACK CHEESE

Bel Babybel, Cheddar (Phases 1–4)
0g carbs per 20g cheese

Bel Babybel, Light (Phases 1–4)
0g carbs per 20g cheese

Bel Babybel, Original (Phases 1–4)
0g carbs per 20g cheese

⚠ **Crosse & Blackwell Branston Cathedral City Dip & Go**
8.6g carbs per 60g pot
Contains added sugars and maize starch

PROCESSED SNACK CHEESE

The Golden Vale Cheese Co., Cheestrings Double Cheddar (Phases 1–4)
Trace carbs per 21g stick

The Golden Vale Cheese Co., Cheestrings Mild Cheddar Tornado (Phases 1–4)
Trace carbs per 21g stick

The Golden Vale Cheese Co., Original Cheestrings (Phases 1–4)
Trace carbs per 21g stick

FYI **Kraft Dairylea Dunkers Original Sticks (Phases 3–4)**
14g carbs per 50g pot
Contains wheat flour

Kraft Dairylea STRIP CHEESE (Phases 1–4)
0.2g carbs per 21g strip

FYI **Kraft Dairylea Tri Bites (Phases 3–4)**
0.6g carbs per 20g portion
Contains wheat flour

FYI **Kraft Light Philadelphia Snack with Italian Bread Sticks (Phases 3–4)**
12g carbs per 50g serving
Contains wheat flour

Ⓕ**Ⓨ**Ⓘ **The Laughing Cow Original Cheez Dippers (Phases 2–4)**
8.9g carbs per 35g portion
Contains wheat flour

⚠ **SCOOBY-DOO Dippers with Primula**
15.7g carbs per 50g pack
Contains added sugars, maize starch and wheat flour

CRISPS

Crisps

Don't be fooled by 'natural' crisps: they may contain fewer additives, but they're about the same in grams of carbs. If you don't have a set of scales to weigh out 25 grams, look to see if the number of crisps is listed in the serving size. If it is, count out that number – or half the number for half the carbs.

The best-tasting potato crisps rarely have more than three ingredients: potatoes, vegetable oil and salt. If the bag you've picked up has anything else, put it back and continue your search – more often than not, buried in the ingredients list will be terms like 'partially hydrogenated oils' and 'modified maize starch', neither of which you want or need. As you can imagine, this is one food you'll want to eat rarely and in very small quantities and only in the maintenance phases of Atkins. Servings are usually given in ounces – there are approximately 19 crisps in an ounce, which is the equivalent of 25 grams.

Soy- and vegetable-based crisps can be a great alternative to traditional salty snacks. However, not all are low in carbs or free of unacceptable ingredients.

(FYI) Atkins Crunchables Herb Flavour (Phases 2–4)
1g Net Carbs per 25g bag
Contains maize flour and wheat flour

**Atkins Crunchables Hot 'N' Spicy Flavour
(Phases 2–4)**
1g Net Carbs per 25g bag

**Cape Cod Reduced Fat Lightly Salted Potato
Chips (Phases 3–4)**
13.4g carbs per 25g serving

Ellert Classic Sea Salt Crinkles (Phases 3–4)
15.7g carbs per 25g serving

⚠ **Kettle Chips, Mature Cheddar and Chive**
13.6 carbs per 25g serving
Contains added sugars

⚠ **Kettle Chips, Salsa with Mesquite**
13.5g carbs per 25g serving
Contains added sugars

⚠ **Kettle Chips, Sea Salt and Balsamic Vinegar**
13.4g carbs per 25g serving
Contains added sugars

⚠ **Kettle Chips, Sea Salt with Crushed Black
Peppercorns**
13.4g carbs per 25g serving
Contains added sugars

Kettle Organics, Lightly Salted (Phases 3–4)
13.4g carbs per 25g serving

⚠ **Own Brand Cheese and Onion Crisps**
12–12.1g carbs per 25g bag
Contains added sugars

Own Brand Ready Salted Crisps (Phases 3–4)
12g carbs per 25g bag

FYI **Own Brand Salt and Vinegar Crisps
(Phases 3–4)**
12.5g carbs per 25g bag
May contain added sugars and trans fats

**Seabrook Original Crinkle Cut Sea Salt
Flavour (Phases 3–4)**
17.3g carbs per 31g bag

⚠ **Walkers Cheese & Onion Lites**
17.1g carbs per 28g bag
Contains added sugars, trans fats and MSG

FYI **Walkers Cheese Quavers (Phases 3–4)**
12g carbs per 20g bag
Contains MSG and wheat flour

Walkers Salt & Shake (Phases 3–4)
11.8g carbs per 24g bag

FYI **Walkers Salt & Vinegar Crisps (Phases 3–4)**
17.3g carbs per 34.5g bag
Contains MSG

**Walkers Sensations Sea Salt and Cracked
Black Pepper (Phases 3–4)**
21.6g carbs per 40g bag

Vegetable Crisps

Kettle Chips, Golden Parsnip (Phases 3–4)
9.8g carbs per 25g serving

Kettle Chips, Sweet Potato (Phases 3–4)
11.1g carbs per 25g serving

Origins, English Country Garden, Hand Cooked Beetroot & Parsnip Vegetable Crisps (Phases 3–4)
7.2g carbs per 25g serving

Origins, Luxury Oven Baked Five Variety, Vegetable Crisps (Phases 3–4)
7.5g carbs per 25g serving

The Stamp Collection: Sweet Potatoes, Carrots & Beetroot Vegetable Chips (Phases 3–4)
8.5g carbs per 25g serving

Corn Crisps

(FYI) Doritos, Chilli Heat Wave Corn Chips (Phases 3–4)
19.1g carbs per 33g bag
Contains aspartame and MSG

(FYI) Doritos, Cool Original Corn Chips (Phases 3–4)
19.1g carbs per 33g bag
Contains MSG

FYI **Doritos Latinos, Chargrilled BBQ (Phases 3–4)**
14.7g carbs per 25g serving
Contains maize starch and MSG

FYI **Doritos, Latinos Mexican Grill Corn Chips
(Phases 3–4)**
14.7g carbs per 25g serving
Contains aspartame, maize starch and MSG

⚠ **Doritos, Latinos, Sour Cream & Sweet Pepper**
15g carbs per 25g serving
Contains added sugars, maize starch and MSG

FYI **Doritos, Tangy Cheese Corn Chips (Phases 3–4)**
18.8g carbs per 33g bag
Contains MSG

Tortilla Chips

⚠ **Own Brand Nacho Cheese Chips**
14.7–16.7g carbs per 25g serving
Contains added sugars, MSG and wheat flour

DIPS

⚠ **Doritos Extra Hot Salsa Dippas Dip**
8.5g carbs per 100g
Contains added sugars

⚠ **Doritos Hot Salsa Dippas Dip**
8.5g carbs per 100g
Contains added sugars

⚠ **Doritos Mild Indian Dippas Dip**
9g carbs per 100g
Contains added sugars

Doritos Mild Salsa Dippas Dip
8.5g carbs per 100g
Contains added sugars

 Doritos Sweet & Zesty Dippas Dip
8g carbs per 100g
Contains added sugars

DRIED FRUIT & FRUIT MIXES

Apricots

> **Humdinger Dried Chopped Apricots (Phases 3–4)**
> 14.3g carbs per 25g serving

> **Sundora Mini Apricots (Phases 3–4)**
> 9g carbs per 25g serving

Compotes & Jellies

 Del Monte Fruitini, Strawberry Jelly with Peach Pieces
18.4g carbs per 120g pot
Contains added sugars

 Hartley's Chunky Fruit Compote, Apple & Summer Fruit
14.7g carbs per 95g pot
Contains added sugars

 Hartley's Smooth Fruit Compote
14g carbs per 90g pouch
Contains added sugar

Currants, Sultanas & Raisins

 Crazy Jack Organic Sultanas (Phases 3–4)
17.3g carbs per 25g serving

⚠ **Crazy Jack Organic Sun-Dried Raisins (Phases 3–4)**
17.2g carbs per 25g serving

Mixed Raisins (Phases 3–4)
21.4g carbs per 30g bag

Own Brand Currants (Phases 3–4)
17g carbs per 25g serving

Own Brand Raisins (Phases 3–4)
16–18g carbs per 25g serving

Raisins & Apricots (Phases 3–4)
18.2g carbs per 30g bag

⚠ **Whitworths Luxury Dried Mixed Fruit**
16.3g carbs per 25g serving
Contains added sugars

Dates

Humdinger Dried Stone-out Dates (Phases 3–4)
18g carbs per 25g serving

⚠ **Whitworths Chopped Dates**
17.2g carbs per 25g serving
Contains added sugars

⚠ **Whitworths Chopped Dates and Walnuts**
14g carbs per 25g serving
Contains added sugars

Fruit Flakes

⚠ **Fruit Bowl Fruit Flakes, Blackcurrant**
19.9g carbs per 25g serving
Contains added sugars

⚠ **Fruit Bowl Fruit Flakes, Strawberry**
19.9g carbs per 25g serving
Contains added sugars

⚠ **Fruit Bowl Fruit Flakes, Strawberry with Yoghurt Coating**
18.2g carbs per 25g serving
Contains added sugars and trans fats

⚠ **Fruit Bowl Fruit Flakes, Tropical**
20g carbs per 25g serving
Contains added sugars

Mixed

Del Monte Fruit Express No Added Sugar Peach & Pear Pieces in Fruit Juice (Phases 3–4)
20g carbs per 185g pot

Del Monte Fruit Express No Added Sugar Tropical Mixed Fruit in Juice (Phases 3–4)
20.7g carbs per 185g pot

Del Monte Fruit in Juice, Mixed Fruit Pieces in Fruit Juice (Phases 3–4)
14.4 carbs per 120g pot

Whitworths Dried Fruit Salad (Phases 3–4)
10g carbs per 25g serving

Others

⚠ **Fruit Bowl School Bars, Strawberry**
16.6g carbs per 20g serving
Contains added sugars

Humdinger Stem Ginger
21g carbs per 25g serving
Contains added sugar

Own Brand Desiccated Coconut (Phases 1–4)
1.6g carbs per 25g serving

 Sundora Apple Slices
13.6g carbs per 25g serving
Contains added sugars

 Sundora Mini Pineapple Pieces
22.2g carbs per 25g serving
Contains added sugars

Sundora Mini Prunes (Phases 3–4)
8.5g carbs per 25g serving

 Whitworths Honey Coated Banana Chips
15g carbs per 25g serving
Contains added sugars

MEAT SNACKS

 Mr Porky Pork Crackles
0g carbs per 40g serving
Contains added sugars, trans fats and MSG

 Peperami, Hot Pork Salami Sausage
0.6g carbs per 25g stick
Contains added sugars, MSG and nitrates

 Peperami, Spicy Pork Salami Sausage
0.4g carbs per 25g stick
Contains added sugars, MSG and nitrates

⚠ **Reinert Snakx Salami on the Go, Original**
0.4g carbs per 50g bag
Contains added sugars and nitrates

⚠ **Reinert Snakx Salami on the Go, Spicy Hot**
0.4g carbs per 50g bag
Contains added sugars and nitrates

⚠ **Rocking JC Beef Jerky**
5.5g carbs per 28g
Contains added sugars, MSG and nitrates

POPCORN

Commercial brands of popcorn came out badly in our reviews, being full of sugar and other unacceptable ingredients as well as being unreasonably high in carbs – a real pity, since a little popped corn goes a long way, and makes a wonderfully filling snack. Search out popping corn and pop it yourself – 15g makes sufficient for a decent-sized portion.

Cypressa Popping Corn (Phases 3–4)
11.4g carbs per 100g

NUTS & SEEDS
Peanuts

KP Original Salted Peanuts (Phases 2–4)
1.9g carbs per 25g serving

FYI **KP Salt & Vinegar Flavour Peanuts (Phases 2–4)**
3.6g carbs per 25g serving
Contains MSG

FYI Own Brand Dry Roasted Peanuts
2.8–3.5g carbs per 25g serving
Some may contain added sugars, maize starch,
modified potato starch and MSG

Own Brand Salted Peanuts (Phases 2–4)
2–2.2g carbs per 25g serving

⚠ **Planters Nutcases Crispy Coated Peanuts,
Thai Sweet Chilli Flavour**
8.7g carbs per 25g serving
Contains added sugars and maize starch

Almonds

Own Brand Flaked Almonds (Phases 2–4)
1.8g carbs per 25g serving

Own Brand Whole Almonds (Phases 2–4)
1.6g carbs per 25g serving

Mixtures

Clearspring Roasted Snack Mix (Phases 2–4)
2.7g carbs per 25g serving

**Own Brand Mixed Nuts and Raisins
(Phases 3–4)**
7–7.7g carbs per 25g serving

Own Brand Salted Nut Selection (Phases 2–4)
2.4g carbs per 25g serving

Others

⚠ **Crazy Jack Organic Brazil Nuts (Phases 2–4)**
1.8g carbs per 25g serving

⚠ **Heartys Soy Nuts, BBQ**
9.15g carbs per 30g bag
Contains added sugars

Own Brand Pine Nuts (Phases 2–4)
1g carbs per 25g serving

Own Brand Salted Cashews (Phases 2–4)
5g carbs per 25g serving

Own Brand Salted Pistachios (Phases 2–4)
2–2.8g carbs per 25g serving

Own Brand Walnuts (Phases 2–4)
Trace carbs per 25g serving

**Own Brand Whole Blanched Hazelnuts
(Phases 2–4)**
1.5g carbs per 25g serving

Seeds

**Clearspring Roasted Pumpkin Seeds
(Phases 2–4)**
1.2g carbs per 55g bag

**Cypressa Roasted and Salted Pumpkin Seeds,
Unshelled (Phases 2–4)**
3.8g carbs per 25g serving

Own Brand Sunflower Seeds (Phases 2–4)
18.6g carbs per 100g

Whitworths Poppy Seeds (Phases 2–4)
4.6g carbs per 25g serving

RICE & CORN CAKES

While these once had a reputation as 'diet food', if you've looked on a package lately, you know that these lighter-than-air snacks are hardly low in carbs. You'll also want to check the ingredients labels carefully, avoiding those that are made with white rice, which is highly refined, and caramel, as well as other sweet-flavoured versions.

⚠ **Kallo Gluten Free Thick Slice Rice Cakes, Caramel**
   7.5g carbs per 10g rice cake
   Contains added sugars

⚠ **Kallo Organic Rice Cakes, Milk Chocolate**
 6.2g carbs per 11g rice cake
   · Contains added sugars

⚠ **Kallo Organic Rice Cakes, Thick Slice, Savoury (Phases 3–4)**
   6.5g carbs per 9g rice cake

⚠ **Kallo Organic Snack Size Rice Cakes, No Added Salt (Phases 3–4)**
   15.7g carbs per 20g serving

⚠ **Kallo Organic Snack Size Rice Cakes, Savoury (Phases 3–4)**
   17.8g carbs per 25g serving

⚠ **Kallo Organic Thin Slice Lightly Salted Corn Cakes (Phases 3–4)**
   3.6g carbs per 4.8g rice cake

⚠ **Kallo Snack Size Gluten Free Rice Cakes, Caramel**
15.8g carbs per 20g serving
Contains added sugars

⚠ **Kallo Snack Size Low Fat Rice Cakes, Apple & Cinnamon**
16.6g carbs per 20g serving
Contains added sugars

Real Foods Corn Thins Original (Phases 3–4)
4.7g carbs per slice

Real Foods Corn Thins Sesame (Phases 3–4)
4.5g carbs per slice

RICE SNACKS

⚠ **Imperial Japanese Style Rice Crackers**
19.8g carbs per 25g serving
Contains added sugars, cornflour and wheat flour

⚠ **Quaker, Snack-a-Jacks Jumbo, Barbecue**
8g carbs per 10g cake
Contains added sugars

⚠ **Quaker, Snack-a-Jacks Jumbo, Cheese**
8.1g carbs per 10g cake
Contains added sugars and MSG

Soups

A bowl of soup can be so nourishing and comforting. It is quick and easy to prepare, handy when you are in a hurry, and a useful way of taking the edge off your appetite before a meal, thus helping you not to overeat. The range of soups that can be found on supermarket shelves is extensive, whether tinned, fresh or dried, which is testament to soup's popularity. Unfortunately, however, a large percentage of popular brand soups contain added sugars, and many also contain modified starch and wheat flour, which, though not unacceptable on later phases of Atkins, should be consumed in moderation. (Refined white flour is unacceptable at any phase.)

By far the best of the bunch are fresh soups, and within those the organic ranges, which contain no additives and very rarely have added sugars. If you choose carefully among those available in the chilled cabinet, you will also find products with lower carb counts than their tinned counterparts.

Of the soups we reviewed, fresh mushroom soups were among the lowest in carbs, lentil soups the highest. And if you fancy a bowl of one of the chunky vegetable soups, be careful as often they are bulked out with potatoes, which can raise carb levels.

You will notice that there are no dried or instant pot soups within our listings. Not only are their carb levels too high for any phase of Atkins, but they contain added sugars and a long list of ingredients best avoided, such as MSG, white flour and many additives.

FRESH SOUPS

Carrot & Coriander

⚠ **Own Brand Fresh Soup Carrot & Coriander**
3.6–4.8g carbs per 100g
Contains added sugars and maize starch

⚠ **Simply Organic Carrot & Coriander Fresh Organic Soup (Phases 2–4)**
3.3g carbs per 100g

Chicken

⚠ **Baxter's Fresh Soup Chicken with Vegetables**
5.5g carbs per 100g
Contains added sugars, modified cornflour and wheat flour

Haddock

New Covent Garden Food Co. Smoked Haddock Chowder (Phases 3–4)
6.7g carbs per 100g

Mushroom

FYI **New Covent Garden Food Co. Wild Mushroom (Phases 3–4)**
3.8g carbs per 100g
Contains wheat flour

FYI **Own Brand Cream of Mushroom (Phases 3–4)**
4–4.7g carbs per 100g
Contains modified maize starch and wheat flour

Own Brand Fresh Mushroom Soup (Phases 2–4)
3.8–4.7g carbs per 100g

Tomato

⚠ **Baxters Fresh Soup Tomato Mediterranean Flavour**
7.7g carbs per 100g
Contains added sugars and modified cornflour

⚠ **Own Brand Tomato and Basil Soup**
6–6.5g carbs per 100g
Contains added sugars and maize starch

Vegetable

⚠ **Baxters Fresh Soup Parsnip, Carrot and Sweet Potato**
8.5g carbs per 100g
Contains added sugars

⚠ **Simply Organic Chunky Vegetable Fresh Organic Soup (Phases 3–4)**
7.8g carbs per 100g

⚠ **Simply Organic Lentil & Parsley Fresh Organic Soup (Phases 3–4)**
9.1g carbs per 100g

JARS, TETRA PAKS & TINNED SOUPS

Asparagus

⚠ **Baxters Luxury Cream of Asparagus Soup**
6g carbs per 100g
Contains added sugars, modified cornflour and wheat flour

Carrot & Coriander

Campbell's Selection Carrot & Coriander Soup (Phases 3–4)
6.4g carbs per 100ml

⚠ **Crosse & Blackwell Waistline Carrot & Coriander Soup**
6.8g carbs per 100g
Contains added sugars, modified maize starch and wheat flour

⚠ **Heinz Carrot & Coriander Soup**
6.2g carbs per 100g
Contains added sugars and modified cornflour

⚠ **Knorr Carrot & Coriander Soup**
3.9g carbs per 100ml
Contains added sugars and modified maize starch

Loyd Grossman Carrot & Coriander Soup (Phases 2–4)
5.4g carbs per 100g

FYI **Own Brand Carrot and Coriander Soup**
4.5–5.5g carbs per 100g
Some may contain added sugars, trans fats, modified maize starch and wheat flour

Chicken

⚠ **Baxters Healthy Choice Chicken & Vegetable Soup**
6.1g carbs per 100g
Contains added sugars and modified cornflour

(FYI) **Campbell's Classics Cream of Chicken Soup (Phases 3–4)**
3.5g carbs per 100g
Contains modified maize starch, MSG and wheat flour

(FYI) **Campbell's Special Choice Cream of Chicken and Mushroom Soup (Phases 3–4)**
3.5g carbs per 100g
Contains modified maize starch and MSG

(FYI) **Loyd Grossman Chicken & Vegetable Soup (Phases 3–4)**
2.6g carbs per 100g
Contains maize starch

⚠ **Own Brand Cream of Chicken Soup**
5–5.7g carbs per 100g
Contains added sugars, modified maize starch and wheat flour

(FYI) **Weight Watchers from Heinz Chicken Soup (Phases 3–4)**
4.4g carbs per 100g
Contains cornflour and wheat flour

Consommé

⚠ **Baxters Luxury Beef Consommé**
0.7g carbs per 100g
Contains added sugars

⚠ **Campbell's Beef Consommé**
0.5g carbs per 100g
Contains added sugars, trans fats and MSG

Lobster

⚠ **Baxters Luxury Lobster Bisque**
3.6g carbs per 100g
Contains added sugars and modified cornflour

Mushroom

[FYI] **Campbell's Classics Cream of Mushroom Soup (Phases 3–4)**
5.3g carbs per 100g
Contains modified maize starch, MSG and wheat flour

[FYI] **Campbell's Selection Country Mushroom Soup (Phases 3–4)**
3.4g carbs per 100g
Contains modified maize starch

⚠ **Crosse & Blackwell Waistline Mushroom & Crème Fraîche Soup**
2.8g carbs per 100g
Contains added sugars and wheat flour

⚠ **Heinz Cream of Mushroom Soup**
5.2g carbs per 100g
Contains added sugars, modified cornflour and wheat flour

⚠ **Loyd Grossman Four Mushroom Soup**
2.5g carbs per 100g
Contains added sugars, modified maize starch and wheat flour

FYI **Own Brand Cream of Mushroom Soup
(Phases 3–4)**
1.4–4.6g carbs per 100g
Contains modified maize starch and wheat flour

Tomato

⚠ **Baxters Organic Tomato and Vegetable**
 6.8g carbs per 100g
Contains added sugars and wheat flour

⚠ **Baxters Vegetarian Mediterranean Tomato
Soup**
6.8g carbs per 100g
Contains added sugars and modified cornflour

⚠ **Campbell's Cream of Tomato Soup**
8.5g carbs per 100g
Contains added sugars and modified maize starch

⚠ **Campbell's Italian Tomato Soup with Basil**
5.3g carbs per 100g
Contains added sugars and modified maize starch

⚠ **Go Organic Italian Tomato & Basil Soup
(Phases 2–4)**
3.3g carbs per 100g

⚠ **Heinz Cream of Tomato Soup**
7.3g carbs per 100g
Contains added sugars and modified cornflour

⚠ **Heinz Organic Cream of Tomato Soup**
 6.9g carbs per 100g
Contains added sugars and modified cornflour

⚠ **Knorr Vie Tomato & Basil Soup**
5.5g carbs per 100ml
Contains added sugars and modified maize starch

⚠ **Loyd Grossman Tomato & Basil Soup**
5.3g carbs per 100g
Contains added sugars and modified maize starch

⚠ **Own Brand Cream of Tomato Soup**
8.7–9.4g carbs per 100g
Contains added sugars and modified maize starch

(FYI) **Weight Watchers from Heinz Mediterranean
Tomato & Red Pepper Soup (Phases 3–4)**
2.4g carbs per 100g
Contains modified cornflour

(FYI) **Weight Watchers from Heinz Mediterranean
Tomato & Vegetable Soup (Phases 3–4)**
3g carbs per 100g
Contains modified cornflour

⚠ **Weight Watchers from Heinz Tomato Soup**
4.6g carbs per 100g
Contains added sugars and modified cornflour

Vegetable

⚠ **Baxters Organic Broccoli and Potato**
 6.2g carbs per 100g
Contains added sugars, cornflour and wheat flour

⚠ **Baxters Organic Carrot and Parsnip with
 Nutmeg**
6.6g carbs per 100g
Contains added sugars and wheat flour

⚠ **Campbell's Classics Vegetable Soup**
6.2g carbs per 100g
Contains added sugars, modified maize starch and MSG

⚠ **Campbell's Selection Mediterranean Minestrone Soup**
6.1g carbs per 100g
Contains added sugars and maize starch

FYI **Campbell's Spring Vegetable Soup (Phases 3–4)**
4.6g carbs per 100g
Contains modified maize starch and MSG

⚠ **Go Organic Carrot Orange & Ginger Soup (Phases 2–4)**
3.6g carbs per 100g

⚠ **Go Organic Creamy Potato & Leek Soup (Phases 3–4)**
5.6g carbs per 100g

⚠ **Knorr Vie Smooth Autumn Vegetable Soup with Crème Fraîche**
4.3g carbs per 100ml
Contains added sugars

⚠ **Own Brand Broccoli & Stilton Soup**
3.7–4.6g carbs per 100g
Contains trans fats, modified maize starch and wheat flour

FYI **Weight Watchers from Heinz Carrot & Lentil Soup (Phases 3–4)**
6g carbs per 100g
Contains modified cornflour

FYI **Weight Watchers from Heinz Country Vegetable Soup (Phases 3–4)**
6g carbs per 100g
Contains modified cornflour and wheat flour

Tinned and Jarred Food

Contrary to popular belief, tinned food can form part of a healthy diet. Just because a food is tinned doesn't mean it is inferior to fresh: in many cases the vitamin and mineral content is equivalent to its fresh counterpart and in some instances it can be better. The majority of tinned vegetables and fruits are packed minutes after harvesting, when nutrient concentrations and eating quality are at their highest, whereas some vitamins in fresh foods can decrease by 50 per cent within the first seven days after harvest when stored at ambient temperatures.

Tinned foods can be more convenient than fresh, especially when time is at a premium. Tinned beans and legumes are particularly useful, as the dried ones must be soaked and then cooked – a process that can take the better part of a day, even when using a quick-soak method. Tinned meats and fish can be handy for fast and tasty salads, casseroles and simple suppers.

It is now possible to find many tinned goods that have no added sugars and are tinned in natural juice or in water rather than syrup, which must be avoided when following Atkins.

Salt is often added when foods are processed; it adds flavour, of course, and acts as a preservative. If you find that tinned foods, such as beans, taste too salty, simply rinse them before using.

One clear benefit of tinned foods: they have nutrition labels and ingredients lists, so you can be sure what you're getting.

Best Bites

Tinned fruits that are packed in water can sometimes be difficult to find. Don't be tempted to buy anything in syrup, even light syrup.

Soup is a great appetite controller. Sip a cup of miso soup or reduced-salt chicken, beef or vegetable broth (add a tablespoon or two of tomato juice for body, if you like) before dinner to fill you up. You won't be tempted to eat as much. Tinned cream soups usually have lower carb counts, but beware: they often contain hydrogenated oils.

FISH

Tinned seafood is wonderfully convenient for making delicious low-carb salads. Combine tinned crab, tuna or prawns with mayonnaise, herbs, seasonings and chopped celery and you have a five-minute lunch or light supper.

Tinned tuna usually comes as chunks or steaks and is packed in oil, brine or spring water. Use tuna packed in oil for heated dishes and water-packed tuna for salads.

Since these foods taste savoury, it can be hard to believe that many contain sugar. Be on the lookout for added sugars in the ingredients lists.

Where naturally occurring carbs are observed when you might have expected to find a zero rating, we have alerted you with an FYI symbol **FYI**. For more information please refer to page 126 in the introduction to the Listings Section.

ANCHOVIES

Admiral Anchovy Paste with Olive Oil (Phases 1–4)
1.8g carbs per 100g

Gia Anchovy Paste (Phases 1–4)
2.1g carbs per 100g

⒡ John West Flat Fillets of Anchovies in Olive Oil (Phases 1–4)
Trace carbs per 10g serving

⒡ Own Brand Anchovies in Olive Oil with Garlic and Parsley (Phases 1–4)
Trace carbs per 100g

⒡ Own Brand Anchovy Fillets in Olive Oil, Jarred (Phases 1–4)
Trace carbs per 100g

⒡ Own Brand Anchovy Fillets in Olive Oil, Tinned (Phases 1–4)
Trace carbs per 100g

CAVIAR

Marina Lumpfish Caviar (Phases 1–4)
2g carbs per 100g

CLAMS

⚠ John West Baby Clams in Brine
3g carbs per 100g
Contains added sugars

COCKLES

⚠ **Van Smirren Seafoods Cockles Cooked and Pickled**
9g carbs per 100g
Contains added sugars

COD & HERRING ROE

John West Pressed Cod Roe (Phases 1–4)
2.3g carbs per 100g

John West Soft Cod Roes (Phases 1–4)
Trace carbs per 100g

John West Soft Herring Roes (Phases 1–4)
Trace carbs per 100g

CRAB

(FYI) **John West Dressed Crab (Phases 3–4)**
2g carbs per 100g
Contains added wheat flour

⚠ **Kingfisher Crabmeat in Brine**
1.7g carbs per 100g
Contains added sugars and MSG

⚠ **Kingfisher De-Luxe Lump Crabmeat in Brine**
1.7g carbs per 100g
Contains added sugars and MSG

Shippam's Crab Spread (Phases 2–4)
5.4g carbs per 100g

HERRINGS

⚠ **John West Herring Fillets in Tomato Sauce**
4.8g carbs per 95g serving
Contains added sugars and modified cornflour

⚠ **Princes Marinated Herring**
1.6g carbs per 100g
Contains added sugars

KIPPERS

(FYI) **John West Kipper Fillets in Brine (Phases 1–4)**
Trace carbs per 100g

(FYI) **John West Kipper Fillets in Sunflower Oil
(Phases 1–4)**
Trace carbs per 100g

(FYI) **Princes Kippers in Lightly Salted Water
(Phases 1–4)**
Trace carbs per 100g
Contains MSG

Princes Kippers in Sunflower Oil (Phases 1–4)
0g carbs per 100g

LOBSTER

(FYI) **John West Dressed Lobster (Phases 3–4)**
2g carbs per 100g
Contains added wheat flour

MACKEREL

⚠ **John West Mackerel Fillets in Curry Sauce**
3.5g carbs per 100g
Contains added sugars and modified cornflour

⚠ **John West Mackerel Fillets in Green Peppercorn Sauce**
2.6g carbs per 100g
Contains added sugars and modified cornflour

⚠ **John West Mackerel Fillets in Mustard Sauce**
4.7g carbs per 100g
Contains added sugars and modified cornflour

(FYI) **John West Traditional Wood Smoked Peppered Mackerel Fillets in Sunflower Oil (Phases 1–4)**
0.5g carbs per 100g

(FYI) **Princes Mackerel Fillets in a Hot Chilli Dressing (Phases 1–4)**
Trace carbs per 100g

Princes Mackerel Fillets in Lightly Salted Water (Phases 1–4)
0g carbs per 100g

⚠ **Princes Mackerel Fillets in Mustard Sauce**
6g carbs per 100g
Contains added sugars, trans fats, modified maize starch and wheat flour

Princes Mackerel Fillets in Olive Oil (Phases 1–4)
0g carbs per 100g

⚠ **Princes Mackerel Fillets in a Rich Spicy Tomato Sauce**
4.7g carbs per 100g
Contains added sugars

Princes Mackerel Fillets in a Rich Tomato Sauce (Phases 1–4)
3.3g carbs per 100g

MUSSELS

John West Smoked Mussels in Sunflower Oil (Phases 2–4)
10g carbs per 100g

Palacio de Oriente Mussels in Galician Sauce (Phases 1–4)
5.5g carbs per 100g

Van Smirren Seafoods Mussels in Brine (Phases 1–4)
1g carbs per 100g

⚠ **Van Smirren Seafoods Mussels Cooked and Pickled**
1g carbs per 100g
Contains added sugars

OYSTERS

John West Smoked Oysters in Sunflower Oil (Phases 2–4)
10g carbs per 100g

PILCHARDS

Glenryck Atlantic Pilchards in Brine (Phases 1–4)
0g carbs per 100g

⚠ Glenryck South Atlantic Pilchard Fillets in Spicy Tomato Sauce
3.5g carbs per 100g
Contains added sugars

(FYI) Glenryck South Atlantic Pilchards in Tomato Sauce (Phases 3–4)
2.3g carbs per 100g
Contains modified maize starch

PRAWNS

⚠ John West Prawns in Brine
1g carbs per 100g
Contains added sugars and MSG

⚠ Kingfisher Prawns in Brine
0.5g carbs per 100g
Contains added sugars and MSG

SALMON

Glenryck Medium Red Salmon in Brine (Phases 1–4)
0g carbs per 100g

(FYI) Glenryck Medium Red Salmon, Skinless and Boneless (Phases 1–4)
0.3g carbs per 100g

(FYI) **John West Pink Salmon (Phases 1–4)**
Trace carbs per 100g

(FYI) **John West Red Salmon (Phases 1–4)**
Trace carbs per 100g

(FYI) **La Piara Smoked Salmon Paté (Phases 1–4)**
1.5g carbs per 100g

Princes Wild Medium Red Salmon (Phases 1–4)
0g carbs per 100g

Princes Wild Pink Salmon (Phases 1–4)
0g carbs per 100g

⚠ **Shippam's Finest Potted Salmon**
1g carbs per 100g
Contains added sugars

Shippam's Salmon Spread (Phases 2–4)
4.2g carbs per 100g

⚠ **Weight Watchers from Heinz Salmon in Lemon Mayonnaise Dressing Made with John West Salmon**
6.4g carbs per 100g
Contains added sugars and modified cornflour

SARDINES

Bela Sardines in Hot Sauce (Phases 1–4)
0g carbs per 100g

Bela Sardines in Lemon Sauce (Phases 1–4)
0g carbs per 100g

FYI **John West Boneless Sardines in Sunflower Oil (Phases 1–4)**
Trace carbs per 100g

John West Boneless Sardines in Tomato Sauce (Phases 1–4)
1.5g carbs per 100g

⚠ **Princes Sardine and Tomato Paste**
3.1g carbs per 100g
Contains added sugars

Princes Sardines in a Rich Tomato Sauce (Phases 1–4)
1.6g carbs per 100g

SHRIMPS

⚠ **John West Shrimps in Brine**
1g carbs per 100g
Contains added sugars

SILD

FYI **John West Sild in Sunflower Oil (Phases 1–4)**
Trace carbs per 100g

⚠ **John West Sild in Tomato Sauce**
2.5g carbs per 100g
Contains added sugars and cornflour

SKIPPERS

⚠ **John West Traditional Smoked Skippers Brisling in Tomato Sauce**
3g carbs per 100g
Contains added sugars and cornflour

John West Traditional Wood Smoked Skippers Brisling in Sunflower Oil (Phases 1–4)
Trace carbs per 100g

TROUT

⚠ **Shippam's Trout and Lemon Paté**
6.2g carbs per 100g
Contains added sugars

TUNA

⚠ **John West Skipjack Tuna in Mayonnaise with Sweet Corn**
4.5g carbs per 100g
Contains added sugars

⚠ **John West Skipjack Tuna Salad with Three Bean Mix in Vinaigrette Dressing**
9.6g carbs per 100g
Contains added sugars

⚠ **John West Skipjack Tuna in Thousand Island Dressing**
5.1g carbs per 100g
Contains added sugars and modified cornflour

FYI **John West Yellowfin Tuna Steak in Olive Oil (Phases 1–4)**
Trace carbs per 100g

FYI **John West Yellowfin Tuna Steak in Springwater (Phases 1–4)**
Trace carbs per 100g

La Piara Tuna with Olive Oil Paté (Phases 2–4)
5.1g carbs per 100g

⚠ **Princes Slimming World Tuna in a Light Lemon Mayonnaise**
3.5g carbs per 100g
Contains added sugars

⚠ **Princes Slimming World Tuna in a Lime and Black Pepper Dressing**
3.5g carbs per 100g
Contains added sugars

⚠ **Princes Slimming World Tuna in a Red Chilli and Lime Dressing**
1g carbs per 100g
Contains added sugars

Princes Tuna & Mayonnaise Paste (Phases 1–4)
1g carbs per 100g

⚠ **Princes Tuna & Red Onion Paste**
5.4g carbs per 100g
Contains added sugars

⚠ **Weight Watchers from Heinz Tuna in Coronation Style Dressing Made with John West Tuna**
6.5g carbs per 100g
Contains added sugars

⚠ **Weight Watchers from Heinz Tuna in Mayonnaise Style Dressing with Sweet Corn Made with John West Tuna**
6.1g carbs per 100g
Contains added sugars

⚠ **Weight Watchers from Heinz Tuna in Tomato and Herb Dressing Made with John West Tuna**
5.1g carbs per 100g
Contains added sugars and modified cornflour

FRUIT

Choose fruit that has been canned in its own juice rather than in sugar syrup, which is unacceptable on any phase of Atkins. Both are higher in carbs than raw fruit, but the fruit doesn't have sugar or other sweetener added to it. Drain off the juice to reduce carbs even further.

APPLES

John West Apple Slices (Phases 3–4)
5g carbs per 100g

⚠ **Morton Fruit Fillings Apple & Blackberry**
22.2g carbs per 100g
Contains added sugars and modified maize starch

Morton Fruit Fillings Bramley Apple
21.1g carbs per 100g
Contains added sugars and modified maize starch

Own Brand Apple Slices No Added Sugar (Phases 3–4)
7.8–9g carbs per 100g

APRICOTS

 Own Brand Apricot Halves in Fruit Juice (Phases 3–4)
8–10g carbs per 100g
Some may contain added sugars

BLACKBERRIES

 Hartley's Blackberries in Apple Juice
8.2g carbs per 100g
Contains added sugars

 John West Blackberries in Fruit Juice (Phases 2–4)
7.1g carbs per 100g

 Own Brand Blackberries in Fruit Juice (Phases 3–4)
7–8.6g carbs per 100g
Contains added sugars

BLACKCURRANTS

 Hartley's Blackcurrants in Apple Juice
9g carbs per 100g
Contains added sugars

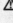 **Own Brand Blackcurrants in Fruit Juice (Phases 3–4)**
8–9.2g carbs per 100g
Some may contain added sugars

CHERRIES

⚠ **Hartley's Black Cherries in Apple Juice**
11.4g carbs per 100g
Contains added sugars

⚠ **Morton Red Cherry Fruit Fillings**
23.9g carbs per 100g
Contains added sugars and modified maize starch

⚠ **Own Brand Black Cherry Pie Filling**
17.7g carbs per 100g
Contains added sugars and modified maize starch

CITRUS FRUITS

Del Monte Mandarin Oranges Whole Segments in Own Juice (Phases 3–4)
10g carbs per 100g

Opies Sliced Lemons in Lemon Juice (Phases 3–4)
7.8g carbs per 100g

Own Brand Mandarin Segments in Fruit/Orange/Natural Juice (Phases 3–4)
7.7–10g carbs per 100g

FRUIT COCKTAIL

Del Monte Fruit Cocktail in Juice (Phases 3–4)
11.2g carbs per 100g

(FYI) **Own Brand Fruit Cocktail in Fruit/Apple Juice**
10–12g carbs per 100g
Contains added sugars

GOOSEBERRIES

⚠ **Hartley's Gooseberries in Apple Juice**
9.4g carbs per 100g
Contains added sugars

GRAPEFRUIT

**Del Monte Grapefruit Segments in Juice
(Phases 3–4)**
10.5g carbs per 100g

**Own Brand Grapefruit Segments in
Fruit/Natural Juice (Phases 3–4)**
8.7–10g carbs per 100g

OLIVES, JARRED

(FYI) **Belazu Black Olives with Herbs (Phases 1–4)**
5.8g carbs per 100g

**Belazu Green Olives with Basil and Garlic
(Phases 1–4)**
1.6g carbs per 100g

Fora Domat Turkish Olives (Phases 1–4)
0.7g carbs per 100g

Karyatis Garlic Stuffed Olives in Extra Virgin Oil (Phases 1–4)
1g carbs per 100g

Karyatis Kalamata Olives in Extra Virgin Oil (Phases 1–4)
0.8g carbs per 100g

Karyatis Mixed Olives in Extra Virgin Oil (Phases 1–4)
0.8g carbs per 100g

(FYI) **McIlhenny Tabasco Spiced Spanish Olives (Phases 1–4)**
0.5g carbs per 100g
Contains MSG

(FYI) **Own Brand Black Olives (Phases 1–4)**
3.3–6g carbs per 100g

(FYI) **Own Brand Green Olives (Phases 1–4)**
3.6g carbs per 100g

Own Brand Green Olives Stuffed with Jalapeño Paste (Phases 1–4)
3.5g carbs per 100g

Own Brand Green Olives Stuffed with Pimento Paste (Phases 1–4)
3.5g carbs per 100g

OLIVES, TINNED

(FYI) **Own Brand Green Tinned Olives (Phases 1–4)**
Trace–0.6g carbs per 100g
Contains MSG

Own Brand Pitted Black Tinned Olives in Brine (Phases 1–4)
Trace–7g carbs per 100g

PEACHES

Del Monte Peach Slices in Juice (Phases 3–4)
11.2g carbs per 100g

⚠ **Own Brand Peach Slices in Fruit/Grape Juice**
10–12g carbs per 100g
All contain added sugars

PEARS

Del Monte Pear Halves in Juice (Phases 3–4)
10.5g carbs per 100g

(FYI) **Own Brand Pear Halves/Quarters in Fruit/Natural/Pear Juice (Phases 3–4)**
9–11g carbs per 100g
Some may contain added sugars

PINEAPPLE

Own Brand Pineapple Slices/Chunks in Natural/Pineapple Juice (Phases 3–4)
12–12.2g carbs per 100g

Princes Pineapple Crushed in Juice (Phases 3–4)
12.2g carbs per 100g

PRUNES

⚠ **Del Monte Prunes in Juice**
25g carbs per 100g
Contains added sugars

Own Brand Prunes in Fruit Juice (Phases 3–4)
19–25.7g carbs per 100g

RASPBERRIES

⚠ **Hartley's Raspberries in Apple Juice**
8.1g carbs per 100g
Contains added sugars

⚠ **John West Raspberries in Fruit Juice**
6.7g carbs per 100g
Contains added sugars

RHUBARB

Own Brand Rhubarb (Phases 1–4)
1–7g carbs per 100g

SUMMER FRUITS

⚠ **Hartley's Summer Fruits in Apple Juice**
8.6g carbs per 100g
Contains added sugars

⚠ Morton Fruit Fillings Summer Fruits
19g carbs per 100g
Contains added sugars and modified maize starch

MEAT & POULTRY

Like many tinned goods, tinned meats and poultry are handy if you're short of time, but be aware that many contain added sugars, which makes them unacceptable on any phase of Atkins. Lurking elsewhere in tinned meats are nitrates, which are used as a preservative, to inhibit the growth of germs or to enhance colour. It's best to seek alternatives where possible. Many also contain monosodium glutamate (MSG), a preservative and flavour enhancer. MSG can cause water retention and headaches in individuals sensitive to it.

You will notice that some products have merited a food alert icon, FYI, even though the carb levels fall within acceptable limits. Further, they have been coded for phases 3–4. We have done this because these products contain maize flour or starch, or wheat flour and we have drawn your attention to this fact in case you wish to choose a product that is free from those additives.

BEEF

Corned Beef

⚠ Fray Bentos Corned Beef
0.8g carbs per 100g
Contains added sugars and nitrates

⚠ Own Brand Corned Beef
1g carbs per 100g
Contains added sugars and nitrates

(FYI) **Princes Corned Beef and Onion Paste (Phases 1–4)**
2.8g carbs per 100g
Contains nitrates

⚠ **Princes Delicious Corned Beef Hash**
5.1g carbs per 100g
Contains added sugars and nitrates

⚠ **Princes Lean Corned Beef**
1g carbs per 100g
Contains added sugars and nitrates

Shippam's Corned Beef and Onion (Phases 1–4)
2.8g carbs per 100g

Beef & Stews

⚠ **Own Brand Irish Stew**
5.9–7g carbs per 100g
Contains added sugars, trans fats, modified maize starch and wheat flour

⚠ **Own Brand Minced Beef & Onions**
2.8–3.1g carbs per 100g
Contains added sugars, trans fats, cornflour and wheat flour

⚠ **Own Brand Stewed Steak**
1.6–4.5g carbs per 100g
Contains added sugars, cornflour and wheat flour

⚠ **Princes Chunky Premium Lean Steak**
3g carbs per 100g
Contains added sugars and wheat flour

(FYI) Princes Full Flavour Beef 'n' Beer (Phases 3–4)
5.5g carbs per 100g
Contains cornflour and wheat flour

⚠ Princes Goulash
5g carbs per 100g
Contains added sugars, modified cornflour and
wheat flour

⚠ Princes Minced Beef with Onions in Gravy
5.5g carbs per 100g
Contains added sugars, modified flour and wheat
flour

⚠ Princes Premium Lean Steak
3g carbs per 100g
Contains added sugars and wheat flour

⚠ Princes Rich & Tasty Beef in Red Wine
5g carbs per 100g
Contains added sugars, modified cornflour and
wheat flour

(FYI) Princes Slices of Beef in Gravy (Phases 3–4)
2g carbs per 100g
Contains wheat flour

**(FYI) Princes Succulent Steak and Kidney
(Phases 3–4)**
4g carbs per 100g
Contains added cornflour, MSG and wheat flour

(FYI) Princes Tender Stewed Steak (Phases 3–4)
3.1g carbs per 100g
Contains cornflour and wheat flour

⚠ **Stagg Classic Chili Con Carne**
8.6g carbs per 100g
Contains added sugars and cornflour

⚠ **Stagg Dynamite Hot Chili Con Carne**
9.6g carbs per 100g
Contains added sugars and cornflour

⚠ **Stagg Silverado Beef Chili Con Carne**
10.9g carbs per 100g
Contains added sugars, cornflour and modified
starch

Hamburgers

⚠ **Goblin Hamburgers**
4.6g carbs per 100g
Contains added sugars and wheat flour

Meat Balls

⚠ **Campbell's Meat Balls in 'Brilliant' Bolognese
Sauce**
12.1g carbs per 100g
Contains added sugars, cornflour and wheat flour

⚠ **Campbell's Meat Balls in 'Gorgeous' Gravy**
9.6g carbs per 100g
Contains added sugars, cornflour, MSG and wheat
flour

⚠ **Campbell's Meat Balls in 'Tasty' Tomato
Sauce**
11.6g carbs per 100g
Contains added sugars, cornflour and wheat flour

CHICKEN

John West Chicken Light Lunch French Style (Phases 2–4)
6.7g carbs per 100g

⚠ **John West Chicken Light Lunch Italian Style**
9.6g carbs per 100g
Contains added sugars

(FYI) **Princes Chicken Roll (Phases 3–4)**
12.5g carbs per 100g
Contains MSG

(FYI) **Princes Chicken Roll with Sage & Onion (Phases 3–4)**
12.5g carbs per 100g
Contains MSG

Shippam's Chicken Spread (Phases 1–4)
2.2g carbs per 100g

⚠ **Stagg Less Than 3% Fat Chicken Grande**
10.2g carbs per 100g
Contains added sugars, modified starch and wheat flour

HAM

⚠ **Own Brand Ham**
0.2g carbs per 100g
Contains added sugars and nitrates

FYI **Princes Bacon Grill (Phases 3–4)**
11g carbs per 100g
Contains nitrates and wheat starch

⚠ Princes Ham
2g carbs per 100g
Contains added sugars and nitrates

PASTES & SPREADS

FYI **La Piara Paté with Provence Herbs (Phases 1–4)**
1g carbs per 100g
Contains MSG and nitrates

⚠ Princes Chicken and Ham Paste
4.5g carbs per 100g
Contains trans fats and nitrates

FYI **Princes Ham and Beef Paste (Phases 2–4)**
3.7g carbs per 100g
Contains nitrates

Shippam's Beef Spread (Phases 1–4)
3g carbs per 100g

Shippam's Chicken Spread (Phases 1–4)
2.2g carbs per 100g

⚠ Shippam's Classic Lamb and Mint Paté
2.9g carbs per 100g
Contains added sugars

PORK

⚠ Own Brand Pork and Ham
2.2g carbs per 100g
Contains added sugars and nitrates

ⓕⓨⓘ PEK Braised Pork Kidneys in Gravy (Phases 3–4)
4g carbs per 100g
Contains modified starch and wheat flour

ⓕⓨⓘ PEK Chopped Pork (Phases 1–4)
1.8g carbs per 100g
Contains nitrates

⚠ Princes Pork Luncheon Meat
7.4g carbs per 100g
Contains added sugars, nitrates and wheat starch

⚠ Spam Lite
2.1g carbs per 100g
Contains added sugars, nitrates and starch

SAUSAGES

ⓕⓨⓘ Princes American Style Hot Dogs (Phases 2–4)
4.5g carbs per 100g
Contains nitrates

⚠ Princes Authentic Bockwurst German Sausages
1.5g carbs per 100g
Contains added sugars and nitrates

⚠ **Princes Hot Dogs in Brine**
4.5g carbs per 100g
Contains added sugars, nitrates and wheat starch

TONGUE

⚠ **Princes Finest Hand Packed Ox Tongue**
0.3g carbs per 100g
Contains added sugars and nitrates

(FYI) **Princes Lunch Tongue (Phases 1–4)**
0.3g carbs per 100g
Contains nitrates

SOUP

Some tinned soups may be low in carbs but still thickened with unacceptable ingredients, such as refined white flour and cornflour, or loaded with added sugars. Very few tinned soups pass the test, so read the labels and ingredients lists on individual soups within brands.

Asparagus

⚠ **Baxters Luxury Cream of Asparagus Soup**
6g carbs per 100g
Contains added sugars, modified cornflour and wheat flour

Carrot & Coriander

⚠ **Heinz Carrot & Coriander Soup**
6.2g carbs per 100g
Contains added sugars and modified cornflour

(FYI) Own Brand Carrot and Coriander Soup (Phases 3–4)

4.5–5.5g carbs per 100g

Some may contain added sugars, trans fats, modified maize starch and wheat flour

Chicken

⚠ Baxters Healthy Choice Chicken & Vegetable Soup

6.1g carbs per 100g

Contains added sugars and modified cornflour

(FYI) Campbell's Classics Cream of Chicken Soup (Phases 3–4)

3.5g carbs per 100g

Contains modified maize starch, MSG and wheat flour

(FYI) Campbell's Special Choice Cream of Chicken and Mushroom Soup (Phases 3–4)

3.5g carbs per 100g

Contains modified maize starch and MSG

(FYI) Own Brand Cream of Chicken Soup (Phases 3–4)

5–5.7g per 100g

Can contain added sugars, modified maize starch, MSG and wheat flour

Consommé

⚠ Baxters Luxury Beef Consommé

0.7g carbs per 100g

Contains added sugars

⚠ **Campbell's Beef Consommé**
0.5g carbs per 100g
Contains added sugars, trans fats and MSG

Lobster

⚠ **Baxters Luxury Lobster Bisque**
3.6g carbs per 100g
Contains added sugars and modified cornflour

Mushroom

Ⓕ **Campbell's Cream of Mushroom Soup (Phases 3–4)**
5.3g per 100g
Contains modified maize starch, MSG and wheat flour

Ⓕ **Campbell's Cream of Mushroom & Chicken Soup (Phases 3–4)**
3.5g carbs per 100g
Contains modified maize starch and MSG

⚠ **Heinz Cream of Mushroom Soup**
5.2g per 100g
Contains added sugars, modified cornflour and wheat flour

Ⓕ **Own Brand Cream of Mushroom Soup (Phases 3–4)**
1.4–4.6g carbs per 100g
Contains modified maize starch and wheat flour

Tomato

⚠ **Baxters Organic Tomato and Vegetable**
⚠ 6.8g carbs per 100g
Contains added sugars and wheat flour

⚠ Baxters Vegetarian Mediterranean Tomato Soup
6.8g carbs per 100g
Contains added sugars and modified cornflour

⚠ Campbell's Cream of Tomato Soup
8.5g carbs per 100g
Contains added sugars and modified maize starch

⚠ Campbell's Italian Tomato Soup with Basil
5.3g carbs per 100g
Contains added sugars and modified maize starch

⚠ Go Organic Italian Tomato & Basil Soup with Onion (Phases 1–4)
3.3g carbs per 100g

⚠ Heinz Cream of Tomato Soup
7.3g carbs per 100g
Contains added sugars and modified cornflour

⚠ Heinz Organic Cream of Tomato Soup
⚠ 6.9g carbs per 100g
Contains added sugars and cornflour

⚠ Own Brand Cream of Tomato Soup
8.7–9.4g carbs per 100g
Contains added sugars and modified maize starch

ⓕⓨⓘ Weight Watchers from Heinz Mediterranean Tomato & Red Pepper Soup (Phases 3–4)
2.4g carbs per 100g
Contains modified cornflour

(FYI) **Weight Watchers from Heinz Mediterranean Tomato & Vegetable Soup (Phases 3–4)**
3g carbs per 100g
Contains modified cornflour

Vegetable

⚠ **Baxters Organic Broccoli and Potato**
⚠ 6.2g carbs per 100g
Contains added sugars, cornflour and wheat flour

⚠ **Baxters Organic Carrot and Parsnip with Nutmeg**
⚠ 6.6g carbs per 100g
Contains added sugars and wheat flour

⚠ **Campbell's Classics Vegetable Soup**
6.2g carbs per 100g
Contains added sugars, modified maize starch and MSG

(FYI) **Campbell's Spring Vegetable Soup (Phases 3–4)**
4.6g carbs per 100g
Contains modified maize starch and MSG

⚠ **Go Organic Carrot Orange & Ginger Soup (Phases 2–4)**
3.6g per 100g

⚠ **Go Organic Creamy Potato & Leek Soup (Phases 3–4)**
5.6g per 100g

⚠ **Own Brand Broccoli & Stilton Soup**
3.7–4.6g carbs per 100g
Contains trans fats, modified maize starch and wheat flour

FYI **Weight Watchers from Heinz Carrot & Lentil Soup (Phases 3–4)**
6g carbs per 100g
Contains modified cornflour

VEGETABLES

When it comes to the nutritional value of tinned vegetables, there are trade-offs. Exposure to oxygen can decrease the amount of some vitamins in a food; the more time that elapses between the field and your table, the fewer nutrients a vegetable retains. Large commercial food companies have processing plants adjacent to their fields. Foods are harvested and tinned within hours, preserving freshness and flavour.

Heat, whether used in the canning process or from cooking at home, can also decrease the amount of nutrients, particularly vitamin C, in a food. While you might think that eating fresh raw vegetables is the answer, heat also helps to break down cell walls in vegetables and increase the availability of other nutrients.

Wherever possible, aim to use fresh, local vegetables. But when they are not available or you are in a rush, tinned vegetables are a useful solution.

ARTICHOKE HEARTS

Cofrusa Artichoke Hearts in Brine (Phases 1–4)
2.5g carbs per 100g

Own Brand Artichoke Hearts in Salted Water (Phases 1–4)
4.9–6g carbs per 100g

Sacla' Artichoke Antipasto (Phases 1–4)
1.8g carbs per 100g

ASPARAGUS, CUT

Green Giant Cut Green Asparagus (Phases 1–4)
1.7g carbs per 100g

**Own Brand Cut Green Asparagus Spears
(Phases 1–4)**
1.4g carbs per 100g

ASPARAGUS, WHOLE SPEARS

**Green Giant Green Asparagus Spears
(Phases 1–4)**
1.7g carbs per 100g

**Own Brand Whole Green Asparagus Spears
(Phases 1–4)**
1.4g carbs per 100g

**Sol Produce Green Asparagus Spears
(Phases 1–4)**
1.4g carbs per 100g

Sol Produce White Asparagus Spears (Phases 1–4)
2.2g carbs per 100g

BEANS & LEGUMES

Tinned beans and legumes are a good source of calcium, which is vital for healthy bones; phosphorus, which is an essential component for of all cells; and thiamin, which is required for energy metabolism.

Draining off the soaking liquid reduces the sodium and accompanying salty taste of tinned beans; rinsing the beans reduces them even further. Introduce beans to your eating plan by tossing a few into a fresh green salad.

Biona Organic Butter Beans (Phases 3–4)
16.8g carbs per 100g

⚠ **Biona Organic Chilli Beans**
12.5g carbs per 100g
Contains added sugars

Biona Organic Green Lentils (Phases 3–4)
15.4g carbs per 100g

Ⓕ**Ⓨ**Ⓘ **Own Brand Borlotti Beans (Phases 3–4)**
16–17.4g carbs per 100g
Some may contain added sugars

⚠ **Own Brand Butter Beans**
11–18.9g carbs per 100g
Contains added sugars

Ⓕ**Ⓨ**Ⓘ **Own Brand Cannellini Beans (Phases 3–4)**
13.5–17.5g carbs per 100g
Some may contain added sugars

Own Brand Chick Peas (Phases 3–4)
14.1–16.1g carbs per 100g

Ⓕ**Ⓨ**Ⓘ **Own Brand Flageolet Beans (Phases 3–4)**
15.7–16.9g carbs per 100g
Some may contain added sugars

Own Brand Green Lentils (Phases 3–4)
10.2–16.9g carbs per 100g

Own Brand Red Kidney Beans (Phases 3–4)
15–17.4g carbs per 100g

BAKED BEANS IN TOMATO SAUCE

Unfortunately, commercially produced baked beans are always filled with added sugars.

⚠ **Crosse & Blackwell Baked Beans in Tomato Sauce**
15.8g carbs per 100g
Contains added sugars and modified maize starch

⚠ **Crosse & Blackwell Waistline Healthy Baked Beans**
13.6g carbs per 100g
Contains added sugars and modified maize starch

⚠ **Heinz Baked Beans in Tomato Sauce**
13.1g carbs per 100g
Contains added sugars and modified cornflour

⚠ **Heinz Healthy Balance Baked Beans in Tomato Sauce**
11.7g carbs per 100g
Contains added sugars and modified cornflour

⚠ **Heinz Organic Baked Beans in Tomato Sauce**
 13.7g carbs per 100g
Contains added sugars and cornflour

⚠ HP Baked Beans in Tomato Sauce
15g carbs per 100g
Contains added sugars and modified maize starch

⚠ Own Brand Baked Beans in Tomato Sauce
14–15.9g carbs per 100g
Contains added sugars and modified maize starch

⚠ Own Brand Economy Baked Beans in Tomato Sauce
10.4–14g carbs per 100g
Contains added sugars and modified maize starch

⚠ Own Brand Healthy Option Baked Beans in Tomato Sauce
13–15.1g carbs per 100g
Contains added sugars and modified maize starch

⚠ Weight Watchers from Heinz Baked Beans in Tomato Sauce
11.3g carbs per 100g
Contains added sugars and modified cornflour

BEANS BAKED WITH FLAVOURINGS

⚠ Heinz BBQ Beans
14.9g carbs per 100g
Contains added sugars and modified cornflour

⚠ Heinz Cheezy Beans
12.5g carbs per 100g
Contains added sugars and modified potato starch

Heinz Curried Beans
17.9g carbs per 100g
Contains added sugars and modified cornflour

 Own Brand Curried Beans
16.5g carbs per 100g
Contains added sugars and modified maize starch

CARROTS, BABY

 Noliko Organic Baby Carrots
 6g carbs per 100g
Contains added sugars

 Own Brand Baby Carrots
3.9–4.4g carbs per 100g
Contains added sugars

CARROTS, SLICED

**Own Brand Economy Sliced Carrots
(Phases 3–4)**
3.9–4.4g carbs per 100g

**Own Brand Sliced Carrots No Added Salt
Range (Phases 3–4)**
4.2–4.4g carbs per 100g

**Own Brand Sliced Carrots in Salted Water
(Phases 3–4)**
4.2–4.4g carbs per 100g

CARROTS, WHOLE

Own Brand No Added Salt Range Whole Carrots (Phases 3–4)
3.9–4.4g carbs per 100g

Own Brand Whole Carrots in Salted Water (Phases 3–4)
4.2–4.4g carbs per 100g

CELERY HEARTS

Bonduelle Whole Celery Hearts (Phases 1–4)
2.1g carbs per 100g

Own Brand Celery Hearts in Salted Water (Phases 1–4)
1.1g carbs per 100g

GARLIC

Gia Garlic Cloves in Brine (Phases 1–4)
1.9g carbs per 100g

GREEN BEANS, CUT

Own Brand Cut Green Beans (Phases 2–4)
3.8–4g carbs per 100g

GREEN BEANS, WHOLE

Own Brand Whole Green Beans (Phases 1–4)
1.6–4.8g carbs per 100g

HEARTS OF PALM

Trout Hall Hearts of Palm (Phases 1–4)
4.4g carbs per 100g

MUSHROOMS, WHOLE

Cooked mushrooms concentrate carbs, so it is important to pay attention to portion size.

Borde Forest Mushroom Mix (Phases 1–4)
6.3g carbs per 100g

Own Brand Whole Button Button Mushrooms (Phases 1–4)
0.5–0.6g carbs per 100g

MUSHROOMS, SLICED

Own Brand Economy Sliced Mushrooms (Phases 1–4)
0.6g carbs per 100g

Own Brand Sliced Mushrooms (Phases 1–4)
0.5–0.6g carbs per 100g

ONIONS

Eazy Fried Spanish Onions in Olive Oil (Phases 1–4)
9g carbs per 100g

PEAS, GARDEN

Peas are high in carbs and you need to exercise caution with portion size. Remember that the phasing information is for the serving size, not for the entire tin.

⚠ **Own Brand Economy Garden Peas**
7–9.4g carbs per 100g
Contains added sugars

⚠ **Own Brand Garden Peas**
7.2–8g carbs per 100g
Contains added sugars

Own Brand No Added Sugar or Salt Range Garden Peas (Phases 3–4)
5.5–9.4g carbs per 100g

PEAS, MUSHY

⚠ **Batchelors Mushy Peas Chip Shop**
13.8g carbs per 100g
Contains added sugars

⚠ **Batchelors Mushy Peas Original**
13.5g carbs per 100g
Contains added sugars

⚠ **Crosse & Blackwell Mushy Processed Peas**
13.1g carbs per 100g
Contains added sugars

Foresight Pease Pudding (Phases 3–4)
15.9g carbs per 100g

⚠ **Own Brand Economy Mushy Peas**
12.1–14g carbs per 100g
Contains added sugars

⚠ **Own Brand Mushy Peas**
12.4–12.8g carbs per 100g
Contains added sugars

PEAS, PETITS POIS

⚠ **Own Brand Petits Pois**
5.5–11g carbs per 100g
Contains added sugars

PEAS, PROCESSED

⚠ **Batchelors Bigga Marrowfat Processed Peas**
10.1g carbs per 100g
Contains added sugars

⚠ **Farrows Giant Marrowfat Processed Peas**
12.3g carbs per 100g
Contains added sugars

⚠ **Natura Organic Processed Peas (Phases 3–4)**
13.5g carbs per 100g

⚠ **Own Brand Economy Processed Peas**
14–17.5g carbs per 100g
Contains added sugars

⚠ **Own Brand Processed Marrowfat Peas**
14–17.5g carbs per 100g
Contains added sugars

POTATOES

⚠ **Noliko Organic Baby Potatoes (Phases 3–4)**
11.5g carbs per 100g

Own Brand Economy Potatoes (Phases 3–4)
9.2–13g carbs per 100g

Own Brand Potatoes (Phases 3–4)
13–15.1g carbs per 100g

RATATOUILLE

⚠ **Own Brand Ratatouille Provencale**
4.2–7g carbs per 100g
Contains added sugars and modified maize starch

SPINACH LEAF

Crosse & Blackwell Spinach Leaf (Phases 1–4)
0.8g carbs per 100g

Own Brand Spinach Leaf (Phases 1–4)
1–3.4g carbs per 100g

SWEETCORN, CREAMED

⚠ **Green Giant**
11.9g carbs per 100g
Contains added sugars and cornflour

SWEETCORN, KERNELS

⚠ **Bonduelle Organic Sweetcorn**
 22.9g carbs per 100g
Contains added sugars

⚠ **Green Giant Niblets Original**
20.8g carbs per 100g
Contains added sugars

Green Giant No Added Salt or Sugar Sweetcorn (Phases 3–4)
16.7g carbs per 100g

⚠ **Green Giant Organic Sweetcorn**
 20.8g carbs per 100g
Contains added sugars

Green Giant Salad Crisp Sweetcorn (Phases 3–4)
13.3g carbs per 100g

⚠ **Own Brand Economy Sweetcorn**
15.5–18.8g carbs per 100g
Contains added sugars

Own Brand No Added Salt or Sugar Sweetcorn (Phases 3–4)
10.6–20.1g carbs per 100g

⚠ **Own Brand Sweetcorn**
15.5–21.8g carbs per 100g
Contains added sugars

SWEETCORN, WHOLE COBS

Green Giant Baby Cobs (Phases 3–4)
2.4g carbs per 100g

Own Brand Baby Corn Cobs (Phases 3–4)
3.4g carbs per 100g

SWEETCORN WITH EXTRA INGREDIENTS

⚠ **Green Giant Sweetcorn with Peppers**
17.9g carbs per 100g
Contains added sugars

TOMATOES

Pay attention to serving sizes. Yes, you can eat up to 175g of raw tomatoes a day during Induction. However, keep in mind that tomatoes cook down considerably, and you won't be allowed as much of the concentrated forms, such as purée and paste; 90g can quickly account for one-quarter of your daily carbs. All tomatoes, with the exception of those with added flavourings, are coded for Induction, but in most cases you will need to eat a smaller amount than the serving sizes listed below.

TOMATOES, CHOPPED

Dettori's Chopped Tomatoes (Phases 1–4)
3.5g carbs per 100g

Heinz Chopped Tomatoes with Herbs (Phases 1–4)
2.9–3g carbs per 100g

Napolina Chopped Tomatoes (Phases 1–4)
3.5g carbs per 100g

Own Brand Chopped Tomatoes (Phases 1–4)
3.5–6g carbs per 100g

Own Brand Economy Chopped Tomatoes (Phases 1–4)
2.9–3.5g carbs per 100g

⚠ **Own Brand Flavoured Chopped Tomatoes (Basil/Herbs/Garlic/Chilli, etc.)**
3.5–6.3g carbs per 100g
Contains added sugar

⚠ **Tarantella Organic Chopped Tomatoes (Phases 1–4)**
3.2g carbs per 100g

TOMATOES, PASSATA

⚠ **Cirio Italian Home Style Passata with Chili & Peppers**
8.6g carbs per 100g
Contains added sugars

Heinz Passata (Phases 1–4)
2.9g carbs per 100g

⚠ **Heinz Tomato Frito**
7.7g carbs per 100g
Contains added sugars and modified cornflour

Napolina Crushed Tomatoes with Basil (Phases 1–4)
6.1g carbs per 100g

Napolina Crushed Tomatoes with Onion & Garlic (Phases 1–4)
6.8g carbs per 100g

Napolina Crushed Tomatoes with Peppers & Chilli (Phases 1–4)
5.7g carbs per 100g

Own Brand Passata (Phases 1–4)
4.2–6.4g carbs per 100g

⚠ **Own Brand Passata with Herbs/Garlic/Basil**
5.5–7.7g carbs per 100g
Contains added sugars

Valfruta Passata di Campagna Thick Country Style Sieved Tomatoes (Phases 1–4)
4.2g carbs per 100g

TOMATOES, WHOLE CHERRY

Cirio Pomodorini Cherry Tomatoes (Phases 1–4)
7g carbs per 100g

Heinz Cherry Tomatoes (Phases 1–4)
2.9g carbs per 100g

TOMATOES, WHOLE PLUM

Dettori's Peeled Plum Tomatoes (Phases 1–4)
3.5g carbs per 100g

Heinz Whole Peeled Tomatoes (Phases 1–4)
2.9g carbs per 100g

⚠ **Napolina Organic Peeled Plum Tomatoes (Phases 1–4)**
3.5g carbs per 100g

Napolina Peeled Plum Tomatoes (Phases 1–4)
3.5g carbs per 100g

Own Brand Economy Plum Tomatoes (Phases 1–4)
2.9–4g carbs per 100g

Own Brand Plum Tomatoes (Phases 1–4)
3–4g carbs per 100g

Vegetables

Vegetables are an essential component of the ANA™ and the primary source of carbohydrates. Not only do they complement the protein and fat elements of your meals, they also supply essential vitamins, minerals, antioxidants and fibre. All vegetables are acceptable in the later phases of Atkins, when you are close to or maintaining your weight, although not everyone will have a carb threshold that allows them to eat every type of vegetable. Sometimes you might find that certain vegetables should only be eaten infrequently.

Where possible, choose fresh produce. Supermarkets nowadays offer the added choice of fresh organic vegetables, which will be stocked in a separate section to avoid contamination. If fresh is not an option, frozen or tinned vegetables are useful alternatives.

FRESH VEGETABLES

Unless stated otherwise, all carb listings are given for uncooked vegetables. Remember that, although we usually list carb values for 100g, this is not a serving size, just the British standard method of listing nutritional data. Therefore, in some cases, 100g will be too large a portion, especially in the early stages of the ANA™.

Artichokes (Phases 1–4)
6.9g carbs per medium artichoke

Asparagus (Phases 1–4)
2g carbs per 100g

Aubergine (Phases 1–4)
2.2g carbs per 100g

Beetroot (Phases 3–4)
7.6g carbs per 100g

Broad Beans (Phases 3–4)
33.2g carbs per 100g

Broccoli (Phases 1–4)
1.5g carbs per 100g

Broccoli Rabe (Phases 1–4)
1.8g carbs per 100g

Brussels Sprouts (Phases 1–4)
4.1g carbs per 100g

Cabbage, Green (Phases 1–4)
4g carbs per 100g

Cabbage, Red (Phases 1–4)
7.4g carbs per 100g

Cabbage, Savoy (Phases 1–4)
6.1g carbs per 100g

Cardoon (Phases 1–4)
4.9g carbs per 100g

Carrots (Phases 3–4)
7.4g carbs per 100g

Cauliflower (Phases 1–4)
3g carbs per 100g

Celeriac (Phases 1–4)
7.2g carbs per 100g

Celery (Phases 1–4)
0.9g carbs per 100g

Chicory (Phases 1–4)
2.8g carbs per 100g

Chinese Cabbage (Pe-tsai) (Phases 1–4)
3.2g carbs per 100g

Chinese Mustard Greens (Phases 1–4)
4.9g carbs per 100g

Chives (Phases 1–4)
4.3g carbs per 100g

Courgettes (Phases 1–4)
1.8g carbs per 100g

Cucumber (Phases 1–4)
1.5g carbs per 100g

Dandelion Greens (Phases 1–4)
5.7g carbs per 100g

Endive (Phases 1–4)
3.3g carbs per 100g

Fennel (Phases 1–4)
1.8g carbs per 100g

Garlic (Phases 1–4)
1.6g carbs per 100g

Green Beans (Phases 1–4)
3.2g carbs per 100g

Jerusalem Artichoke (Phases 3–4)
17.4g carbs per 100g

Jicama (Phases 1–4)
3.9g carbs per 100g

Kale (Phases 1–4)
1.4g carbs per 100g

Kohlrabi (Phases 1–4)
6.2g carbs per 100g

Leeks (Phases 1–4)
2.9g carbs per 100g

Lettuce, Butterhead (Phases 1–4)
2.3g carbs per 100g

Lettuce, Cos (Phases 1–4)
3.3g carbs per 100g

Lettuce, Iceberg (Phases 1–4)
2.1g carbs per 100g

Mangetouts (Phases 1–4)
4.2g carbs per 100g

Mushrooms, Button (White) (Phases 1–4)
0.4g carbs per 100g

Mushrooms, Oyster (Phases 1–4)
3.8g carbs per 100g

Mushrooms, Portobello (Phases 1–4)
4.1g carbs per 100g

Mushrooms, Shiitake (Phases 1–4)
12.1g carbs per 100g cooked (see also Dried Vegetables)

Okra (Phases 1–4)
3g carbs per 100g

Onions (Phases 1–4)
7.9g carbs per 100g

Pak Choi (Phases 1–4)
2.2g carbs per 100g

Parsnips (Phases 3–4)
12.5g carbs per 100g

Peas, shelled (Phases 3–4)
11.3g carbs per 100g

Peppers, Chilli (Phases 1–4)
0.7g carbs per 100g

Peppers, Green (Phases 1–4)
2.6g carbs per 100g

Peppers, Red (Phases 1–4)
6.4g carbs per 100g

Peppers, Yellow (Phases 1–4)
6.4g carbs per 100g

Potatoes, White (Phases 3–4)
16.6g carbs per 100g

Pumpkin (Phases 1–4)
2.2g carbs per 100g

Radicchio (Phases 1–4)
4.9g carbs per 100g

Radishes (Phases 1–4)
1.9g carbs per 100g

Rocket (Phases 1–4)
2g carbs per 100g

Sauerkraut (Phases 1–4)
1.1g carbs per 100g

Shallots (Phases 1–4)
3.3g carbs per 100g

Spinach (Phases 1–4)
1.6g carbs per 100g

Spring Greens (Phases 1–4)
3.1g carbs per 100g

Spring Onions (Phases 1–4)
3g carbs per 100g

Sprouts, Alfalfa (Phases 1–4)
3.8g carbs per 100g

Sprouts, Mung Bean (Phases 1–4)
2.2g carbs per 100g

Squash, Acorn (Phases 3–4)
10.4g carbs per 100g

Squash, Butternut (Phases 3–4)
11.7g carbs per 100g

Squash, Chayote (Phases 1–4)
2.2g carbs per 100g

Squash, Spaghetti (Phases 1–4)
6.9g carbs per 100g

Sugar Snaps (Phases 1–4)
3.4g carbs per 100g

Swede (Phases 2–4)
5g carbs per 100g

Sweetcorn (Phases 3–4)
2.3g carbs per 100g

Sweet Potatoes (Phases 3–4)
21.3g carbs per 100g

Swiss Chard (Phases 1–4)
3.7g carbs per 100g

Taro (Phases 3–4)
26.5g carbs per 100g

Tomatoes, Cherry (Phases 1–4)
3.9g carbs per 100g

Tomatoes, Plum (Phases 1–4)
3.9g carbs per 100g

Tomatoes, Red (Phases 1–4)
3.1g carbs per 100g

Turnips (Phases 1–4)
4.5g carbs per 100g

Watercress (Phases 1–4)
0.4g carbs per 100g

FROZEN VEGETABLES

As with fresh vegetables, most frozen vegetables are acceptable for certain phases of Atkins – provided that what you're buying is *just* vegetables. Avoid frozen vegetables swimming in sauces that include starches; also, butter-flavoured and cheese-flavoured sauces usually contain partially hydrogenated vegetable oils. As a result, we have not included such products, with the exception of that old favourite, creamed spinach. Choose plain vegetables and cook them in stock for added flavour, then dress them with butter or olive oil.

You may find that frozen vegetables are higher in carbs than fresh ones. This is because frozen vegetables are always cooked, which frequently concentrates their nutrients.

Asparagus Spears (Phases 1–4)
2.2g carbs per 100g

Broccoli (Phases 1–4)
2g carbs per 100g

Brussels Sprouts (Phases 1–4)
4g carbs per 100g

Carrots (Phases 3–4)
5g carbs per 100g

Cauliflower (Phases 1–4)
2.3g carbs per 100g

Courgettes (Phases 3–4)
2.2g carbs per 100g

Green Beans (Phases 1–4)
4.8g carbs per 100g

Kale (Phases 1–4)
2.9g carbs per 100g

Mixed Vegetables (Phases 3–4)
6.8g carbs per 100g

Mixed Vegetables Stir-Fry (Phases 3–4)
6.4g carbs per 100g

Onions (Phases 1–4)
5g carbs per 100g

Peas, Green (Phases 3–4)
9.5g carbs per 100g

Petit Pois (Phases 3–4)
7g carbs per 100g

Spinach, Leaf (Phases 1–4)
1.2g carbs per 100g

Sweetcorn (Phases 3–4)
20g carbs per 100g

TINNED & JARRED VEGETABLES

Advances in technology have meant that the quality of tinned and jarred vegetables has improved significantly, so that they are a good alternative to fresh. Steer clear of those with added sugars.

ARTICHOKE HEARTS

Cofrusa Artichoke Hearts in Brine (Phases 1–4)
2.5g carbs per 100g

Own Brand Artichoke Hearts in Salted Water (Phases 1–4)
4.9–6g carbs per 100g

Sacla' Artichoke Antipasto (Phases 1–4)
1.8g carbs per 100g

ASPARAGUS, CUT

Green Giant Cut Green Asparagus (Phases 1–4)
1.7g carbs per 100g

Own Brand Cut Green Asparagus Spears (Phases 1–4)
1.4g carbs per 100g

ASPARAGUS, WHOLE SPEARS

Green Giant Green Asparagus Spears (Phases 1–4)
1.7g carbs per 100g

Own Brand Whole Green Asparagus Spears (Phases 1–4)
1.4g carbs per 100g

Sol Produce Green Asparagus Spears (Phases 1–4)
1.4g carbs per 100g

Sol Produce White Asparagus Spears (Phases 1–4)
2.2g carbs per 100g

BEANS & LEGUMES

Biona Organic Butter Beans (Phases 3–4)
16.8g carbs per 100g

⚠ Biona Organic Chilli Beans
12.5g carbs per 100g
Contains added sugars

Biona Organic Green Lentils (Phases 3–4)
15.4g carbs per 100g

Ⓕ Own Brand Borlotti Beans (Phases 3–4)
16–17.4g carbs per 100g
Some may contain added sugars

⚠ Own Brand Butter Beans
11–18.9g carbs per 100g
Contains added sugars

Ⓕ Own Brand Cannellini Beans (Phases 3–4)
13.5–17.5g carbs per 100g
Some may contain added sugars

Own Brand Chick Peas (Phases 3–4)
14.1–16.1g carbs per 100g

(FYI) **Own Brand Flageolet Beans (Phases 3–4)**
15.7–16.9g carbs per 100g
Some may contain added sugars

Own Brand Green Lentils (Phases 3–4)
10.2–16.9g carbs per 100g

Own Brand Red Kidney Beans (Phases 3–4)
15–17.4g carbs per 100g

BAKED BEANS IN TOMATO SAUCE

Unfortunately, commercially produced baked beans are
always filled with added sugars.

⚠ **Crosse and Blackwell Baked Beans in Tomato
Sauce**
15.8g carbs per 100g
Contains added sugars and modified maize starch

⚠ **Crosse and Blackwell Waistline Healthy Baked
Beans**
13.6g carbs per 100g
Contains added sugars and modified maize starch

⚠ **Heinz Baked Beans in Tomato Sauce**
13.1g carbs per 100g
Contains added sugars and modified cornflour

⚠ **Heinz Healthy Balance Baked Beans in Tomato Sauce**
11.7g carbs per 100g
Contains added sugars and modified cornflour

⚠ **Heinz Organic Baked Beans in Tomato Sauce**
⚠ 13.7g carbs per 100g
Contains added sugars and cornflour

⚠ **HP Baked Beans in Tomato Sauce**
15g carbs per 100g
Contains added sugars and modified maize starch

⚠ **Own Brand Baked Beans in Tomato Sauce**
14 –15.9g carbs per 100g
Contains added sugars and modified maize starch

⚠ **Own Brand Economy Baked Beans in Tomato Sauce**
10.4–14g carbs per 100g
Contains added sugars and modified maize starch

⚠ **Own Brand Healthy Option Baked Beans in Tomato Sauce**
13–15.1g carbs per 100g
Contains added sugars and modified maize starch

⚠ **Weight Watchers from Heinz Baked Beans in Tomato Sauce**
11.3g carbs per 100g
Contains added sugars and modified cornflour

BEANS BAKED WITH FLAVOURINGS

⚠ Heinz BBQ Beans
14.9g carbs per 100g
Contains added sugars and modified cornflour

⚠ Heinz Cheezy Beans
12.5g carbs per 100g
Contains added sugars and modified potato starch

⚠ Heinz Curried Beans
17.9g carbs per 100g
Contains added sugars and modified cornflour

⚠ Own Brand Curried Beans
16.5g carbs per 100g
Contains added sugars and modified maize starch

CARROTS, BABY

⚠ Noliko Organic Baby Carrots
⚠ 6g carbs per 100g
Contains added sugars

⚠ Own Brand Baby Carrots
3.9–4.4g carbs per 100g
Contains added sugars

CARROTS, SLICED

Own Brand Economy Sliced Carrots (Phases 3–4)
3.9–4.4g carbs per 100g

**Own Brand Sliced Carrots No Added Salt
Range (Phases 3–4)**
4.2–4.4g carbs per 100g

**Own Brand Sliced Carrots in Salted Water
(Phases 3–4)**
4.2–4.4g carbs per 100g

CARROTS, WHOLE

**Own Brand No Added Salt Range Whole
Carrots (Phases 3–4)**
3.9–4.4g carbs per 100g

**Own Brand Whole Carrots in Salted Water
(Phases 3–4)**
4.2–4.4g carbs per 100g

CELERY HEARTS

Bonduelle Whole Celery Hearts (Phases 1–4)
2.1g carbs per 100g

**Own Brand Celery Hearts in Salted Water
(Phases 1–4)**
1.1g carbs per 100g

GARLIC

Gia Garlic Cloves in Brine (Phases 1–4)
1.9g carbs per 100g

GREEN BEANS, CUT

Own Brand Cut Green Beans (Phases 1–4)
3.8–4g carbs per 100g

GREEN BEANS, WHOLE

Own Brand Whole Green Beans (Phases 1–4)
1.6–4.8g carbs per 100g

HEARTS OF PALM

Trout Hall Hearts of Palm (Phases 1–4)
4.4g carbs per 100g

MUSHROOMS, SLICED

Own Brand Economy Sliced Mushrooms (Phases 1–4)
0.6g carbs per 100g

Own Brand Sliced Mushrooms (Phases 1–4)
0.5–0.6g carbs per 100g

MUSHROOMS, WHOLE

Borde Forest Mushroom Mix (Phases 1–4)
6.3g carbs per 100g

Own Brand Whole Button Button Mushrooms (Phases 1–4)
0.5–0.6g carbs per 100g

ONIONS

**Eazy Fried Spanish Onions in Olive Oil
(Phases 1–4)**
9g carbs per 100g

PEAS, GARDEN

⚠ **Own Brand Economy Garden Peas**
7–9.4g carbs per 100g
Contains added sugars

⚠ **Own Brand Garden Peas**
7.2–8g carbs per 100g
Contains added sugars

**Own Brand No Added Sugar or Salt Range
Garden Peas (Phases 3–4)**
5.5–9.4g carbs per 100g

PEAS, MUSHY

⚠ **Batchelors Mushy Peas Chip Shop**
13.8g carbs per 100g
Contains added sugars

⚠ **Batchelors Mushy Peas Original**
13.5g carbs per 100g
Contains added sugars

⚠ **Crosse and Blackwell Mushy Processed Peas**
13.1g carbs per 100g
Contains added sugars

Foresight Pease Pudding (Phases 3–4)
15.9g carbs per 100g

⚠ **Own Brand Economy Mushy Peas**
12.1g–14g carbs per 100g
Contains added sugars

⚠ **Own Brand Mushy Peas**
12.4–12.8g carbs per 100g
Contains added sugars

PEAS, PETITS POIS

⚠ **Own Brand Petits Pois**
5.5–11g carbs per 100g
Contains added sugars

PEAS, PROCESSED

⚠ **Batchelors Bigga Marrowfat Processed Peas**
10.1g carbs per 100g
Contains added sugars

⚠ **Farrows Giant Marrowfat Processed Peas**
12.3g carbs per 100g
Contains added sugars

⚠ **Natura Organic Processed Peas (Phases 3–4)**
13.5g carbs per 100g

⚠ **Own Brand Economy Processed Peas**
14–17.5g carbs per 100g
Contains added sugars

Own Brand Processed Marrowfat Peas
14–17.5 g carbs per 100g
Contains added sugars

POTATOES

 Noliko Organic Baby Potatoes (Phases 3–4)
11.5g carbs per 100g

Own Brand Economy Potatoes (Phases 3–4)
9.2–13g carbs per 100g

Own Brand Potatoes (Phases 3–4)
13–15.1g carbs per 100g

RATATOUILLE

 Own Brand Ratatouille Provencale
4.2–7g carbs per 100g
Contains added sugars and modified maize starch

SPINACH LEAF

Crosse & Blackwell Spinach Leaf (Phases 1–4)
0.8g carbs per 100g

Own Brand Spinach Leaf (Phases 1–4)
1–3.4g carbs per 100g

SWEETCORN, CREAMED

 Green Giant Creamed Sweetcorn
11.9g carbs per 100g
Contains added sugars and cornflour

SWEETCORN, KERNELS

⚠ **Bonduelle Organic Sweetcorn**
 22.9g carbs per 100g
Contains added sugars

⚠ **Green Giant Niblets Original**
20.8g carbs per 100g
Contains added sugars

Green Giant No Added Salt or Sugar Sweetcorn (Phases 3–4)
16.7g carbs per 100g

⚠ **Green Giant Organic Sweetcorn**
 20.8g carbs per 100g
Contains added sugars

Green Giant Salad Crisp Sweetcorn (Phases 3–4)
13.3g carbs per 100g

⚠ **Own Brand Economy Sweetcorn**
15.5–18.8g carbs per 100g
Contains added sugars

Own Brand No Added Salt or Sugar Sweetcorn (Phases 3–4)
10.6–20.1g carbs per 100g

⚠ **Own Brand Sweetcorn**
15.5–21.8g carbs per 100g
Contains added sugars

SWEETCORN, WHOLE COBS

Green Giant Baby Cobs (Phases 3–4)
2.4g carbs per 100g

Own Brand Baby Corn Cobs (Phases 3–4)
3.4g carbs per 100g

SWEETCORN WITH EXTRA INGREDIENTS

⚠ **Green Giant Sweetcorn with Peppers**
17.9g carbs per 100g
Contains added sugars

TOMATOES, CHOPPED

Dettori's Chopped Tomatoes (Phases 1–4)
3.5g carbs per 100g

**Heinz Chopped Tomatoes with Herbs
(Phases 1–4)**
2.9–3g carbs per 100g

Napolina Chopped Tomatoes (Phases 1–4)
3.5g carbs per 100g

Own Brand Chopped Tomatoes (Phases 1–4)
3.5–6g carbs per 100g

**Own Brand Economy Chopped Tomatoes
(Phases 1–4)**
2.9–3.5g carbs per 100g

⚠ **Own Brand Flavoured Chopped Tomatoes (Basil/Herbs/Garlic/Chilli, etc.)**
3.5–6.3g carbs per 100g
Contains added sugars

⚠ **Tarantella Organic Chopped Tomatoes (Phases 1–4)**
3.2g carbs per 100g

TOMATOES, PASSATA

⚠ **Cirio Italian Home Style Passata with Chilli & Peppers**
8.6g carbs per 100g
Contains added sugars

Heinz Passata (Phases 1–4)
2.9g carbs per 100g

⚠ **Heinz Tomato Frito**
7.7g carbs per 100g
Contains added sugars and modified cornflour

Napolina Crushed Tomatoes with Basil (Phases 1–4)
6.1g carbs per 100g

Napolina Crushed Tomatoes with Onion & Garlic (Phases 1–4)
6.8g carbs per 100g

Napolina Crushed Tomatoes with Peppers & Chilli (Phases 1–4)
5.7g carbs per 100g

Own Brand Passata (Phases 1–4)
4.2–6.4g carbs per 100g

 Own Brand Passata with Herbs/Garlic/Basil
5.5–7.7g carbs per 100g
Contains added sugar

**Valfruta Passata di Campagna Thick Country
Style Sieved Tomatoes (Phases 1–4)**
4.2g carbs per 100g

TOMATOES, SUN-DRIED

Sun-dried tomatoes are acceptable in Induction but you
must pay attention to portion size because the natural
sugars in tomatoes are even more concentrated. Use
reconstituted sun-dried tomatoes as a salad topping
rather than a main ingredient.

Gia Sun Dried Tomatoes in Oil (Phases 1–4)
7.5g carbs per 100g

Own Brand Sun-Dried Tomatoes (Phases 1–4)
11g carbs per 100g

**Sacla' Sun-Dried Tomato Antipasto
(Phases 1–4)**
8.1g carbs per 100g

TOMATOES, WHOLE CHERRY

**Cirio Pomodorini Cherry Tomatoes
(Phases 1–4)**
7g carbs per 100g

Heinz Cherry Tomatoes (Phases 1–4)
2.9g carbs per 100g

TOMATOES, WHOLE PLUM

Dettori's Peeled Plum Tomatoes (Phases 1–4)
3.5g carbs per 100g

Heinz Whole Peeled Tomatoes (Phases 1–4)
2.9g carbs per 100g

⚠ **Napolina Organic Peeled Plum Tomatoes
(Phases 1–4)**
3.5g carbs per 100g

Napolina Peeled Plum Tomatoes (Phases 1–4)
3.5g carbs per 100g

**Own Brand Economy Plum Tomatoes
(Phases 1–4)**
2.9–4g carbs per 100g

Own Brand Plum Tomatoes (Phases 1–4)
3–4g carbs per 100g

DRIED VEGETABLES

Dried vegetables are a storecupboard favourite for
making soups and stews. A little goes a long way. Be
sure to be sparing in your portions or else you will
unwittingly load up on carbs.

MIXED

Whitworths Dried Country Vegetables (Phases 3–4)
22.1g carbs per 25g

MUSHROOMS, SLICED

You must be sparing in your portions of dried mushrooms or else you will exceed your carb count, especially with shiitake or mixed varieties.

Whitworths Dried Sliced Mushrooms (Phases 1–4)
1.2g carbs per 25g

MUSHROOMS, WHOLE

Borde Girolles (Phases 1–4)
12.7g carbs per 25g

Borde Porcini (Phases 1–4)
7.8g carbs per 25g

Borde Shiitake (Phases 1–4)
14.1g carbs per 25g

Merchant Gourmet Mixed Mushrooms (Phases 1–4)
14.5g carbs per 25g

Merchant Gourmet Porcini (Phases 1–4)
1.25g carbs per 25g

⚠ Unique Organic Porcini (Phases 1–4)
1.25g carbs per 25g

ONIONS

Whitworths Dried Onions (Phases 1–4)
17.1g carbs per 25g

PEAS

Batchelors Bigga Dried Peas (Phases 3–4)
9.4g carbs per 25g

Batchelors Quick Soak Dried Peas (Phases 3–4)
10.5g carbs per 25g

**Whitworths Dried Marrowfat Peas
(Phases 3–4)**
12.5g carbs per 25g

POTATOES

⚠ **Smash Original with Smoked Bacon/Cheddar
& Onion/Fried Onion**
3.4–3.5g carbs per 25g
Contains trans fats and potato starch

TOMATOES

**Merchant Gourmet Italian Sun Dried
Tomatoes (Phases 1–4)**
5.1g carbs per 25g

**Merchant Gourmet Mi-Cuit Semi Dried
Tomatoes Ready to Eat (Phases 1–4)**
5.7g carbs per 25g

Vegetarian

Contrary to misconceptions, it is perfectly possible for non-meat-eaters to follow Atkins successfully. More importantly, vegetarianism is no longer considered in the UK to be an alternative eating lifestyle, and even confirmed carnivores enjoy vegetarian products and meals as an occasional change to their diet.

With 26 per cent of households in the UK eating less meat or avoiding it altogether, supermarket chains have responded by increasing the range of non-meat products they stock. As a result, the days of consuming only nut loaf, brown rice and dry veggie burgers – long synonymous with being a vegetarian – have gone. Improvements in food manufacturing processes and an ever-widening range of ingredients have resulted in an array of foods that look appetizing and offer great texture and flavour, and there is a substitute for virtually every type and style of food typically made with meat.

The majority of alternatives on the supermarket shelves and in the chiller or freezer cabinets are made from soya, in its various forms, or Quorn.

SOYA

The soya bean is the seed of the leguminous soya bean plant. It has been a staple part of the Chinese diet for over 4,000 years but has been widely consumed in the West only since the 1960s. Soya foods include tofu, tempeh, textured vegetable protein, miso, soya sauces, soya oil and margarine and soya dairy alternatives.

Soya protein contains isoflavones, plant compounds that have been linked to cardiovascular health, particularly lower levels of blood cholesterol, and are thought to alleviate symptoms of menopause and reduce the risk of cancers caused by hormonal irregularities.

- **Tofu**, or soya bean curd, is available in a variety of textures, from extra-firm to soft to silken. Firm tofu is better for stir-fries and grilling because it retains its shape and texture. Soft tofu, on the other hand, works best for blending and adding to soups. Silken tofu makes a dairy-free, protein-rich addition to smoothies.
- **Flavoured tofus** are a good alternative for quick meals – you won't need to add spices or flavourings – but avoid those that come with sauces. Flavoured tofu without sauce has about 2g carbs per serving; those with a sauce can have 5–7g carbs and usually contain added sugars.
- **Tempeh** is made of cooked, fermented soya beans. It is higher in protein than tofu and it also has more flavour. Tempeh is always firm in texture
- **Textured vegetable protein** is basically de-fatted soya flour that has been processed and dried to produce a substance with a sponge-like texture, which may be flavoured to resemble meat.
- **Quorn** products are made with mycoprotein, a fungus and a relative of mushrooms, truffles and morels.

If you are going to use meat alternatives in your diet you need to approach this carefully when following Atkins, as healthy alternatives do not always equate with low carbs. Many of the products will be bulked out with breadcrumbs, beans, potatoes or rice. Be aware that although the carb count might be low, if the product contains such ingredients it may not necessarily be suitable for all phases. In such cases, we have drawn your attention to it with an FYI alert.

Further, when reviewing Own Brand products, some – but not all – of them *may* contain ingredients that would normally merit an unacceptable symbol △. Because not *all* will contain trans fats or added sugars, we have used an FYI symbol **FYI** to advise you to study the ingredients panel before buying.

No matter how healthy some of these products purport to be, many of the most popular brands available in UK supermarkets contain added sugars and trans fats, which should be avoided on all phases of Atkins.

BEEF, POULTRY & BACON SUBSTITUTES

Frozen

△ **Morningstar Farms Meat-free Streaky Strips**
13.4g carbs per 100g
Contains added sugars and modified cornflour

Quorn Chicken Style Roast (Phases 1–4)
4g carbs per 100g

△ **Quorn Crispy Fillets**
14.2g carbs per 100g
Contains added sugars, trans fats and wheat flour

Quorn Fillets (Phases 1–4)
5.9g carbs per 100g

△ **Quorn Garlic & Herb Fillets**
16.7g per 100g
Contains wheat flour

⚠ **Quorn Pork Style Ribsters**
4.8g carbs per 100g
Contains trans fats

Quorn Swedish Style Balls (Phases 1–4)
5.4g carbs per 100g

Realeat Vege Mince (Phases 1–4)
6g carbs per 100g

Chilled

Quorn Chicken Style Pieces (Phases 1–4)
5.8g carbs per 100g

⚠ **Quorn Deli Mini Fillets Chargrilled BBQ Style**
10.5g carbs per 100g
Contains added sugars

⚠ **Quorn Deli Style Bacon**
8.1g carbs per 100g
Contains trans fats

Quorn Deli Style Chicken (Phases 1–4)
4.5g carbs per 100g.

Quorn Fillets (Phases 1–4)
5.9g carbs per 100g

FYI **Quorn Fillets in a White Wine Sauce with Mushrooms & Chives (Phases 3–4)**
4.7g carbs per 100g
Contains modified maize starch

⚠ **Quorn Lamb Style Grills**
7.6g carbs per 100g
Contains trans fats

🄵🄸 **Quorn Lemon & Black Pepper Fillets (Phases 3–4)**
16.2g carbs per 100g
Contains wheat flour

Quorn Mince (Phases 1–4)
4.5g carbs per 100g

⚠ **Quorn Mini Fillets Chargrilled Chinese Style**
15.6g carbs per 100g
Contains added sugars and trans fats

⚠ **Quorn Peppered Steaks**
7.4g carbs per 100g
Contains added sugars and trans fats

Quorn Swedish Style Balls (Phases 1–4)
5.4g carbs per 100g

⚠ **The Redwood Co. Meat Free Streaky-Style Vegetarian Rashers**
12.4g carbs per 100g
Contains added sugars

⚠ **The Redwood Co. Vegetarian Cheatin' 'Chicken'**
7.8g carbs per 100g
Contains added sugars

⚠ **The Redwood Co. Vegetarian Cheatin' 'Turkey'**
8.1g carbs per 100g
Contains added sugars

⚠ **The Redwood Co. Vegideli Organic Meat Free**
⚠ **Bio Rashers**
13.3g carbs per 100g
Contains added sugars

INTERNATIONAL

The Really Interesting Food Co. Thai Green Curry (Phases 2–4)
7.9g carbs per 100g

The Really Interesting Food Co. Tofu and Vegetable Curry (Phases 2–4)
7.8g carbs per 100g

Mother Hemp Green Pesto (Phases 2–4)
2.9g carbs per 100g

Mother Hemp Red Pesto (Phases 1–4)
3g carbs per 100g

DRIED

⚠ **Bacos Bacon Flavour Soya Chips**
1.8g carbs per serving, 25.6g carbs per 100g
Contains added sugar and trans fats

⚠ **Direct Foods Burgamix**
19g carbs per 100g
Contains trans fats

Realeat Vegebanger Mix (Phases 1–4)
4.4g carbs per sausage shape, 40g carbs per 100g

Realeat Vegeburger Mix (Phases 3–4)
12.5g carbs per burger, 40g carbs per 100g

SAUSAGES

Frozen

⚠ **Linda McCartney Sausages**
8.6g carbs per 100g
Contains added sugars and trans fats

(FYI) **Own Brand Vegetarian/Meatfree Hot Dog Sausages (Phases 1–4)**
6g carbs per 100g
Some may contain added sugars

(FYI) **Own Brand Vegetarian Sausage (Phases 3–4)**
2–20.5g carbs per 100g
Some may contain added sugars and wheat

Chilled

⚠ **Cauldron Organic Glamorgan Leek & Cheese**
⚠ **Veggie Sausages**
11.2g carbs per 100g
Contains added sugars and wheat flour

⚠ **Cauldron Peppery & Succulent Cumberland Veggie Sausages**
14.4g carbs per 100g
Contains added sugars and trans fats

⚠ **Cauldron Succulent Lincolnshire Veggie Sausages**
10.5g carbs per 100g
Contains added sugars, trans fats and wheat flour

⚠ **Cauldron Sun-dried Tomato & Black Olive Sausages**
9.4g carbs per 100g
Contains added sugars

⚠ **GranoVita Vegetable Frankfurters**
2.6g carbs per 100g
Contains trans fats and wheat flour

Quorn Leek & Pork Style Sausages (Phases 1–4)
5.5g carbs per 100g

Quorn Sausages (Phases 1–4)
4.5g carbs per 100g

Quorn Spinach & Gruyère Sausages (Phases 1–4)
6.5g carbs per 100g

The Redwood Co. Vegideli Meat Free Sage & Marjoram Sausages (Phases 1–4)
9.1g carbs per 100g

(FYI) **Tivall Vegetarian Spicy Sausages (Phases 3–4)**
5g carbs per 100g
Contains modified starch

⚠ **Wicken Fen Vegetarian Gourmet Sausages Mushroom and Tarragon**
17g carbs per 100g
Contains trans fats

BURGERS

Frozen

(FYI) **Birds Eye Captain's Vegetable Burgers (Phases 3–4)**
25.5g carbs per 100g
Contains wheat flour

(FYI) **Birds Eye Crunchy Vegetable Quarter Pounders (Phases 3–4)**
24.9g carbs per 100g
Contains wheat flour

⚠ **Dalepak Vegetable Quarter Pounders**
20.8g carbs per 100g
Contains added sugars, trans fats and wheat flour

⚠ **Goodlife Organic Vegetable Burgers (Phases 3–4)**
26.3g carbs per 100g

⚠ **Linda McCartney Flame Grilled Burgers**
2.9g carbs per 100g
Contains trans fats

⚠ **Own Brand Vegetable & Spicy Bean Quarter Pounders**
28–35g carbs per 100g
Contains added sugars, trans fats and wheat flour

(FYI) **Own Brand Vegetarian/Meatfree Burgers (Phases 1–4)**
3.9–7g carbs per 100g
Some may contain added sugars

(FYI) Own Brand Vegetarian/Meatfree Quarterpounders (Phases 1–4)
0.3–7g carbs per 100g
Some may contain added sugars and trans fats

(FYI) Quorn Burgers (Phases 3–4)
8.8g carbs per 100g
Contains starch

⚠ Quorn Premium Burgers
5.5g carbs per 100g
Contains trans fats

⚠ Quorn Southern Style Burgers
17g carbs per 100g
Contains trans fats and wheat flour

Chilled

Cauldron Chilli-flavour Brown Rice & Tofu Burgers (Phases 3–4)
13.5g carbs per 100g

⚠ Cauldron Crunchy Carrot, Peanut & Onion Nut Burgers
26.8g carbs per 100g
Contains added sugars

⚠ Cauldron Organic Juicy Mushroom Burgers
⚠ 15.1g carbs per 100g
Contains added sugars

⚠ Cauldron Roast Vegetable & Sweet Basil Crisp Burgers
24.3g carbs per 100g
Contains added sugars and wheat flour

Cauldron Savoury Burgers (Phases 3–4)
13.2g carbs per 100g

Dried

⚠ Direct Foods Sosmix
12.4g carbs per sausage, 33g carbs per 100g
Contains added sugars and trans fats

NUT PRODUCTS
Cutlets, frozen

Ⓕⓨⓘ Goodlife Nut Cutlets (Phases 3–4)
21.8g carbs per 100g
Contains wheat flour

Ⓕⓨⓘ Own Brand Vegetable and Nut Cutlets (Phases 3–4)
22g carbs per 100g
Some may contain added sugars, trans fats and wheat flour

Nuggets, frozen

⚠ Own Brand Vegetarian Nuggets
10.5–14.7g carbs per 100g
Contains added sugars, breadcrumbs and wheat flour

Ⓕⓨⓘ Quorn Southern Style Nuggets (Phases 3–4)
18.8g carbs per 100g
Contains wheat flour

Roast, dried

Granose Nut Roast Mix Loaf (Phases 3–4)
23g carbs per 100g

DELI

Paté

⚠ **Cauldron Organic Aromatic Herb & Soya Bean Paté (Phases 3–4)**
14.1g carbs per 100g

⚠ **Cauldron Organic Fragrant Moroccan**
⚠ **Chickpea Paté**
9.4g carbs per 100g
Contains added sugars

⚠ **Cauldron Organic Soft & Creamy Mushroom Paté (Phases 2–4)**
4.3g carbs per 100g

⚠ **Cauldron Organic Spinach, Cheese & Crunchy Almond Paté (Phases 2–4)**
6.3g carbs per 100g

⚠ **Cauldron Organic Sweet Roasted Parsnip &**
⚠ **Carrot Paté**
9.8g carbs per 100g
Contains added sugars

Quorn Deli Farmhouse Style Paté (Phases 2–4)
7.8g carbs per 100g

Quorn Paté Brussels Style (Phases 2–4)
5.7g carbs per 100g

CHILLED MEAT & POULTRY ALTERNATIVES

Quorn Deli Florentine (Phases 2–4)
5.8g carbs per 100g

Quorn Deli Smokey Ham Style (Phases 2–4)
5.7g carbs per 100g

FYI ### Quorn Deli Turkey Style with Stuffing (Phases 3–4)
6.6g carbs per 100g
Contains wheat flour

Quorn Deli Wafer Thin Chicken Style (Phases 1–4)
4g carbs per 100g

⚠ ### Quorn Deli Wafer Thin Ham Style
8.4g carbs per 100g
Contains added sugars

FALAFEL

Frozen

Goodlife Falafel with Yogurt and Mint Dip (Phases 3–4)
22.4g carbs per 100g

Chilled

⚠ ### Cauldron Organic Spicy Middle Eastern Falafel
 23.3g carbs per 100g
Contains added sugars and wheat flour

TOFU

Chilled

⚠ ### Cauldron Organic Golden Marinated Tofu
 ### Pieces
2.4g carbs per 100g
Contains added sugars

⚠ **Cauldron Organic Savoury Beech Smoked Tofu (Phases 1–4)**
1g carbs per 100g

⚠ **Cauldron Organic Tofu Natural Soya Bean Curd (Phases 1–4)**
1.2g carbs per 100g

Cauldron Tofu Plain and Simple (Phases 1–4)
1.3g carbs per 100g

Marigold Braised Tofu (Phases 2–4)
6.7g carbs per 100g

Tetra Pak

Blue Dragon Tofu Firm Silken Style (Phases 1–4)
2.4g per 100g

Mori Nu Tofu Firm Silken Style (Phases 1–4)
2.4g per 100g

READY MEALS

Frozen

⚠ **Linda McCartney Lasagne**
14.6g carbs per 100g
Contains added sugars, modified maize starch and wheat flour

Chilled

⚠ **Quorn Cottage Pie**
9g carbs per 100g
Contains added sugars and modified maize starch

Tinned

⚠ **Crosse & Blackwell Hunger Breaks Big Brunch Meat Free**
16.7g carbs per 100g
Contains added sugars and maize starch

⚠ **Heinz Meat Free Spaghetti Bolognese**
13.1g carbs per 100g
Contains added sugars, cornflour and wheat flour

PASTA & RICE

Frozen

⚠ **Own Brand Spinach and Ricotta Cannelloni**
12.5–17.3g carbs per 100g
Contains added sugars, trans fats, modified maize starch and wheat flour

⚠ **Ross Spinach and Ricotta Cannelloni**
13.2g carbs per 100g
Contains modified maize starch and wheat flour

FROZEN VEGETABLE PRODUCTS

ⓕⓥⓘ **Birds Eye Captain's Vegetable Fingers (Phases 3–4)**
23.8g carbs per 100g
Contains wheat flour

ⓕⓥⓘ **Dalepak Cauliflower Cheese Grills**
20.1g carbs per 100g
Contain added sugars, trans fats, maize starch and wheat flour

⚠ **Dalepak Vegetable Fingers**
26.7g carbs per 100g
Contains added sugars, trans fats and wheat flour

⚠ **Dalepak Vegetable Grills**
22.5g carbs per 100g
Contains added sugars and wheat flour

⚠ **Own Brand Potato & Cheese Bakes**
22.4–24.5g carbs per 100g
Contains trans fats, modified maize starch and
wheat flour

SOYA PRODUCTS

Milks

Holland & Barrett Unsweetened Soya
(Phases 1–4)
0.6g carbs per 100ml

⚠ **Provamel Alpro Chilled Soya**
2.8g carbs per 100ml
Contains added sugars

⚠ **Provamel Alpro Soya Sweetened Organic UHT**
Soya
2.8g carbs per 100ml
Contains added sugars

 Provamel Alpro Soya Unsweetened Organic
UHT Soya (Phases 1–4)
0.4g carbs per 100 ml

⚠ **Provamel Alpro Sweetened**
2.8g carbs per 100ml
Contains added sugars

Provamel Alpro Unsweetened (Phases 1–4)
2.8g carbs per 100ml

So Good Soya Chilled (Phases 2–4)
5.3g carbs per 100ml

So Good Soya Life (Phases 2–4)
5g carbs per 100ml

Cream Alternative

⚠ **Provamel Alpro Soya Dream**
1.8g carbs per 100ml
Contains added sugars

Yogurts

(FYI) **Granovita Deluxe Soyage, Black Cherry (Phases 3–4)**
16.5g carbs per 100g
Contains cornflour

⚠ **Provamel Alpro Soya Plain Organic Low Fat**
⚠ 3.2g carbs per 100g
Contains added sugars

⚠ **Provamel Alpro Soya Plain Organic Low Fat**
⚠ **Summer Fruits**
14.7g carbs per 100g
Contains added sugars and cornflour

Atkins Products

Advantage

Atkins Advantage™ Bar Chocolate Decadence
Atkins Advantage™ Bar Chocolate Hazelnut Crunch
Atkins Advantage™ Bar Chocolate Orange Sensation
Atkins Advantage™ Bar Fruits of the Forest
Atkins Advantage™ Ready-to-Drink Shake Chocolate
    Flavour
Atkins Advantage™ Ready-to-Drink Shake Strawberry
    Flavour
Atkins Advantage™ Ready-to-Drink Shake Vanilla
    Flavour
Atkins Advantage™ Shake Mix Chocolate Flavour
Atkins Advantage™ Shake Mix Strawberry Flavour
Atkins Advantage™ Shake Mix Vanilla Flavour

Bake Mix

Atkins Quick Quisine™ Bake Mix

Bread

Atkins™ Sliced White Loaf

Crunchables

Atkins Crunchables™ Herb Flavour
Atkins Crunchables™ Hot 'n' Spicy Flavour

Endulge

Atkins Endulge™ Caramel Hazelnut Bar
Atkins Endulge™ Caramel Wafer Crisp
Atkins Endulge™ Chocolate Crème Wafer Crisp
Atkins Endulge™ Crispy Milk Chocolate Bar

Atkins Endulge™ Milk Chocolate Bar
Atkins Endulge™ Mint Wafer Crisp

Flavoured Drinks

Atkins™ Apple & Cranberry Flavoured Drink
Atkins™ Grapefruit & Lime Flavoured Drink

Fromage Frais

Atkins™ Fromage Frais Peaches & Cream
Atkins™ Fromage Frais Raspberries & Cream
Atkins™ Fromage Frais Strawberries & Cream

Low-Carb Milk

Atkins™ Low-Carb Semi-Skimmed Milk

Morning Shine

Atkins Morning Shine™ Apple Crisp Breakfast Bar
Atkins Morning Shine™ Chocolate Chip Crisp
    Breakfast Bar
Atkins Morning Shine™ Tropical Juice Drink
Atkins Morning Shine™ Cinnamon Breakfast Flakes
Atkins Morning Shine™ Mixed Berry Granola Cereal
    Bar
Atkins Morning Shine™ Strawberry Crisp Breakfast Bar

Salads & Wraps*

Atkins Gourmet™ Chargrilled Chicken Salad
Atkins Gourmet™ Chargrilled Chicken & Bacon Salad
Atkins Gourmet™ Crayfish & Salsa Salad
Atkins Gourmet™ Prawn & Poached Salmon Salad
Atkins Gourmet™ Chicken & Bacon Wrap
Atkins Gourmet™ Roast Chicken & Salad Wrap
Atkins Gourmet™ Chargrilled Chicken Strips

Available at Boots the Chemist

Index

Make
www.thorsonselement.com
your online sanctuary

www.thorsonselement.com

Get online information, inspiration and guidance to help you on the path to physical and spiritual well-being. Drawing on the integrity and vision of our authors and titles, and with health advice, articles, astrology, tarot, a meditation zone, author interviews and events listings, www.thorsonselement.com is a great alternative to help create space and peace in our lives.

So if you've always wondered about practising yoga, following an allergy-free diet, using the tarot or getting a life coach, we can point you in the right direction.

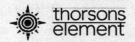

thorsons
element